Study Guide for Ricci and Kyle's

Maternity and Pediatric Nursing

Wolters Kluwer | Lippincott Williams & Wilkins
Health

Philadelphia · Baltimore · New York · London
Buenos Aires · Hong Kong · Sydney · Tokyo

Managing Editor: Annette Ferran
Senior Production Editor: Tom Gibbons
Director of Nursing Production: Helen Ewan
Senior Managing Editor/Production: Erika Kors
Manufacturing Coordinator: Karin Duffield
Compositor: Aptara Inc. Corp.

9 8 7 6 5 4 3 2 1

Printed in the United States of America

ISBN-13: 978-1-6054-7629-2

Care has been taken to confirm the accuracy of the information presented and to describe generally accepted practices. However, the authors, editors, and publisher are not responsible for errors or omissions or for any consequences from application of the information in this book and make no warranty, expressed or implied, with respect to the currency, completeness, or accuracy of the contents of the publication. Application of this information in a particular situation remains the professional responsibility of the practitioner; the clinical treatments described and recommended may not be considered absolute and universal recommendations.

The authors, editors, and publisher have exerted every effort to ensure that drug selection and dosage set forth in this text are in accordance with the current recommendations and practice at the time of publication. However, in view of ongoing research, changes in government regulations, and the constant flow of information relating to drug therapy and drug reactions, the reader is urged to check the package insert for each drug for any change in indications and dosage and for added warnings and precautions. This is particularly important when the recommended agent is a new or infrequently employed drug.

Some drugs and medical devices presented in this publication have Food and Drug Administration (FDA) clearance for limited use in restricted research settings. It is the responsibility of the health care provider to ascertain the FDA status of each drug or device planned for use in his or her clinical practice.

Preface

This Study Guide was developed by the Instructional Design firm of LearningMate and reviewed by Kathleen Beebe, RNC, PhD, Jo Anne Kirk, MSN, RN, and Susan Miovech, PhD, RNC, to accompany *Maternity and Pediatric Nursing* by Susan Scott Ricci and Terri Kyle. The Study Guide is designed to help you practice and retain the knowledge you have gained from the textbook, and it is structured to integrate that knowledge and give you a basis for applying it in your nursing practice. The following types of exercises are provided in each chapter of the Study Guide.

ASSESSING YOUR UNDERSTANDING

The first section of each Study Guide chapter concentrates on the basic information of the textbook chapter and helps you to remember key concepts, vocabulary, and principles.

- *Fill in the Blanks*

Fill in the blank exercises test important chapter information, encouraging you to recall key points.

- *Labeling*

Labeling exercises are used where you need to remember certain visual representations of the concepts presented in the textbook.

- *Match the Following*

Matching questions test your knowledge of the definition of key terms.

- *Sequencing*

Sequencing exercises ask you to remember particular sequences or orders, for example, testing processes and prioritizing nursing actions.

- *Short Answers*

Short answer questions cover facts, concepts, procedures, and principles of the chapter. These questions ask you to recall information as well as demonstrate your comprehension of the information.

APPLYING YOUR KNOWLEDGE

The second section of each Study Guide chapter consists of case study–based exercises that ask you to begin to apply the knowledge you've gained from the textbook chapter and reinforced in the first section of the Study Guide chapter. A case study scenario based on the chapter's content is presented, and then you are asked to answer some questions, in writing, related to the case study. The questions cover the following areas:

- Assessment
- Planning Nursing Care
- Communication
- Reflection

PRACTICING FOR NCLEX

The third and final section of the Study Chapters helps you practice NCLEX-style questions while further reinforcing the knowledge you have been gaining and testing for yourself through the textbook chapter and the first two sections of the study guide chapter. In keeping with the NCLEX, the questions presented are multiple-choice and scenario-based, asking you to reflect, consider, and apply what you know and to choose the best answer out of those offered.

ANSWER KEYS

The answers for all of the exercises and questions in the Study Guide are provided at the back of the book, so you can assess your own learning as you complete each chapter.

We hope you will find this Study Guide to be helpful and enjoyable, and we wish you every success in your studies toward becoming a nurse.

The Publishers

Contents

CHAPTER 1

Perspectives on Maternal and Child Health Care

SECTION I: LEARNING OBJECTIVES

1. Identify the key milestones in the evolution of maternal and child health nursing.

2. Describe the major components, concepts, and influences associated with the nursing management of women, children, and their families.

3. Compare the past definitions of health and illness to the current definitions as well as the measurement of health and illness in children.

4. Identify the factors that impact maternal and child health.

5. Delineate the structures, roles, and functions of the family and how they impact the health of women and children.

6. Evaluate how society and culture can influence the health of women, children, and families.

7. Appraise the health care barriers affecting women, children, and their families.

8. Debate the ethical and legal issues that may arise when caring for women, children, and their families.

SECTION II: ASSESSING YOUR UNDERSTANDING

Activity A *Fill in the blanks.*

1. A _____ is a lay birth assistant who provides quality emotional, physical, and educational support to the woman and family during childbirth and the postpartum period.

2. _____ fetal surgery is a procedure that involves opening the uterus during pregnancy, performing a surgery, and replacing the fetus in the uterus.

3. The use of oral contraceptives makes a woman susceptible to _____ cancer.

4. The _____ is considered the basic social unit.

5. Under certain conditions, a minor can be considered _____ and can make health care decisions independently of parents.

6. Overall plans in the health care delivery system improve access to preventive services but may limit the access to _____ care, which greatly impacts women and children with chronic or long-term illnesses.

7. The process of increasing desirable behavior and decreasing or eliminating undesirable behavior is known as _____.

8. The ability to apply knowledge about a client's culture to adapt his or her health care accordingly is known as cultural _____.

9. With the emphasis on reducing costs and on preventive care and services, _____ guidance and education by nurses has become ever more important.

10. _____ is the measure of prevalence of a specific illness in a population at a particular time.

Activity B *Match the terms in Column A with their descriptions in Column B.*

Column A

____ 1. Asian-Americans

____ 2. African-Americans

____ 3. Arab-Americans

____ 4. Native-Americans

____ 5. Hispanic

Column B

a. Newborn not given colostrum

b. Liberal use of oil on newborn's and infant's scalp and skin

c. Quiet, stoic appearance of woman during labor

d. Wrapping of newborn's stomach at birth to prevent cold or wind from entering baby's body

e. Mother's legs brought together after birth of newborn to prevent air from entering uterus

Activity C *Put the acts or programs in correct sequence by writing the letters in the boxes provided below.*

Given below are the federal programs in support of the health of women and children. Indicate the proper order of enactment of these programs.

a. Omnibus Budget Reconciliation Act

b. Child Health Assessment Program

c. U.S. Children's Bureau

d. Education for All Handicapped Children Act

e. Title V of the Social Security Act

☐ → ☐ → ☐ → ☐ → ☐

Activity D *Briefly answer the following.*

1. What are the risk factors the nurse should monitor for in women that could lead to CVD?

_____

_____

_____

2. What are the components of case management?

_____

_____

_____

3. What are the protective factors that boost resilience in children?

_____

_____

_____

4. What is evidence-based nursing practice?

_____

_____

_____

5. What does maternal mortality rate measure?

_____

_____

_____

6. What are the predictors of infant mortality?

_____

_____

_____

SECTION III: APPLYING YOUR KNOWLEDGE

Activity E *Consider this scenario and answer the questions.*

An eight-year-old child is brought to the clinic for his annual exam. During the health history, the nurse learns that the child's parents have been divorced for several years and his mother recently married a man who has two children from a previous marriage. The child's mother states, "His stepfather is a wonderful man, but we have different discipline beliefs. He firmly believes the child should obey the family rules without questioning them, and he doesn't see anything wrong with a spanking now and then."

1. How should the nurse address the mother's concerns?

_____

_____

_____

2. Later during your assessment, the mother expresses concern about how the divorce and now the remarriage may affect her child. How should the nurse respond?

_____

_____

_____

SECTION IV: PRACTICING FOR NCLEX

Activity F *Answer the following questions.*

1. A female client who has just given birth has been reading health reports and is alarmed at the high rate of infant mortality. She seems anxious about the health of her child and wants to know ways to keep her baby from getting an infection. Which of the following instructions should the nurse offer?

a. Place infant on his or her back to sleep

b. Breastfeed the infant

c. Feed the infant foods high in starch

d. Feed the infant liquids frequently

2. A group of nurses are running a campaign initiated by the Maternal and Child Health Bureau to educate women about better maternal and infant care. Which of the following measures should they advocate for the prevention of neural defects in infants?

a. Take folic acid supplements

b. Take vitamin E supplements

c. Perform mild exercises during pregnancy

d. Regularly eat citrus fruits during pregnancy

3. A nurse is caring for a client who wishes to undergo abortion. The nurse has concerns because abortion is against her personal convictions, and this is interfering with her professional duty. Which of the following should the nurse do to follow ANA's code of ethics for nurses?

a. Provide emotional support to the client while caring for her

b. Not allow her personal convictions to interfere with her profession

c. Involve the client's family in convincing the client against an abortion

d. Make arrangements for alternate care providers

4. A female client who has just given birth arrives in a health care facility wanting to know of ways to prevent sudden infant death syndrome (SIDS). Which of the following instructions should the nurse provide?

a. Drape the infant in warm clothes

b. Feed a mixture of salts, sugar, and water

c. Provide very soft bedding

d. Place the infant on his or her back to sleep

5. A nurse is caring for a critically ill female client who has recently been diagnosed with advanced lung cancer. Which of the following could have contributed to the late detection and diagnosis?

a. Women have a stronger resistance against lung cancer

b. Lung cancer has no early symptoms

c. Lung cancer is considered more deadly in men than women

d. Lung cancer is more challenging to diagnose in women than in men

6. A ten-year-old girl is living with her grandparents. Which nursing intervention is necessary with this family structure?

   a. Teaching the grandparents basic child care skills

   b. Determining who the decision-maker is

   c. Assessing the child for emotional problems

   d. Helping to assess the need for financial aid

7. The nurse is caring for an Arab-American child. Which approach would be most successful?

   a. Inquiring about folk remedies used

   b. Coordinating care through the mother

   c. Dealing exclusively with the father

   d. Promoting preventive health care

8. The nurse is teaching discipline to the parents of a nine-year-old girl. Which of the following topics is an example of extinction discipline?

   a. Going out for ice cream

   b. Ignoring the child's temper tantrum

   c. Letting the child go to a friend's house

   d. Praising the child for displaying appropriate behavior

9. A client who has two school-age children is getting divorced and is unsure of its impact on her children. Which would be the best instruction for the nurse to give the client?

   a. Treat your children like adults

   b. Make your side of the disagreement clear

   c. Move out when the children are in school

   d. Discuss how things will work after the divorce

10. A nurse is caring for a 31-year-old pregnant female client who is subjected to abuse by her partner. The client has developed a feeling of hopelessness and does not feel confident in dealing with the situation at home, which makes her feel suicidal. Which of the following nursing interventions should the nurse offer to help the client deal with her situation?

    a. Counsel client's partner to refrain from subjecting his partner to abuse

    b. Help client know the legal impact of her situation to protect her

    c. Provide emotional support to empower the client to help herself

    d. Introduce the client to a women's rights group

11. A nurse has been caring for a female client who requires follow-up care in a health care facility for breast cancer. How can the nurse ensure that the client keeps her appointments?

    a. Avoid long delays before examination

    b. Schedule appointments to match client's comfort

    c. Avoid a hurried examination

    d. Encourage telephone consultation services

12. A nurse is caring for a 54-year-old critically ill female client who has been diagnosed with cardiovascular disease. The management of CVD in the client is challenging because the disease was not diagnosed in a timely manner. Which of the following reasons could have contributed to the difficulty in diagnosing this client's CVD? Select all that apply.

    a. CVD is considered more deadly in males

    b. CVD is still thought of as a "man's disease"

    c. Symptoms of CVD present differently in females than in males

    d. CVD has no early symptoms, making the diagnosis difficult

13. A female client who has a positive family history of cardiovascular disease comes to a health care facility to learn about preventive measures against the disease. On which of the following prevention efforts should the nurse educate the client to reduce the client's chance of developing CVD? Select all that apply.

    a. Stress management

    b. Increased fluid intake

    c. Consumption of simple carbohydrates

    d. Daily exercise

14. A female client comes to a health care facility complaining of nausea and discomfort in her stomach. Initial interview reveals that the client has experienced unexplained fatigue and cold sweats in the past. The physician suspects cardiovascular disease. Which of the following questions should the nurse ask the client when assessing for cardiovascular disease? Select all that apply.

    a. "Do you experience weight fluctuations or have diabetes?"

    b. "Do you smoke regularly?"

    c. "Are you consuming a diet high in starch?"

    d. "Did you have your first child after the age of 30?"

15. A fourteen-year-old pregnant client is undergoing assessment in a health care facility. Which of the following teenage pregnancy–related complications should the nurse be aware of during assessment? Select all that apply.

    a. Dystocia

    b. Anemia

    c. Preterm labor

    d. Cephalopelvic disproportion

    e. Cardiovascular disease

CHAPTER 2

Family-Centered Community-Based Care

SECTION I: LEARNING OBJECTIVES

1. Examine the major components and key elements of family-centered home health care.

2. Explain the factors that have influenced an increased emphasis on community-based care.

3. Differentiate community-based nursing from that of acute care settings.

4. Explain the different levels of prevention in community-based nursing, providing examples of each.

5. Formulate examples of cultural issues that may be faced when providing community-based nursing.

6. Provide culturally competent care to women, children, and their families.

7. Identify the variety of settings available for providing community-based care to women, children, and their families.

8. Outline the various roles and functions assumed by the community health nurse.

9. Demonstrate the ability to use excellent therapeutic communication skills when interacting with women, children, and their families.

10. Explain the process of health teaching as it relates to women, children, and their families.

11. Examine the importance of discharge planning and case management in providing community-based care.

SECTION II: ASSESSING YOUR UNDERSTANDING

Activity A *Fill in the blanks.*

1. _____ communication, also referred to as body language, includes attending to others and active listening.

2. _____ management focuses on coordinating health care services while balancing quality and cost outcomes.

3. _____ may be defined as a "specific group of people, often living in a defined geographic area, who share a common culture, values, and norms."

4. _____ clinics offer a community-based site for the childbearing family to access services.

5. Primary _____ involves avoiding the disease or condition before it occurs through health promotion activities, environmental protection, and specific protection against disease or injury.

6. _____ is the study of the causes, distribution, and control of disease in populations.

7. Cultural _____ is defined as the knowledge, willingness, and ability to adapt health care to enhance its acceptability to and effectiveness with patients from diverse cultures.

8. Cultural _____ involve participating in cross-cultural interactions with people from culturally diverse backgrounds.

9. _____ literacy is the ability to read, understand, and use health care information.

10. Medically _____ children have medically complex needs that require skilled nursing interventions.

Activity B *Consider the following figures.*

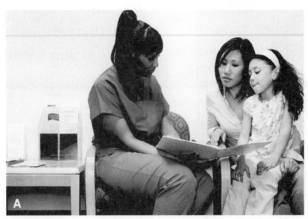

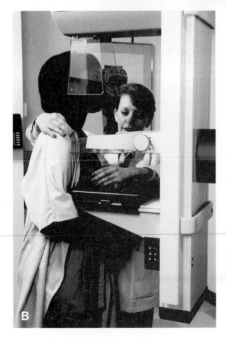

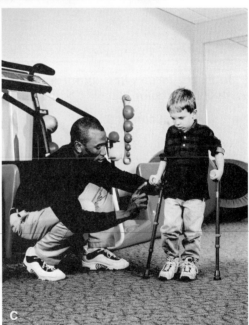

1. What does the figure depict?

   _____

   _____

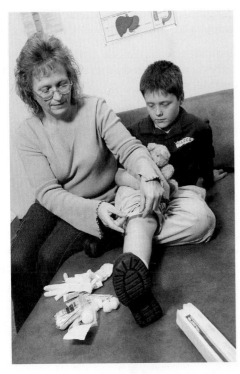

2. Identify the figure.

_____

_____

Activity C *Match the locales in Column A with their purpose in Column B.*

Column A

___ **1.** Counseling centers

___ **2.** Wellness centers

___ **3.** Retail centers

___ **4.** Wholeness healing centers

___ **5.** Educational centers

Column B

a. Offer stress reduction techniques

b. Provide acupuncture, aromatherapy, and herbal remedies

c. Provide women's health lectures, instruction on breast self-examinations and Pap smears, and computers for research

d. Offer various support groups

e. Offer specialty equipment for rental and purchase

Activity D *Put the activities in correct sequence by writing the letters in the boxes provided below.*

1. Given below, in random order, are steps of patient and family education. Arrange them in the correct sequence.

   a. Intervening to enhance learning

   b. Planning education

   c. Evaluating learning

   d. Documenting teaching and learning

   e. Assessing teaching and learning needs

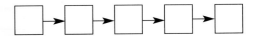

Activity E *Briefly answer the following.*

1. What techniques can the nurse use to enhance learning?

_____

_____

_____

2. What is school nursing?

_____

_____

_____

3. What are the duties of a triage nurse in a pediatric office?

_____

_____

_____

4. What is an individualized health plan (IHP)?

_____

_____

_____

5. What are the factors that have influenced an increased emphasis on health promotion and illness prevention?

_____

_____

_____

6. What is a birthing center?

_____

_____

_____

SECTION III: APPLYING YOUR KNOWLEDGE

Activity F *Consider this scenario and answer the questions.*

By the year 2050, people of African, Asian, and Latino backgrounds will make up one-half of the American population. This growing diversity has strong implications for the provision of health care. A nurse is employed in a clinic that provides prenatal services to a multicultural community predominated by African and Latino families.

1. How should the nurse adapt to different cultural beliefs and practices?

_____

_____

_____

2. List examples of cultural characteristics that would be important for a nurse to understand.

_____

_____

_____

3. What activities would help ensure that a nurse delivers culturally competent nursing care to diverse families?

_____

_____

_____

SECTION IV: PRACTICING FOR NCLEX

Activity G *Answer the following questions.*

1. Nurses in community care settings spend more time in management and supervisory roles than their counterparts in the acute care setting. Which of the following activities is part of case management?

  a. Helping a grandmother to learn a procedure

  b. Assessing the sanitary conditions of the home

  c. Establishing eligibility for a Medicaid waiver

  d. Scheduling speech and respiratory therapy services

2. The nurse is caring for a three-year-old boy who must have a lumbar puncture. Which of the following actions would provide the greatest contribution toward atraumatic care?

  a. Having a child life specialist play with the child

  b. Explaining the lumbar puncture procedure

  c. Letting the child take his teddy bear with him

  d. Keeping the parents calm in front of the child

3. The nurse is educating the family of a two-year-old Chinese boy with bronchiolitis about the disorder and its treatment. Which of the following actions, involving an interpreter, can jeopardize the family's trust?

  a. Allowing too little appointment time for the translation

  b. Using a person who is not a professional interpreter

  c. Asking the interpreter questions not meant for the family

  d. Using an older sibling to communicate with the parents

4. The nurse is striving to form a partnership with the family of a medically fragile child being cared for at home. Which of the following activities is part of family-centered home care?

  a. Recognizing unique family strengths

  b. Ensuring a safe, nurturing environment

  c. Managing information given to parents

  d. Correcting inadequate coping methods

5. Nurses play important roles in a variety of community settings. Which of the following goals is common to all community settings?

  a. Remove or minimize health barriers to learning

  b. Promote the health of a specific group of children

c. Determine initially the type of care a child needs

d. Ensure the health and well-being of children and families

6. A nurse is assigned to take care of a high-risk newborn in the home environment after discharge. Which of the following conditions should the nurse monitor for in the infant?

a. Anencephaly

b. Hydrocephalus

c. Fetal distress syndrome

d. Spina bifida

7. A pregnant client arrives at the maternity clinic for a routine check-up. The client has been reading books on pregnancy and wants to know ways to prevent the incidence of neural tube defects (NTDs) in her fetus. Which of the following should the nurse suggest to prevent the occurrence of NTDs?

a. Take vitamin E supplements

b. Take folic acid supplements

c. Consume legumes frequently

d. Consume citrus fruits frequently

8. A nurse has to address a group of women on the issue of women's health during their reproductive years. Which of the following reasons does the nurse provide regarding the need for comprehensive, community-centered care to women during their reproductive years?

a. Women have more health problems during their reproductive years

b. Women are more susceptible to stress during their reproductive years

c. Women's immune system weakens immediately after birth

d. Women's health care needs change with their reproductive goals

9. The nurse has to prepare a discharge plan as a part of her postpartum care of a client, whom she is caring for in a home-based setting. Which of the following aspects of care should the nurse include in her postpartum care in this environment?

a. Provide the client with self-help books about infant care

b. Monitor the physical and emotional well-being of family members

c. Recognize infant needs in the discharge plan

d. Identify developing complications in the infant

10. A nurse is caring for a Turkish client. The nurse understands that there could be major cultural differences between her and her client. What could be the consequence of a nurse assigning a client to a staff member who is of the same culture as the client?

a. Exemplifies stereotyping

b. Ensures better care and understanding

c. Helps in assessing client's culture

d. Helps build better nurse–client relationship

11. A nurse is caring for a non-English-speaking immigrant client who is pregnant. The nurse is finding it difficult to communicate with the client because of the language barrier. In this situation, which of the following guidelines should the nurse follow to establish a good relationship with this client? Select all that apply.

a. Convey empathy for what the client is experiencing

b. Listen actively by giving verbal and body language clues

c. Interact with the client only when required to reduce difficulty and awkwardness

d. Show respect by valuing the client and viewing her as special

e. Answer the client with simple answers of "yes" and "no"

12. A nurse who has been working in the acute care setting has to care for a client in a home-based setting. The nurse understands that providing care in a home environment is going to be demanding in terms of time and effort. Which of the following tasks should the nurse plan to maximize her home visits to her client? Select all that apply.

a. Prioritize client's needs by their potential to threaten client's health

b. Make an individualized plan of client care

c. Bear in mind the client's readiness to accept intervention and education

d. Train the family to obtain necessary materials or supplies before the visit

e. Develop goals reflecting primary, secondary, and tertiary prevention

13. The nurse is providing home care services to a five-year-old with multiple medical needs. Which of the following activities is unique to a home care nurse?

    a. Preparing the child to see a physician
    b. Conducting health screenings
    c. Coordinating therapists' visits
    d. Collaborating with teachers and staff

14. The nurse is educating a 15-year-old girl with Graves' disease, and her family, about the disease and its treatment. Which of the following methods of evaluating learning is least effective?

    a. Having the child and family demonstrate skills
    b. Asking closed-ended questions for specific facts
    c. Requesting the parent to teach the child skills
    d. Setting up a scenario for them to talk through

15. A nurse is assessing a client who has been diagnosed as diabetic. Which of the following reactions by the client could indicate poor literacy skills?

    a. Does not comply with treatment regimens
    b. Asks many questions regarding laboratory tests
    c. Keeps appointments regularly
    d. Answers queries regarding medications

Anatomy and Physiology of the Reproductive System

SECTION I: LEARNING OBJECTIVES

1. Define the key terms utilized in this chapter.

2. Explain the structure and function of the major external and internal female genital organs.

3. Outline the phases of the menstrual cycle, dominant hormones involved, and changes taking place in each phase.

4. Classify external and internal male reproductive structures and the function of each in hormonal regulation.

SECTION II: ASSESSING YOUR UNDERSTANDING

Activity A *Fill in the blanks.*

1. The vagina is a tubular, fibromuscular organ lined with mucous membrane that lies in a series of transverse folds called _____.

2. _____ stimulates the production of milk within a few days after childbirth.

3. The _____, which lies against the testes, is a coiled tube almost 20 feet long that collects sperm from the testes and provides the space and environment for sperm to mature.

4. In the male, the _____ is the terminal duct of the reproductive and urinary systems, serving as a passageway for semen and urine.

5. The _____ is the mucosal layer that lines the uterine cavity in nonpregnant women.

6. _____ glands, located on either side of the female urethral opening, secrete a small amount of mucus to keep the opening moist and lubricated for the passage of urine.

7. The incision made into the perineal tissue to provide more space for the presenting part of the delivering fetus is called an _____.

8. In the male, the _____ gland lies just under the bladder in the pelvis and surrounds the middle portion of the urethra.

9. The _____ is a pear-shaped muscular organ at the top of the vagina.

10. The _____ is the thin-skinned sac that surrounds and protects the testes.

Activity B *Consider the following figures.*

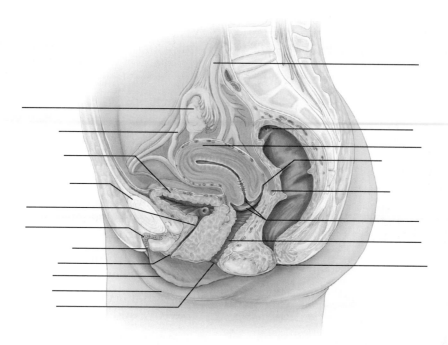

1. a. Identify and label the figure.

_____

_____

b. What are the various parts and their functions?

_____

_____

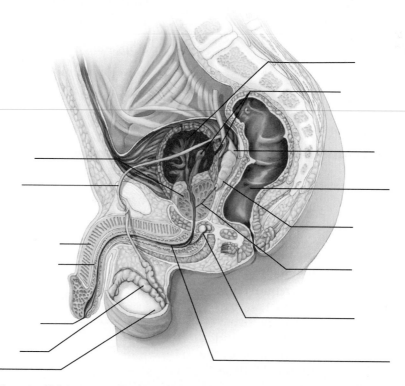

2. a. Identify and label the figure.

_____

_____

b. What are the various parts and their functions?

_____

_____

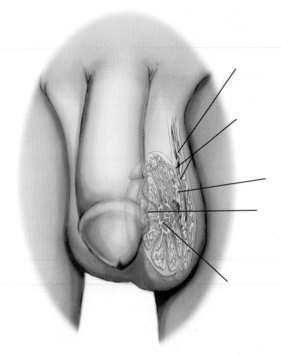

3. Identify and label the figure.

_____

_____

Activity C *Match the hormones in Column A with their functions in Column B.*

Column A

_____ **1.** Gonadotropin-Releasing Hormone (GnRH)

_____ **2.** Follicle-Stimulating Hormone (FSH)

_____ **3.** Luteinizing Hormone (LH)

_____ **4.** Estrogen

_____ **5.** Progesterone

Column B

a. It maintains the uterine decidual lining and reduces uterine contractions, allowing pregnancy to be maintained.

b. It is required for the final maturation of preovulatory follicles and luteinization of the ruptured follicle.

c. It is primarily responsible for the maturation of the ovarian follicle.

d. It inhibits FSH production and stimulates LH production.

e. It induces the release of FSH and LH to assist with ovulation.

Activity D *Put the activities in correct sequence by writing the letters in the boxes provided below.*

1. Given below, in random order, are steps occurring during the endometrial cycle. Arrange them in the correct sequence.

a. The endometrium becomes thickened and more vascular and glandular.

b. Cervical mucus becomes thin, clear, stretchy, and more alkaline.

c. The spiral arteries rupture, releasing blood into the uterus.

d. The ischemia leads to shedding of the endometrium down to the basal layer.

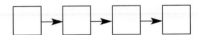

2. Given below, in random order, are pubertal events. Arrange them in the correct sequence.

a. Growth spurt

b. Appearance of pubic and then axillary hair

c. Development of breast buds

d. Onset of menstruation

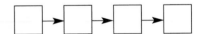

Activity E *Briefly answer the following.*

1. What is the vulva?

_____

_____

_____

2. What is colostrum?

_____

_____

_____

3. What are the physical changes observed in women during their perimenopausal years?

_____

_____

_____

4. What is the role of the nurse when caring for menopausal women?

_____

_____

_____

5. What is the function of the testes?

_____

_____

_____

6. What is the function of the bulbourethral, or Cowper's, glands?

_____

_____

_____

SECTION III: APPLYING YOUR KNOWLEDGE

Activity F *Consider this scenario and answer the questions.*

Susan is a 14-year-old high school student who came to the school nurse's office because she had her first period. She has received health education information in class, but Susan has many questions about her body. She asks the school nurse a lot of questions.

a. Describe what a nurse should teach Susan about the changes in her body and menstruation.

_____

_____

_____

b. Describe the nurse's response when Susan asks how long her cycles will last.

_____

_____

_____

SECTION IV: PRACTICING FOR NCLEX

Activity G *Answer the following questions.*

1. A client is trying to have a baby and wants to know the best time to have intercourse to increase the chances of pregnancy. Which of the following is the ideal time for intercourse, to help her chances of conceiving?

   a. A week after ovulation
   b. One or two days before ovulation
   c. Anytime after ovulation
   d. Anytime during the week before ovulation

2. Which of the following organs is responsible for providing lubrication during intercourse?

   a. Endocrine glands
   b. Pituitary glands
   c. Skene's glands
   d. Bartholin's glands

3. Which of the following is the mucosal layer that lines the uterine cavity in nonpregnant women?

   a. Endometrium
   b. Fundus
   c. Mons pubis
   d. Clitoris

4. A nurse is caring for a client who has given birth. The client reports that her breast milk is dark yellow. Which of the following information should the nurse give to the client regarding the situation?

   a. Modify diet to reduce excess fat intake
   b. The yellow fluid is colostrum and is rich in maternal antibodies
   c. Breastfeeding should be avoided until the breast milk becomes normal
   d. Completely stop breastfeeding and use formula instead

5. A client complains of pain on one side of the abdomen. On further questioning, the nurse discovers that the pain occurs regularly around two weeks before menstruation. The client has not missed a period, and she exercises regularly. Which of the following is the most likely cause of the pain?

   a. Early signs of pregnancy

   b. Irregular menstruation cycle

   c. Pain during ovulation

   d. Exercising regularly

6. A client asks the nurse how she would know if ovulation has occurred. Which of the following is a sign of ovulation that the nurse should inform the client about?

   a. Pain in the vaginal area

   b. Rise in temperature by 0.5–1°F

   c. Uneasiness or sickness

   d. Lack of sleep

7. A nurse is assessing a 45-year-old client. The client asks for information regarding the changes that are most likely to occur with menopause. Which of the following should the nurse tell the client?

   a. Uterus tilts backward

   b. Uterus shrinks and gradually atrophies

   c. Cervical muscle content increases

   d. Outer layer of the cervix becomes rough

8. Which of the following hormones is called the hormone of pregnancy because it reduces uterine contractions during pregnancy?

   a. Luteinizing hormone

   b. Estrogen

   c. Follicle-stimulating hormone

   d. Progesterone

9. During cold conditions, how does the body react to maintain scrotal temperature?

   a. Cremaster muscles relax

   b. Frequency of urination increases

   c. Scrotum is pulled closer to the body

   d. Increase in blood flow to genital area

10. A nurse is screening an elderly client for prostate cancer. What are the effects of aging on the prostate gland?

    a. Prostate gland enlarges with age

    b. Production of semen stops

    c. Prostate gland stops functioning

    d. Prostate gland causes painful erection

11. Which of the following organs provides the space and environment for sperm cells to mature?

    a. Vas deferens

    b. Epididymis

    c. Testes

    d. Cowper's glands

12. A nurse is explaining the menstrual cycle to a 12-year-old client who has experienced menarche. Which of the following should the nurse tell the client?

    a. An average cycle length is about 15 to 20 days

    b. Ovary contains 400,000 follicles at birth

    c. Duration of the flow is about 3 to 7 days

    d. Blood loss averages 120 to 150 mL

13. A nurse is providing information regarding ovulation to a couple who want to have a baby. Which of the following should the nurse tell the clients?

    a. Ovulation takes place 10 days before menstruation

    b. The lifespan of the ovum is only about 48 hours

    c. At ovulation, a mature follicle ruptures, releasing an ovum

    d. When ovulation occurs, there is a rise in estrogen

14. Which of the following hormones is secreted from the hypothalamus in a pulsatile manner throughout the reproductive cycle?

    a. Follicle-stimulating hormone

    b. Gonadotropin-releasing hormone

    c. Luteinizing hormone

    d. Estrogen

CHAPTER 4

Common Reproductive Issues

SECTION I: LEARNING OBJECTIVES

1. Define the key terms utilized in this chapter.

2. Examine common reproductive concerns in terms of symptoms, diagnostic tests, and appropriate interventions.

3. Identify risk factors and outline appropriate client education needed in common reproductive disorders.

4. Compare and contrast the various contraceptive methods available and their overall effectiveness.

5. Explain the physiologic and psychological aspects of menopause.

6. Delineate the nursing management needed for women experiencing common reproductive disorders.

SECTION II: ASSESSING YOUR UNDERSTANDING

Activity A *Fill in the blanks.*

1. _____ involves the in-growth of the endometrium into the uterine musculature.

2. Primary dysmenorrhea is caused by increased _____ production by the endometrium in an ovulatory cycle.

3. _____ is the direct visualization of the internal organs with a lighted instrument inserted through an abdominal incision.

4. During _____, the ovary begins to sputter, producing irregular and missed periods and an occasional hot flash.

5. Male sterilization is accomplished with a surgical procedure known as a _____.

6. In a _____ abortion, the woman takes certain medications to induce a miscarriage to remove the products of conception.

7. _____ is a condition in which bone mass declines to such an extent that fractures occur with minimal trauma.

8. At the onset of ovulation, cervical mucus that is more abundant, clear, slippery, and smooth is known as _____ mucus.

9. The _____ body temperature refers to the lowest body temperature and is reached upon awakening.

10. Oral contraceptives, called _____, contain only progestin and work primarily by thickening the cervical mucus to prevent penetration of the sperm and make the endometrium unfavorable for implantation.

Activity B *Consider the following figures.*

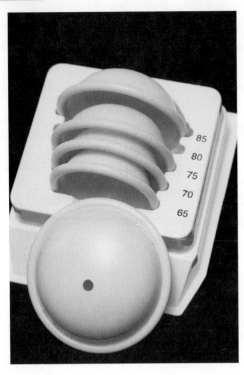

1. What is the purpose of this device?

_____

_____

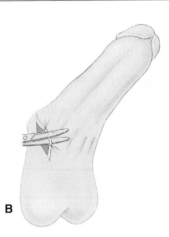

B

2. a. What is being done in this procedure?

_____

_____

b. What is the outcome of this procedure?

_____

_____

Activity C *Match the terms in Column A with the definitions in Column B.*

Column A

____ **1.** Amenorrhea

____ **2.** Dysmenorrhea

____ **3.** Metrorrhagia

____ **4.** Menometrorrhagia

____ **5.** Oligomenorrhea

Column B

a. Bleeding between periods

b. Bleeding occurring at intervals of more than 35 days

c. Absence of menses during the reproductive years

d. Difficult or painful or abnormal menstruation

e. Heavy bleeding occurring at irregular intervals, with flow lasting more than 7 days

Activity D *Put the steps in correct sequence by writing the letters in the boxes provided below.*

1. Given below, in random order, are steps occurring during diaphragm insertion. Write the correct sequence.

a. Hold the diaphragm between the thumb and fingers and compress it to form a "figure-eight" shape.

b. Place a tablespoon of spermicidal jelly or cream in the dome and around the rim of the diaphragm.

c. Select the position that is most comfortable for insertion.

d. Tuck the front rim of the diaphragm behind the pubic bone so that the rubber hugs the front wall of the vagina.

e. Insert the diaphragm into the vagina, directing it downward as far as it will go.

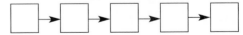

2. Given below, in random order, are steps occurring during cervical cap insertion. Write the correct sequence.

a. Pinch the sides of the cervical cap together.

b. Use one finger to feel around the entire circumference to make sure there are no gaps between the cap rim and the cervix.

c. Pinch the cap dome and tug gently to check for evidence of suction.

d. Insert the cervical cap into the vagina, and place over the cervix.

e. Compress the cervical cap dome.

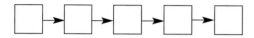

Activity E *Briefly answer the following.*

1. What are the common laboratory tests ordered to determine the cause of amenorrhea?

_____

_____

_____

2. What is menopause?

_____

_____

_____

3. What are the risk factors associated with endometriosis?

_____

_____

_____

4. What is infertility?

_____

_____

_____

5. What is the Two-Day Method for contraception?

_____

_____

_____

6. What are intrauterine systems?

_____

_____

_____

SECTION III: APPLYING YOUR KNOWLEDGE

Activity F *Consider this scenario and answer the questions.*

Alexa is a 14-year-old lacrosse player who has been training vigorously for selection on her high school team. Alexa comes to the health care provider's office to have her health forms for school completed. The office nurse takes her history, and the client describes that she has been experiencing amenorrhea.

1. How should the nurse describe "primary amenorrhea" to Alexa?

_____

_____

_____

2. State the causes of "primary amenorrhea" that may be related to Alexa.

_____

_____

_____

3. What treatments may be considered for Alexa?

_____

_____

_____

4. What counseling and education should the nurse provide for Alexa at this visit?

_____

_____

_____

SECTION IV: PRACTICING FOR NCLEX

Activity G *Answer the following questions.*

1. The nurse is assessing a client for amenorrhea. Which of the following should the nurse document as evidence of androgen excess secondary to a tumor?

   a. Reduced subcutaneous fat

   b. Hypothermia

c. Irregular heart rate and pulse

d. Facial hair and acne

2. A nurse is teaching a female client about fertility awareness as a method of contraception. Which of the following should the nurse mention as an assumption for this method?

a. Sperm can live up to 24 hours after intercourse

b. The "unsafe period" is approximately 6 days

c. The exact time of ovulation can be determined

d. The "safe period" is 3 days after ovulation

3. The nurse is instructing a client with dysmenorrhea on how to manage her symptoms. Which of the following should the nurse include in the teaching plan? Select all that apply.

a. Increase intake of salty foods

b. Increase water consumption

c. Avoid keeping legs elevated while lying down

d. Use heating pads or take warm baths

e. Increase exercise and physical activity

4. A client is to be examined for the presence and extent of endometriosis. Which of the following tests should the nurse prepare the client for?

a. Tissue biopsy

b. Hysterosalpingogram

c. Clomiphene citrate challenge test

d. Laparoscopy

5. A couple is being assessed for infertility. The male partner is required to collect a semen sample for analysis. What instruction should the nurse give him?

a. Abstain from sexual activity for 10 hours before collecting the sample

b. Avoid strenuous activity for 24 hours before collecting the sample

c. Collect a specimen by ejaculating into a condom or plastic bag

d. Deliver sample for analysis within 1 to 2 hours after ejaculation

6. A client needs additional information about the cervical mucus ovulation method after having read about it in a magazine. She asks the nurse about cervical changes during ovulation. Which of the following should the nurse inform the client about?

a. Cervical os is slightly closed

b. Cervical mucus is dry and thick

c. Cervix is high or deep in the vagina

d. Cervical mucus breaks when stretched

7. A female client has undergone a clomiphene citrate challenge test. The FSH level is 16.5. What should the nurse tell this client?

a. "This is a good result; we just need to chart your cycle."

b. "I'm sorry, but adoption seems to be your only option."

c. "You might want to consider the option of using donor eggs."

d. "Artificial insemination might be a solution to your problems."

8. A client has been following the conventional 28-day regimen for contraception. She is now considering switching to an extended Oral Contraceptive (OC) regimen. She is seeking information about specific safety precautions. Which of the following is true for the extended OC regimen?

a. It is not as effective as the conventional regimen

b. It prevents pregnancy for three months at a time

c. It carries the same safety profile as the 28-day regimen

d. It does not ensure restoration of fertility if discontinued

9. A 30-year-old client would like to try using basal body temperature (BBT) as a fertility awareness method. Which of the following instructions should the nurse provide the client?

a. Avoid unprotected intercourse until BBT has been elevated for six days

b. Avoid using other fertility awareness methods along with BBT

c. Use the axillary method of taking the temperature

d. Take temperature before rising and record it on a chart

10. A client who is not well-educated has approached the nurse for information about contraception. She indicates that she is not comfortable about using any barrier methods and would like the option of regaining fertility after a couple of years. Which of the following methods should the nurse suggest to this client?
    a. Basal body temperature
    b. Coitus interruptus
    c. Lactational amenorrhea method
    d. CycleBeads or Depo-Provera

11. A client would like some information about the use of a cervical cap. Which of the following should the nurse include in the teaching plan of this client? Select all that apply.
    a. Inspect the cervical cap prior to insertion
    b. Apply spermicide to the rim of the cervical cap
    c. Wait for 30 minutes after insertion before engaging in intercourse
    d. Remove the cervical cap immediately after intercourse
    e. Do not use the cervical cap during menses

12. A healthy 28-year-old female client who has a sedentary lifestyle and is a chain smoker is seeking information about contraception. The nurse informs this client of the various options available and the benefits and the risks of each. Which of the following should the nurse recognize as contraindicated in the case of this client?
    a. The Lunelle injection or Depo-Provera
    b. Combination oral contraceptives
    c. A copper intrauterine device
    d. Implantable contraceptives

13. A client in her second trimester of pregnancy asks the nurse for information regarding certain oral medications to induce a miscarriage. What information should this client be given about such medications?
    a. They are available only in the form of suppositories
    b. They can be taken only in the first trimester
    c. They present a high risk of respiratory failure
    d. They are considered a permanent end to fertility

14. A client reports that she has multiple sex partners and has a lengthy history of various pelvic infections. She would like to know if there is any temporary contraceptive method that would suit her condition. Which of the following should the nurse suggest for this client?
    a. Intrauterine device
    b. Condoms
    c. Oral contraceptives
    d. Tubal ligation

15. When caring for a client with reproductive issues, the nurse is required to clear up misconceptions. This enables new learning to take hold and a better client response to whichever methods are explored and ultimately selected. Which of the following are misconceptions that the nurse needs to clear up? Select all that apply.
    a. Breastfeeding does not protect against pregnancy
    b. Taking birth control pills protects against STIs
    c. Douching after sex will prevent pregnancy
    d. Pregnancy can occur during menses
    e. Irregular menstruation prevents pregnancy

16. A 52-year-old client is seeking treatment for menopause. She is not very active and has a history of cardiac problems. Which of the following therapy options should the nurse recognize as contraindicated for this client?
    a. Long-term hormone replacement therapy
    b. Selective estrogen receptor modulators
    c. Lipid-lowering agents
    d. Bisphosphonates

17. A 49-year-old client undergoing menopause complains to the nurse of loss of lubrication during intercourse, which she feels is hampering her sex life. Which of the following responses is appropriate for the nurse?
    a. "Don't worry! This is a normal process of aging."
    b. "Have you considered contacting a support group for women your age?"
    c. "You can manage the condition by using OTC moisturizers or lubricants."
    d. "All you need is a positive outlook and a supportive partner."

18. A couple is interested in seeking treatment for infertility. Which of the following should the nurse ensure in the initial stage?

    a. The couple is aware of the risks and benefits of treatments

    b. The couple has access to all the required medical facilities

    c. The couple is financially sound and can handle the treatment costs

    d. The couple's emotional distress level is not unusually high

19. A client has opted to use an intrauterine device for contraception. Which of the following effects of the device on monthly periods should the nurse inform the client about?

    a. Periods become lighter

    b. Periods become more painful

    c. Periods become longer

    d. Periods reduce in number

20. A 30-year-old client tells the nurse that she would like to use a contraceptive sponge but does not know enough about its use and whether it will protect her against sexually transmitted infections. Which of the following information should the nurse provide the client about using a contraceptive sponge? Select all that apply.

    a. Keep the sponge for more than 30 hours to prevent STIs

    b. Wet the sponge with water before inserting it

    c. Insert the sponge 24 hours before intercourse

    d. Leave the sponge in place for at least six hours following intercourse

    e. Replace sponge every two hours for the method to be effective

CHAPTER 5

Sexually Transmitted Infections

SECTION I: LEARNING OBJECTIVES

1. Define the key terms utilized in this chapter.

2. Construct the spread and control of sexually transmitted infections.

3. Identify risk factors and outline appropriate client education needed in common sexually transmitted infections.

4. Judge how contraceptives can play a role in the prevention of sexually transmitted infections.

5. Analyze the physiologic and psychological aspects of sexually transmitted infections.

6. Delineate the nursing management needed for women with sexually transmitted infections.

SECTION II: ASSESSING YOUR UNDERSTANDING

Activity A *Fill in the blanks.*

1. _____ is a common vaginal infection characterized by a heavy yellow, green, or gray frothy discharge.

2. The _____ stage of syphilis is characterized by diseases affecting the heart, eyes, brain, central nervous system, and/or skin.

3. _____ are a common cause of skin rash and pruritus throughout the world.

4. _____ is an intense pruritic dermatitis caused by a mite.

5. Vulvovaginal candidiasis, if not treated effectively during pregnancy, can cause the newborn to contract an oral infection known as _____ during the birth process.

6. _____ is a complex, curable bacterial infection caused by the spirochete *Treponema pallidum.*

7. Hepatitis B virus (HBV) can result in serious, permanent damage to the _____ .

8. Cervicitis, acute urethral syndrome, salpingitis, PID, and infertility are conditions associated with _____ infection.

9. A person is said to be in the last stage of AIDS when the _____ T-cell count is less than or equal to 200.

10. Any woman suspected of having gonorrhea should be tested for _____ also, because co-infection (45%) is extremely common.

Activity B *Consider the following figures.*

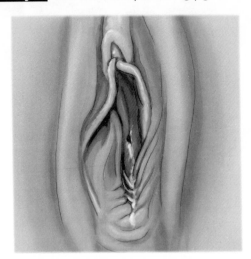

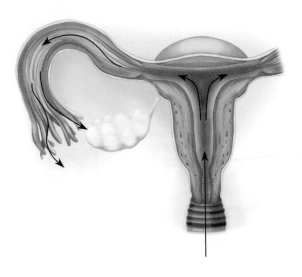

1. a. Identify this disease.

_____

_____

b. What is the consequence if this disease is untreated?

_____

_____

3. a. Identify the disease shown in the figure.

_____

_____

b. What are the causes of this disease?

_____

_____

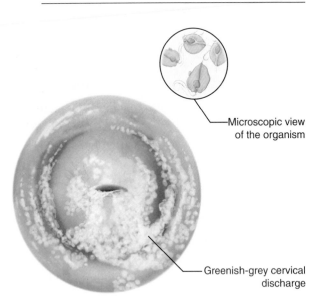

Microscopic view of the organism

Greenish-grey cervical discharge

2. a. Identify this disease.

_____

_____

b. What are the clinical manifestations of this disease?

_____

_____

Activity C *Match the sexually transmitted infections in Column A with their related descriptions in Column B.*

Column A	Column B
____ **1.** Human immuno-deficiency virus (HIV)	**a.** Inflammation and infection of the vagina
____ **2.** Vaginitis	**b.** Acute, systemic viral infection that can be transmitted sexually
____ **3.** Hepatitis	**c.** Retrovirus causes breakdown in immune function, leading to acquired immunodeficiency syndrome (AIDS)
____ **4.** Gonorrhea	
____ **5.** Genital herpes	
____ **6.** Human papillomavirus (HPV)	**d.** A recurrent, life-long viral infection
	e. Cause of essentially all cases of cervical cancer
	f. Very severe bacterial infection in the columnar epithelium of the endocervix

Activity D *Put the activities in correct sequence by writing the letters in the boxes provided below.*

1. Given below, in random order, are the manifestations of syphilis in its various stages. Arrange the stages in their correct order.

   a. Flu-like symptoms; rash on trunk, palms, and soles

   b. Life-threatening heart disease and neurologic disease that slowly destroys the heart, eyes, brain, central nervous system, and skin

   c. Painless ulcer at site of bacterial entry that disappears in 1 to 6 weeks

   d. No clinical manifestations even though serology is positive

   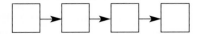

Activity E *Briefly answer the following.*

1. What are the predisposing factors for the occurrence of vulvovaginal candidiasis?

   _____

   _____

   _____

2. What are the symptoms of hepatitis A?

   _____

   _____

   _____

3. How is HIV transmitted?

   _____

   _____

   _____

4. What is acquired immunodeficiency syndrome (AIDS)?

   _____

   _____

   _____

5. What are the causes of vaginitis?

   _____

   _____

   _____

6. What are clinical manifestations of chlamydia?

   _____

   _____

   _____

SECTION III: APPLYING YOUR KNOWLEDGE

Activity F *Consider this scenario and answer the questions.*

1. A nurse is caring for a 22-year-old pregnant client who has been diagnosed with gonorrhea. The client seems to be very apprehensive about seeking treatment and wants to know if her newborn would be at risk for the infection.

   a. What information should the nurse provide the client regarding the transmission of the infection to the newborn?

   _____

   _____

   _____

   b. What factors should a nurse be aware of when caring for the client with gonorrhea or any other STI?

   _____

   _____

   _____

   c. Which groups of clients are at a higher risk for developing gonorrhea?

   _____

   _____

   _____

SECTION IV: PRACTICING FOR NCLEX

Activity G *Answer the following questions.*

1. A nurse is caring for a female client who has a history of recurring vulvovaginal candidiasis. Which of the following instructions should the nurse offer the client to prevent vulvo-vaginal candidiasis?

   a. Use superabsorbent tampons

   b. Douche the affected area regularly

   c. Wear white, 100% cotton underpants

   d. Increase intake of carbonated drinks

2. An HIV-positive client who is on antiretroviral therapy complains of anorexia, nausea, and vomiting. Which of the following suggestions should the nurse offer the client to cope with this condition?

   a. Use high-protein supplements

   b. Eat dry crackers after meals

   c. Limit number of meals to three a day

   d. Constantly drink fluids while eating

3. A client complaining of genital warts has been diagnosed with HPV. The genital warts have been treated, and they have disappeared. Which of the following should the nurse include in the teaching plan when educating the client about the condition?

   a. Applying steroid creams in affected area promotes comfort

   b. Even after warts are removed, HPV still remains

   c. All women above the age of 30 should get themselves vaccinated against HPV

   d. Use of latex condoms is associated with increased risk of cervical cancer

4. A female client is prescribed metronidazole for the treatment of trichomoniasis. Which of the following instructions should the nurse give the client undergoing treatment?

   a. Avoid extremes of temperature to the genital area

   b. Use condoms during sex

   c. Increase fluid intake

   d. Avoid alcohol

5. A nurse is required to assess a client complaining of unusual vaginal discharge for bacterial vaginosis. Which of the following is a classic manifestation of this condition that the nurse should assess for?

   a. Characteristic "stale fish" odor

   b. Heavy yellow discharge

   c. Dysfunctional uterine bleeding

   d. Erythema in the vulvovaginal area

6. A nurse needs to assess a female client for primary stage HSV infection. Which of the following symptoms related to this condition should the nurse assess for?

   a. Rashes on the face

   b. Yellow-green vaginal discharge

   c. Loss of hair or alopecia

   d. Genital vesicular lesions

7. A nurse working in a community health education program is assigned to educate community members about sexually transmitted infections. Which of the following nursing strategies should be adopted to prevent the spread of sexually transmitted infections in the community?

   a. Promote use of oral contraceptives

   b. Emphasize the importance of good body hygiene

   c. Discuss limiting the number of sex partners

   d. Emphasize not sharing personal items with others

8. A nurse who is conducting sessions on preventing the spread of sexually transmitted infections in a particular community discovers that there is a very high incidence of hepatitis B in the community. Which of the following measures should she take to ensure the prevention of hepatitis B?

   a. Ensure that the drinking water is disease-free

   b. Instruct people to get vaccinated for hepatitis B

   c. Educate about risks of injecting drugs

   d. Educate teenagers to delay onset of sexual activity

9. A nurse is caring for a client undergoing treatment for bacterial vaginosis. Which of the following instructions should the nurse give the client to prevent recurrence of bacterial vaginosis? Select all that apply.

a. Practice monogamy

b. Use oral contraceptives

c. Avoid smoking

d. Undergo colposcopy tests frequently

10. A pregnant client arrives at the community clinic complaining of fever blisters and cold sores on the lips, eyes, and face. The primary health care provider has diagnosed it as the primary episode of genital herpes simplex, for which antiviral therapy is recommended. Which of the following information should the nurse offer the client when educating her about managing the infection?

a. Antiviral drug therapy cures the infection completely

b. Kissing during the primary episode does not transmit the virus

c. Safety of antiviral therapy during pregnancy has not been established

d. Recurrent HSV infection episodes are longer and more severe

11. A 19-year-old female client has been diagnosed with pelvic inflammatory disease due to untreated gonorrhea. Which of the following instructions should the nurse offer when caring for the client? Select all that apply.

a. Use an intrauterine device (IUD)

b. Avoid douching vaginal area

c. Complete the antibiotic therapy

d. Increase fluid intake

e. Limit the number of sex partners

12. A client complaining of genital ulcers has been diagnosed with syphilis. Which of the following nursing interventions should the nurse implement when caring for the client? Select all that apply.

a. Have the client urinate in water if urination is painful

b. Suggest the client apply ice packs to the genital area for comfort

c. Instruct the client to wash her hands with soap and water after touching lesions

d. Instruct the client to wear nonconstricting, comfortable clothes

e. Instruct the client to abstain from sex during the latency period

13. A nurse is conducting an AIDS awareness program for women. Which of the following instructions should the nurse include in the teaching plan to empower women to develop control over their lives in a practical manner so that they can prevent becoming infected with HIV? Select the most appropriate responses.

a. Give opportunities to practice negotiation techniques

b. Encourage women to develop refusal skills

c. Encourage women to use female condoms

d. Support youth development activities to reduce sexual risk-taking

e. Encourage women to lead a healthy lifestyle

14. A nurse is caring for an HIV-positive client who is on triple-combination HAART. Which of the following should the nurse include in the teaching plan when educating the client about the treatment? Select all that apply.

a. Exposure of fetus to antiretroviral agents is completely safe

b. Successful antiretroviral therapy may prevent AIDS

c. Unpleasant side effects such as nausea and diarrhea are common

d. Provide written materials describing diet, exercise, and medications

e. Ensure that the client understands the dosing regimen and schedule

15. A nurse is caring for a female client who is undergoing treatment for genital warts due to HPV. Which of the following information should the nurse include when educating the client about the risk of cervical cancer? Select all that apply.

a. Use of broad-spectrum antibiotics increases risk of cervical cancer

b. Obtaining Pap smears regularly helps early detection of cervical cancer

c. Abnormal vaginal discharge is a sign of cervical cancer

d. Recurrence of genital warts increases risk of cervical cancer

e. Use of latex condoms is associated with a lower rate of cervical cancer

16. A nurse is caring for a client who has just delivered a baby. Which of the following information should the nurse give the client regarding hepatitis B vaccination for the baby?

    a. Vaccine may not be safe for underweight or premature babies

    b. Vaccine consists of a series of three injections given within 6 months

    c. Vaccine is administered only after the infant is at least 6 months old

    d. Vaccine is required only if mother is identified as high-risk for hepatitis B

17. A pregnant client has been diagnosed with gonorrhea. Which of the following nursing interventions should be performed to prevent gonococcal ophthalmia neonatorum in the baby?

    a. Administer cephalosporins to mother during pregnancy

    b. Instill a prophylactic agent in the eyes of the newborn

    c. Perform a cesarean operation to prevent infection

    d. Administer an antiretroviral syrup to the newborn

18. A pregnant client is diagnosed with AIDS. Which of the following interventions should the nurse undertake to minimize the risk of transmission of AIDS to the infant?

    a. Ensure that the baby is delivered via cesarean

    b. Begin triple-combination HAART for the newborn

    c. Ensure that the baby is breastfed instead of being given formula

    d. Administer antiretroviral syrup to the infant within 12 hours after birth

CHAPTER 6

Disorders of the Breasts

SECTION I: LEARNING OBJECTIVES

1. Define the key terms utilized in this chapter.

2. Identify the incidence, risk factors, screening methods, and treatment modalities for benign breast conditions.

3. Outline preventive strategies for breast cancer through lifestyle changes and health screening.

4. Explain the incidence, risk factors, treatment modalities, and nursing considerations related to breast cancer.

5. Develop an educational plan to teach breast self-examination to a group of young women.

SECTION II: ASSESSING YOUR UNDERSTANDING

Activity A *Fill in the blanks.*

1. _____ is a useful adjunct to mammography that produces images of the breasts by sending sound waves through a conductive gel applied to the breasts.

2. _____, an alternative to radiation therapy, involves the use of a catheter to implant radioactive seeds into the breast after a tumor has been removed surgically.

3. Hormone therapy is used to block or counter the effect of the hormone _____ while treating breast cancer.

4. _____ is contraindicated for women whose active connective tissue conditions make them especially sensitive to the side effects of radiation.

5. _____ involves taking x-ray pictures of the breasts while they are compressed between two plastic plates.

6. _____, a type of therapy for breast cancer, leads to side effects such as hair loss, weight loss, and fatigue.

7. The removal of all breast tissue, the nipple, and the areola for breast cancer treatment is known as _____.

8. When diagnosing a woman with intraductal papilloma, a _____ card is used to evaluate nipple discharge for the presence of occult blood.

9. _____ is used as an adjunct therapy for breast cancer.

10. _____ are common benign solid breast tumors that occur in about 10% of all women and account for up to half of all breast biopsies.

Activity B   *Consider the following figures.*

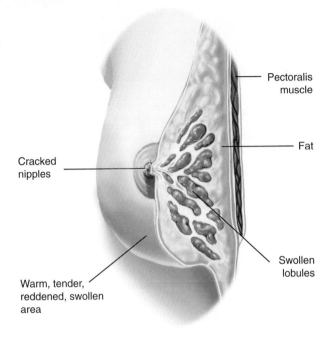

Pectoralis muscle

Fat

Cracked nipples

Swollen lobules

Warm, tender, reddened, swollen area

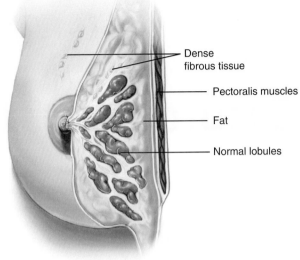

Dense fibrous tissue

Pectoralis muscles

Fat

Normal lobules

A

1.

a. Identify the disease depicted in the figure above.

_____

_____

b. What are the clinical manifestations of this disease?

_____

_____

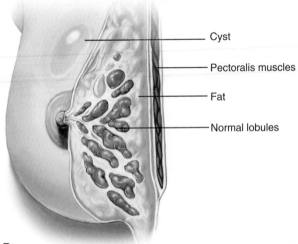

Cyst

Pectoralis muscles

Fat

Normal lobules

B

2. a. Identify the disease and the stage of disease depicted in each figure.

_____

_____

b. What are the clinical manifestations of the depicted disease stages?

_____

_____

Activity C *Match the benign breast disorders in Column A with their related descriptions in Column B.*

Column A

_____ **1.** Fibrocystic breast changes

_____ **2.** Fibroadenomas

_____ **3.** Intraductal papilloma

_____ **4.** Mammary duct ectasia

_____ **5.** Mastitis

Column B

a. An infection of the connective tissue in the breast, occurring primarily in lactating women

b. Dilation and inflammation of the ducts behind the nipple

c. Benign, wart-like growths found in the mammary ducts, usually near the nipple, caused by a proliferation and overgrowth of ductal epithelial tissue.

d. Firm, rubbery, well-circumscribed, freely mobile nodules that might or might not be tender when palpated

e. Lumpy, tender breasts; multiple, smooth, tiny "pebbles" or lumpy "oatmeal" under skin in later stages

Activity D *Briefly answer the following.*

1. What are benign breast disorders?

_____

_____

2. What are the three aspects on which breast cancers are classified?

_____

_____

3. What is breast-conserving surgery?

_____

_____

_____

4. What is adjunct therapy?

_____

_____

_____

5. What are the side effects of chemotherapy?

_____

_____

6. Why is the status of the axillary lymph nodes important in the diagnosis of breast cancer?

_____

_____

_____

SECTION III: APPLYING YOUR KNOWLEDGE

Activity E *Consider this scenario and answer the questions.*

1. Mrs. Taylor, 54, presents to the women's health community clinic, where a nurse assesses her. She is very upset and crying. She tells the nurse that she found one large lump in her left breast and she knows that "it's cancer and I will die." When the nurse asks about her problem, she states that she does not routinely check her breasts and she hasn't had a mammogram for years because "they're too expensive." She also describes the intermittent pain she experiences in her breast.

a. What specific questions should the nurse include in her assessment of Mrs. Taylor?

_____

_____

b. What education does Mrs. Taylor need regarding breast health?

_____

_____

_____

c. Explain what treatment modalities are available if Mrs. Taylor does have a malignancy.

_____

_____

_____

d. What community referrals are needed to meet Mrs. Taylor's future needs?

_____

_____

_____

SECTION IV: PRACTICING FOR NCLEX

Activity F *Answer the following questions.*

1. A client complains of lumpy, tender breasts, particularly during the week before menses. She complains of pain that often dissipates after the onset of menses. The nurse has to examine the client's breasts to confirm fibrocystic breast changes. Which of the following is the best time in the client's menstrual cycle to perform a breast examination?

   a. When the client is ovulating

   b. During the second phase of client's menstrual cycle

   c. A week after the client has completed her menses

   d. Immediately after the client's menses

2. A client arrives at the health care facility complaining of a lump that she felt during her breast self-examination. Upon diagnosis, the physician suspects fibroadenomas. Which of the following questions should the nurse ask when assessing the client?

   a. "Do you consume foods high in fat?"

   b. "Are you lactating?"

   c. "Are you taking oral contraceptives?"

   d. "Do you smoke regularly?"

3. A female client who has a two-month-old baby arrives at a health care facility complaining of flulike symptoms with fever and chills. When examining the breast, the nurse observes an increase in warmth, tenderness, and swelling with abraded nipples. The diagnosis indicates mastitis. Which of the following

instructions should the nurse provide the client to help her cope with the condition?

   a. Increase fluid intake

   b. Avoid breastfeeding for a month

   c. Avoid changing positions while nursing

   d. Apply cold compresses to the affected breast

4. Mammography is recommended for a client diagnosed with intraductal papilloma. Which of the following factors should the nurse ensure when preparing the client for a mammography?

   a. Client has not consumed fluids an hour prior to testing

   b. Client has not applied deodorant on the day of testing

   c. Client is just going to start her menses

   d. Client has taken an aspirin before the testing

5. A female client with a malignant tumor of the breast has to undergo chemotherapy for a period of 6 months. Which of the following side effects should the nurse monitor for when caring for this client?

   a. Vaginal discharge

   b. Headache

   c. Chills

   d. Constipation

6. A client diagnosed with fibroadenoma is worried about her chances of developing breast cancer. She also asks the nurse about various breast disorders and their risks. Which of the following benign breast disorders should the nurse mention as high risk for breast cancer?

   a. Fibrodenomas

   b. Mastitis

   c. Mammary duct ectasia

   d. Intraductal papilloma

7. It is recommended that a 48-year-old female client with breast cancer undergo a sentinel lymph node biopsy before lumpectomy. The client is anxious to know the reason for removing the sentinel lymph node. Which of the following information should the nurse offer the client?

   a. It will prevent lymphedema, which is a common side effect

   b. It will reveal the hormone-receptor status of the cancer

c. It will lessen the aggressiveness of the subsequent chemotherapy

d. It will allow the degree of HER-2/neu oncoprotein to be revealed

8. A client has undergone a mastectomy for breast cancer. Which of the following instructions should the nurse include in the post-surgery client-teaching plan?

   a. Breathe rapidly for an hour

   b. Elevate the affected arm on a pillow

   c. Avoid moving the affected arm in any way

   d. Restrict intake of medication

9. A 62-year-old female client arrives at a health care facility complaining of skin redness in the breast area, along with skin edema. The physician suspects inflammatory breast cancer. Which of the following is a symptom of inflammatory breast cancer that the nurse should assess for?

   a. Palpable mobile cysts

   b. Palpable papilloma

   c. Increased warmth of the breast

   d. Induced nipple discharge

10. A 41-year-old female client arrives at a health care setting complaining of dull nipple pain with a burning sensation, accompanied by pruritus around the nipple. The physician suspects mammary duct ectasia. Which of the following is a manifestation of mammary duct ectasia that the nurse should assess for?

    a. Torturous tubular swellings in the upper half of breast

    b. Increased warmth of the breasts, along with redness

    c. Skin retractions on the breast when the skin is pulled

    d. Green-colored nipple discharge with consistency of toothpaste

11. A 52-year-old female client with an ER+ breast cancer has to undergo hormonal therapy after her initial treatment. The client has to be administered selective estrogen receptor modulator (SERM). Which of the following side effects of SERM should the nurse monitor for when caring for the client?

    a. Fever

    b. Weight loss

    c. Hot flashes

    d. Chills

12. A nurse is assigned to educate a group of women on cancer awareness. Which of the following are the modifiable risk factors for breast cancer? Select all that apply.

    a. Failing to breastfeed for up to a year after pregnancy

    b. Early menarche or late menopause

    c. Postmenopausal use of estrogen and progestins

    d. Not having children until after age 30

    e. Previous abnormal breast biopsy

13. A nurse is educating a client on the technique for performing breast self-examination. Which of the following instructions should the nurse include in the teaching plan with regard to the different degrees of pressure that need to be applied on the breast?

    a. Light pressure midway into the tissue

    b. Medium pressure around the areolar area

    c. Medium pressure on the skin throughout

    d. Hard pressure applied down to the ribs

14. A female client with metastatic breast disease is prescribed trastuzumab as part of her immunotherapy. Which of the following is the adverse effect of trastuzumab that a nurse should monitor for with the first infusion of the antibody?

    a. Stroke

    b. Hepatic failure

    c. Myelosuppression

    d. Dyspnea

15. A nurse is caring for a female client undergoing radiation therapy after her breast surgery. Which of the following is the side effect of radiation therapy that the client is likely to experience?

    a. Anorexia

    b. Infection

    c. Fever

    d. Nausea

16. A nurse is caring for a client who has just had her intraductal papilloma removed through a surgical procedure. What instructions should the nurse give this client as part of her care?

    a. Apply warm compresses to the affected breast

    b. Continue monthly breast self-examinations

    c. Wear a supportive bra 24 hours a day

    d. Refrain from consuming salt in diet

17. Lumpectomy is a treatment option for clients diagnosed with breast cancer with tumors smaller than 5 cm. For which of the following clients is lumpectomy contraindicated? Select all that apply.

    a. Client who has had an early menarche or late onset of menopause

    b. Client who has had previous radiation to the affected breast

    c. Client who has failed to breastfeed for up to a year after pregnancy

    d. Client whose connective tissue is reported to be sensitive to radiation

    e. Client whose surgery will not result in a clean margin of tissue

18. A 38-year-old female client has to undergo lymph node surgery in conjunction with mastectomy. The client is likely to experience lymphedema due to the surgery. Post-surgery, which of the following factors will make the client more susceptible to lymphedema? Select all that apply.

    a. Use of the affected arm for drawing blood or measuring blood pressure

    b. Engaging in activities like gardening without using gloves

    c. Not consuming foods that are rich in phytochemicals

    d. Not wearing a well-fitted compression sleeve

    e. Not consuming a diet high in fiber and protein

19. A 33-year-old female client complains of yellow nipple discharge and a pain in her breasts a week before menses that dissipates on the onset of menses. Diagnosis reveals that the client is experiencing fibrocystic breast changes. Which of the following instructions should the nurse offer the client to help alleviate the condition? Select all that apply.

    a. Increase fluid intake steadily

    b. Avoid caffeine

    c. Practice good hand-washing techniques

    d. Maintain a low-fat diet

    e. Take diuretics as recommended

20. A nurse is educating a 43-year-old female client about required lifestyle changes to help avoid breast cancer. Which of the following instructions regarding diet and food habits should the nurse include in the teaching plan? Select all that apply.

    a. Restrict intake of salted foods

    b. Limit intake of processed foods

    c. Consume seven or more portions of complex carbohydrates daily

    d. Increase liquid intake to 3 liters daily

    e. Consume at least five servings of proteins daily

Benign Disorders of the Female Reproductive Tract

SECTION I: LEARNING OBJECTIVES

1. Define the key terms bolded throughout the chapter.

2. Identify the major pelvic relaxation disorders in terms of etiology, management, and nursing interventions.

3. Outline the nursing management needed for the most common benign reproductive disorders in women.

4. Relate the implications of urinary incontinence to future quality of life and to its pathology, clinical manifestations, and treatment options.

5. Compare the various benign growths to their symptomatology and course of management.

6. Explore the emotional impact on a woman diagnosed with polycystic ovarian syndrome and the nurse's role as a counselor, educator, and advocate.

SECTION II: ASSESSING YOUR UNDERSTANDING

Activity A *Fill in the blanks.*

1. _____ occurs when the posterior bladder wall protrudes downward through the anterior vaginal wall.

2. Uterine _____ occurs when the uterus descends through the pelvic floor and into the vaginal canal.

3. A _____ is a silicone or plastic device that is placed into the vagina to support the uterus, bladder, and rectum as a space-filling device.

4. _____ are small benign growths that may be associated with chronic inflammation, an abnormal local response to increased levels of estrogen, or local congestion of the cervical vasculature.

5. Uterine fibroids, or _____, are benign proliferations composed of smooth muscle and fibrous connective tissue in the uterus.

6. _____ exercises strengthen the pelvic-floor muscles to support the inner organs and prevent further prolapse.

7. Rectocele occurs when the _____ sags and pushes against or into the posterior vaginal wall.

8. Weakened pelvic floor musculature also prevents complete closure of the _____, resulting in urine leakage during moments of physical stress.

9. _____, or irregular, acyclic uterine bleeding, is the most frequent clinical manifestation of women with endometrial polyps.

10. _____ ultrasound is used to distinguish fluid-filled ovarian cysts from a solid malignancy.

Activity B *Consider the following figures.*

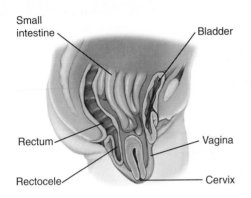

Small intestine

Bladder

Rectum

Vagina

Rectocele

Cervix

1. Identify the disorders, if any, shown in the figure.

_____

_____

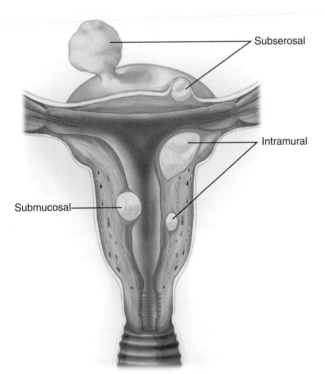

Subserosal

Intramural

Submucosal

2. Identify the disorder in the figure.

_____

_____

Activity C *Match the benign disorders of the female reproductive tract in Column A with their correct definitions in Column B.*

Column A

_____ **1.** Pelvic organ prolapse

_____ **2.** Stress incontinence

_____ **3.** Uterine fibroids

_____ **4.** Polycystic ovarian syndrome

_____ **5.** Urge incontinence

Column B

a. Abnormal descent or herniation of the pelvic organs from their original attachment sites or their normal positions in the pelvis

b. Benign tumors composed of muscular and fibrous tissue in the uterus

c. Presence of multiple inactive follicle cysts within the ovary that interfere with ovarian function

d. Precipitous loss of urine, preceded by a strong urge to void, with increased bladder pressure and detrusor contraction

e. Accidental leakage of urine that occurs with increased pressure on the bladder from coughing, sneezing, laughing, or physical exertion

Activity D *Briefly answer the following.*

1. What are the causes of pelvic organ prolapse?

_____

_____

_____

2. What are Kegel exercises?

_____

_____

_____

3. What are the causes of urinary incontinence?

_____

_____

_____

4. What is the Colpexin™ Sphere?

_____

_____

_____

5. What is uterine artery embolization (UAE)?

_____

_____

_____

6. What are Bartholin's cysts?

_____

_____

_____

SECTION III: APPLYING YOUR KNOWLEDGE

Activity E *Consider this scenario and answer the questions.*

1. Mrs. Scott, age 57, comes in for her yearly gynecological examination and complains of "feeling like something is coming down in her vagina." She has chronic smoker's cough. Upon completion of a pelvic exam, uterine prolapse is diagnosed.

   a. What are the contributing factors to this disorder?

   _____

   _____

   _____

   b. What are the symptoms of uterine prolapse that may affect Mrs. Scott's daily activities?

   _____

   _____

   _____

   c. What are the nonsurgical and surgical interventions available to Mrs. Scott?

   _____

   _____

   _____

SECTION IV: PRACTICING FOR NCLEX

Activity F *Answer the following questions.*

1. A 40-year-old client arrives at the community health center experiencing a strange dragging feeling in the vagina. At times, she feels as if there is a "lump" there as well. Which of the following conditions may be an indication of these symptoms?

   a. Urinary incontinence

   b. Endocervical polyps

   c. Pelvic organ prolapse

   d. Uterine fibroids

2. A nurse is caring for a client for whom estrogen replacement therapy has been recommended for pelvic organ prolapse. Which of the following is the most appropriate nursing intervention the nurse should implement before the start of the therapy?

   a. Discuss the effective dose of estrogen required to treat the client

   b. Evaluate the client to validate her risk for complications

   c. Discuss the dietary modifications following therapy

   d. Discuss the cost of estrogen replacement therapy

3. A nurse is caring for a female client with symptoms of early-stage pelvic organ prolapse. Which of the following instructions related to dietary and lifestyle modifications should the nurse provide to the client to help prevent pelvic relaxation and chronic problems later in life?

   a. Increase dietary fiber

   b. Avoid caffeine products

   c. Avoid excess intake of fluids

   d. Increase high-impact aerobics

4. Myomectomy is recommended to a client for removal of uterine fibroids. The client is concerned about the surgery and wants to know if there are any disadvantages associated with it. Which of the following is a disadvantage of myomectomy?

   a. Fertility is jeopardized

   b. Uterus is scarred and adhesions may form

   c. Uterine walls are weakened

   d. Fibroids may grow back

5. Kegel exercises are recommended for a client with pelvic organ prolapse. Of which of the following should the nurse inform the client about the exercises?

   a. They should be performed after food intake

   b. They alleviate mild prolapse symptoms

   c. They are not recommended after surgery

   d. They increase blood pressure

6. A nurse is assessing a 45-year-old client for uterine fibroids. Which of the following are the predisposing factors for uterine fibroids? Select all that apply.

   a. Age

   b. Nulliparity

   c. Smoking

   d. Obesity

   e. Hyperinsulinemia

7. A nurse is caring for a client who has been prescribed gonadotropin-releasing hormone (GnRH) medication for uterine fibroids. Which of the following is a side effect of GnRH medications that the nurse should monitor the client for?

   a. Increased vaginal discharge

   b. Vaginal dryness

   c. Urinary tract infections

   d. Vaginitis

8. A nurse is caring for a 32-year-old client for whom pessary usage is recommended for uterine prolapse. Which of the following instructions should the nurse include in the teaching plan for the client?

   a. Avoid jogging and jumping

   b. Wear a girdle or abdominal support

   c. Report any discomfort with urination

   d. Avoid lifting heavy objects

9. A nurse is caring for a 45-year-old client using a pessary to help decrease leakage of urine and support a prolapsed vagina. Which of the following is the most common recommendation a nurse should provide to the client regarding pessary care?

   a. Douche vaginal area with diluted vinegar or hydrogen peroxide

   b. Remove the pessary twice weekly, and clean it with soap and water

   c. Use estrogen cream to make the vaginal mucosa more resistant to erosion

   d. Remove the pessary before sleeping or intercourse

10. A client with abnormal uterine bleeding is diagnosed with small ovarian cysts. The nurse has to educate the client on the importance of routine check-ups. Which of the following is the most appropriate assessment for this client's condition?

    a. Monitor gonadotropin level every month

    b. Monitor blood sugar level every 15 days

    c. Schedule periodic Pap smears

    d. Schedule ultrasound every 3 to 6 months

11. A client with large uterine fibroids is scheduled to undergo a hysterectomy. Which of the following interventions should the nurse perform as a part of the preoperative care for the client?

    a. Teach turning, deep breathing, and coughing

    b. Instruct the client to reduce activity level

    c. Educate the client on the need for pelvic rest

    d. Instruct the client to avoid a high-fat diet

12. A 40-year-old client complains of low back pain after standing for a long time. The diagnosis reveals pelvic organ prolapse. The client has doubts regarding her eligibility for surgery. For which if the following clients is surgery for pelvic organ prolapse contraindicated? Select all that apply.

    a. Clients with low back pain and pelvic pressure

    b. Clients at high risk of recurrent prolapse after surgery

    c. Client who is morbidly obese before surgery

    d. Client who has severe pelvic organ prolapse

    e. Client who has chronic obstructive pulmonary disease

13. A nurse is caring for a female client with urinary incontinence. Which of the following instructions should the nurse include in the client's teaching plan to reduce the incidence or severity of incontinence? Select all that apply.

    a. Continue pelvic floor exercises

    b. Increase fiber in the diet

    c. Increase intake of orange juice

    d. Control blood glucose levels

    e. Wipe from back to front

14. A client has undergone an abdominal hysterectomy to remove uterine fibroids. Which of the followings interventions should a nurse perform as a part of the postoperative care for the client? Select all that apply.

   a. Administer analgesics promptly and use a PCA pump

   b. Avoid pillows and changing positions frequently

   c. Avoid intake of excess carbonated beverages in the diet

   d. Change linens and gown frequently to promote hygiene

   e. Administer antiemetics to control nausea and vomiting

15. A client with complaints of interference with normal voiding patterns and altered bowel habits is diagnosed with polycystic ovarian syndrome. Which of the following is the most appropriate instruction the nurse should provide to the client to help alleviate her condition?

   a. Adhere to follow-up care

   b. Increase intake of fiber-rich foods

   c. Increase fluid intake

   d. Perform Kegel exercises

Cancers of the Female Reproductive Tract

SECTION I: LEARNING OBJECTIVES

1. Define the key terms addressed in the chapter.

2. Identify the major modifiable risk factors for reproductive tract cancers.

3. Examine the risk factors, screening methods, and treatment modalities for cancers of the reproductive tract.

4. Outline the nursing management needed for the most common malignant reproductive tract cancers in women.

5. Propose lifestyle changes and recommended health screenings needed to reduce risk or prevent reproductive tract cancers.

6. Investigate community resources available for the women undergoing surgery for a malignant reproductive condition.

7. Relate the psychological distress experienced by women diagnosed with cancer and the information needed to assist them to cope.

SECTION II: ASSESSING YOUR UNDERSTANDING

Activity A *Fill in the blanks.*

1. High-grade _____ can progress to invasive cervical cancer; the progression takes up to 2 years.

2. _____ is a microscopic examination of the lower genital tract with use of a magnifying instrument.

3. _____ is the use of liquid nitrogen to freeze abnormal cervical tissue.

4. _____ or uterine cancer is a malignant neoplastic growth of the uterine lining.

5. Pap smear results are classified by the _____ System.

6. _____ refers to the surgical removal of the uterus.

7. _____ is a biologic tumor marker associated with ovarian cancer.

8. The two major types of vulvar intraepithelial neoplasia (VIN) are classic (undifferentiated) and _____ (differentiated).

9. Ovarian cancer usually originates in the ovarian _____.

10. _____ cell carcinomas that begin in the epithelial lining of the vagina tend to spread early by directly invading the bladder and rectal walls.

Activity B *Consider the following figures.*

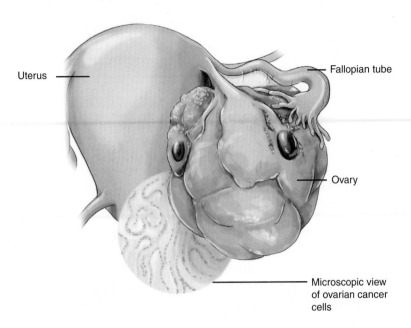

Uterus

Fallopian tube

Ovary

Microscopic view
of ovarian cancer
cells

1. a. Identify the disorder shown in the image.

_____

_____

b. What are the treatment options available
for this disorder?

_____

_____

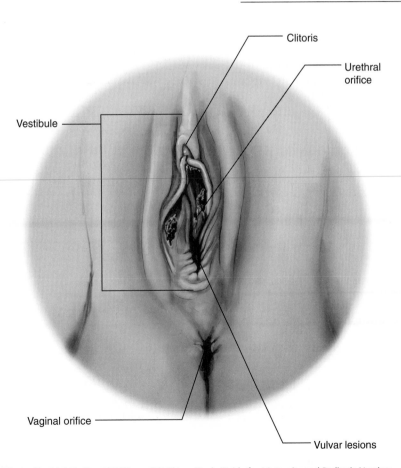

Clitoris

Urethral
orifice

Vestibule

Vaginal orifice

Vulvar lesions

2. a. Identify the disorder shown in the images on the preceding page.

_____

_____

b. What are the treatment options for this disorder?

_____

_____

Activity C *Match the stages of endometrial cancer in Column A with the relevant organs affected during that stage in Column B.*

Column A

____ **1.** Stage I

____ **2.** Stage II

____ **3.** Stage III

____ **4.** Stage IV

Column B

a. Cervix

b. Muscle wall of the uterus

c. Bladder mucosa, with distant metastases to the lungs, liver, and bone

d. Bowel or vagina, with metastases to pelvic lymph nodes

Activity D *Put the items in correct sequence by writing the letters in the boxes provided below.*

Given below, in random order, are some of the steps performed by a nurse while assisting with the collection of a Pap smear. Choose the most likely sequence in which they would have occurred.

a. Provide support to the client as the practitioner obtains a sample

b. Drape the client with a sheet, leaving the perineal area exposed

c. Wash hands thoroughly

d. Transfer the specimen to a container or a slide

e. Position the client in stirrups or foot pedals so that her knees fall outward

f. Assemble the equipment, maintaining sterility of equipment

☐ → ☐ → ☐ → ☐ → ☐ → ☐

Activity E *Briefly answer the following.*

1. What are the risk factors associated with cervical cancer?

_____

_____

_____

2. What are the treatment options for endometrial cancer?

_____

_____

_____

3. What are the risk factors for ovarian cancer?

_____

_____

_____

4. What is a transvaginal ultrasound used for?

_____

_____

_____

5. What are the nursing interventions when caring for clients with cancers of the female reproductive tract?

_____

_____

_____

6. What are the diagnostic options for endometrial cancer?

_____

_____

_____

SECTION III: APPLYING YOUR KNOWLEDGE

Activity F *Consider this scenario and answer the questions.*

1. Amy, age 60, has been diagnosed with ovarian cancer. Because this cancer develops slowly, remains silent, and is without symptoms until the cancer is far advanced, it is considered one of the worst gynecologic malignancies.

   a. What are the most common symptoms of ovarian cancer?

   _____

   _____

   _____

   b. There is still no adequate screening test to identify early cancer of the ovary. What suggestions should a nurse give a client to facilitate early detection of this type of cancer?

   _____

   _____

   _____

   c. State the nursing diagnoses related to malignancies of the reproductive tract.

   _____

   _____

   _____

   d. Explain the four stages of ovarian cancer.

   _____

   _____

   _____

SECTION IV: PRACTICING FOR NCLEX

Activity G *Answer the following questions.*

1. A nurse is educating a 25-year-old client with a family history of cervical cancer. Which of the following tests should the nurse inform the client about to detect cervical cancer at an early stage?
   a. Papanicolaou test
   b. Blood tests for mutations in the BRCA genes
   c. CA-125 blood test
   d. Transvaginal ultrasound

2. A client presents for her annual Pap test. She wants to know about the risk factors that are associated with cervical cancer. Which of the following should the nurse inform the client is a risk factor for cervical cancer?
   a. Early age at first intercourse
   b. Obesity (at least 50 pounds overweight)
   c. Hypertension
   d. Infertility

3. A client is waiting for the results of an endometrial biopsy for suspected endometrial cancer. She wants to know more about endometrial cancer and asks the nurse about the available treatment options. Which of the following treatment information should the nurse give the client?
   a. Surgery involves removal of the uterus only
   b. In advanced cancers, radiation and chemotherapy are used instead of surgery
   c. Surgery involves removal of the uterus, fallopian tubes, and ovaries; adjuvant therapy is used if relevant
   d. Follow-up care after the relevant treatment should last for at least 6 months after the treatment

4. A 65-year-old client presents at a local community health care center for a routine check-up. While obtaining her medical history, the nurse learns that the client had her menarche when she was 13 years old. She experienced menopause at 51. She is between 5 and 10 pounds underweight but is otherwise in good physical condition. The nurse should inform the client of which of the following factors that increase the client's risk of getting ovarian cancer?

   a. The client's age at menarche
   b. The client's present age
   c. The client's age at menopause
   d. The client's weight

5. A client presents at a community health care center for a routine check-up. The client wants to know about any tests that can effectively detect ovarian cancer early. About which of the following tests that can detect ovarian cancer should the nurse inform the client?

   a. Pap smears
   b. Serum CA-125
   c. Yearly bimanual pelvic examinations
   d. Regular x-rays of the pelvic area

6. A client presents for a routine check-up at a local health care center. One of the client's distant relatives died of ovarian cancer, and the client wants to know about measures that can reduce the risk of ovarian cancer. About which of the following measures to reduce the risk of ovarian cancer should the nurse inform the client?

   a. Provide genetic counseling and thorough assessment
   b. Instruct the client to avoid use of oral contraceptives
   c. Instruct the client to avoid breastfeeding
   d. Instruct the client to use perineal talc or hygiene sprays

7. A nurse is caring for a client who has been diagnosed with genital warts due to human papillomavirus (HPV). The nurse explains to the client that HPV increases the risk of vulvar cancer. Which of the following preventive measures to reduce the risk of vulvar cancer should the nurse explain to the client?

   a. Genital examination should be done only by the primary health care provider
   b. Genital examination should be done only by the client
   c. The client should avoid tight undergarments
   d. The client should use OTC drugs for self-medication of suspicious lesions
   e. The client should use oral contraceptives as opposed to barrier methods

8. When working in a local community health care center, a nurse is frequently asked about cervical cancer and ways to prevent it. Which of the following must the nurse advise regarding ways to reduce the risk of cervical cancer? Select all that apply.

   a. Encourage the use of an IUD for contraception
   b. Encourage cessation of smoking and drinking
   c. Encourage prevention of STIs to reduce risk factors
   d. Avoid stress and high blood pressure
   e. Counsel teenagers to avoid early sexual activity

9. The endometrial biopsy of a client reveals cancerous cells, and the primary health care provider has diagnosed it as endometrial cancer. Which of the following are responsibilities of the nurse as part of the treatment of the client? Select all that apply.

   a. Make sure the client understands all the available treatment options
   b. Inform the client that changes in sexuality are normal and need not be reported
   c. Inform the client about the possible advantages of a support group
   d. Offer the family explanations and emotional support throughout the treatment
   e. Inform the client that follow-up care is not required unless something unusual occurs

10. A nurse is conducting a session on education about cancers of the reproductive tract and is explaining the importance of visiting a health care professional if certain unusual symptoms appear. Which of the following should the nurse include in her list of symptoms that merit a visit to a health care professional for diagnosing cancers of the reproductive tract? Select all that apply.

    a. Irregular bowel movements

    b. Irregular vaginal bleeding

    c. Increase in urinary frequency

    d. Persistent low backache not related to standing

    e. Elevated or discolored vulvar lesions

11. A client has been referred for a colposcopy by the physician. The client wants to know more about the examination. Which of the following information regarding a colposcopy should the nurse give to the client?

    a. Client may feel pain in the vaginal area during the exam

    b. The test is conducted because of abnormal results in Pap smears

    c. Intercourse should be avoided for at least a week afterward

    d. Client may experience pain during urination for a week following the test

12. The results of a Pap smear test have been classified as ASC-H as per the 2001 Bethesda system. Which of the following is the correct interpretation of the result?

    a. Repeat the Pap smear in 4 to 6 months, or refer for a colposcopy

    b. Refer for a colposcopy without HPV testing

    c. Immediate colposcopy; follow-up is based on the results of findings

    d. No need for any further Pap smear screenings

13. Which of the following is the major initial symptom of endometrial cancer?

    a. Abnormal and painless vaginal bleeding

    b. Diabetes mellitus

    c. Liver disease

    d. Severe back pain

14. Which of the following risk factors are associated with vaginal cancer? Select all that apply.

    a. Advancing age

    b. HIV infection

    c. Persistent ovulation over time

    d. Smoking

    e. Hormone replacement therapy for more than 10 years

15. Which of the following risk factors has been linked to the development of vulvar cancer?

    a. Lichen sclerosus

    b. Previous pelvic radiation

    c. Exposure to diethylstilbestrol (DES) in utero

    d. Tamoxifen use

11. A nurse is caring for a rape victim who has just arrived at the local health care facility. Which of the following interventions should the nurse perform to minimize risk of pregnancy in this client?

    a. Administer prescribed double dose of emergency contraceptive pills

    b. Wait for first signs of pregnancy before taking action

    c. Apply spermicidal cream or gel near the vaginal area

    d. Administer regular oral contraceptive pills

12. A nurse is caring for a pregnant client and discovers signs of bruises near her neck. On questioning, the nurse learns that the bruises were caused by her husband. The client tells the nurse that her husband had stopped abusing her some time ago, but this was the first time during the pregnancy that she was assaulted. She blames herself because she admits to not paying enough attention to her husband. Which of the following facts about abuse during pregnancy should the nurse tell the client to convince her that the abuse was not her fault? Select all that apply.

    a. Abuse is a result of concern for the unborn child when the mother doesn't fulfill her responsibilities toward the newborn

    b. Abuse is a result of resentment toward the interference of the growing fetus and change in the woman's shape

    c. Abuse is a result of the perception of the partner that the baby will be a competitor after he or she is born

    d. Abuse is a result of insecurity and jealousy of the pregnancy and the responsibilities it brings

    e. Most men exhibit violent reactions during pregnancy as a way of coping with the stress

13. A nurse is caring for a 16-year-old female immigrant. Which of the following questions must she ask the client to assess if she is a victim of human trafficking? Select all that apply.

    a. "Can you leave your job or situation if you wish?"

    b. "Can you come and go as you please?"

    c. "What is your education level?"

    d. "What do your parents and siblings do?"

    e. "Is there a lock on your door so you cannot get out?"

14. A nurse is working in a local community health care facility where she frequently encounters victims of abuse. Which of the following signs should the nurse assess for to find out if a client is a victim of abuse? Select all that apply.

    a. Client is affected by sexually transmitted infections frequently

    b. Client has mental health problems such as depression, anxiety, or substance abuse

    c. Client has injuries on the face, head, and neck

    d. Partner of the suspected victim seems relaxed and not overly worried

    e. The reported history of the injury is inconsistent with the actual presenting problem

15. A nurse is caring for a rape victim. Which of the following questions should the nurse ask the client to know the extent of physical symptoms of posttraumatic stress disorder (PTSD)? Select all that apply.

    a. "Are you having trouble sleeping?"

    b. "Have you felt irritable or experienced outbursts of anger?"

    c. "Do you have heart palpitations or sweating?"

    d. "Do you feel numb emotionally?"

    e. "Do upsetting thoughts and nightmares of the trauma bother you?"

CHAPTER 10

Fetal Development and Genetics

SECTION I: LEARNING OBJECTIVES

1. Identify the process of fertilization, implantation, and cell differentiation.

2. Explain the functions of the placenta, umbilical cord, and amniotic fluid.

3. Outline normal fetal development from conception through birth.

4. Compare the various inheritance patterns, including nontraditional patterns of inheritance.

5. Analyze examples of ethical and legal issues surrounding genetic testing.

6. Delineate the role of the nurse in genetic counseling and genetics-related activities.

SECTION II: ASSESSING YOUR UNDERSTANDING

Activity A *Fill in the blanks.*

1. _____ is one of two or more alternative versions of gene at a given position or locus on a chromosome that imparts the same characteristic of that gene.

2. Any change in gene structure or location leads to a _____, which may alter the type and amount of protein produced.

3. Humans typically have 22 pairs of non-sex chromosomes or _____ and one pair of sex chromosomes.

4. The _____ originates from the ectoderm germ layer during the early stages of embryonic development; it is a thin protective membrane that contains the amniotic fluid.

5. _____ are long continuous strands of deoxyribonucleic acid (DNA) that carry genetic information.

6. The _____ reaches the uterine cavity about 72 hours after fertilization.

7. The pictorial analysis of the number, form, and size of an individual's chromosomes is termed _____.

8. _____ causes an increase in the number of haploid sets (23) of chromosomes in a cell.

9. A genetic disorder is a disease caused by an abnormality in an individual's genetic material, or _____.

10. The genotype, together with environmental variation that influences the individual, determines the _____, or the observed, outward characteristics of an individual.

Activity B *Consider the following figures.*

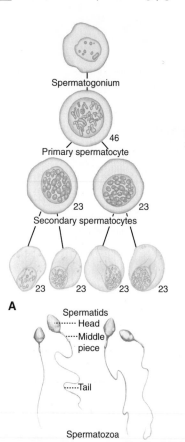

A

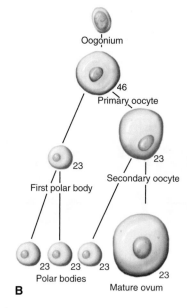

B

1. Identify the figure.

_____

_____

2. Identify the figure.

_____

_____

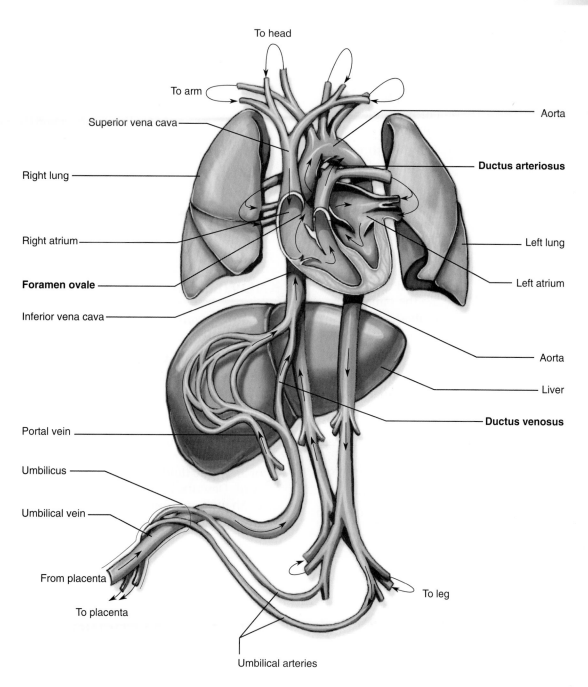

To head

To arm

Superior vena cava

Right lung

Right atrium

Foramen ovale

Inferior vena cava

Portal vein

Umbilicus

Umbilical vein

From placenta

To placenta

Aorta

Ductus arteriosus

Left lung

Left atrium

Aorta

Liver

Ductus venosus

To leg

Umbilical arteries

3. a. Identify the figure.

_____

_____

b. Explain the process in the figure.

_____

_____

Activity C *Match the terms in Column A with their descriptions in Column B.*

Column A

_____ **1.** Monosomies

_____ **2.** Trisomies

_____ **3.** Triploidy

_____ **4.** Mosaicism

_____ **5.** Homozygous

Column B

a. Three whole sets of chromosomes in a single cell

b. There are three copies of a particular chromosome instead of the usual two

c. There is only one copy of a particular chromosome instead of the usual pair

d. Both alleles for a trait are the same in the individual

e. Chromosomal abnormalities that do not show up in every cell

Activity D *Briefly answer the following.*

1. How does conception occur?

_____

_____

_____

2. What are the different stages of fetal development?

_____

_____

_____

3. What determines the sex of a zygote?

_____

_____

_____

4. What happens during differentiation of the zygote?

_____

_____

_____

5. What is amniotic fluid?

_____

_____

_____

6. What are the hormones produced by the placenta?

_____

_____

_____

SECTION III: APPLYING YOUR KNOWLEDGE

Activity E *Consider this scenario and answer the questions.*

1. Shana is 16 weeks pregnant and comes into the prenatal clinic for a routine check-up. She tells the nurse she is worried because she feels the baby moving a lot and has concerns "it might get tangled in its cord." She wants to know if this could be true and, if so, why. Shana also wants to know about the functions of amniotic fluid, placenta, and the umbilical cord. Describe how the nurse should respond to Shana's questions and concerns.

_____

_____

_____

SECTION IV: PRACTICING FOR NCLEX

Activity F *Answer the following questions.*

1. The nurse is counseling a couple who are concerned that the woman has achondroplasia in her family. The woman is not affected. Which of the following statements by the couple indicates the need for more teaching?

a. "If the mother has the gene, then there is a 50% chance of passing it on."

b. "If the father doesn't have the gene, then his son won't have achondroplasia."

c. "If the father has the gene, then there is a 50% chance of passing it on."

d. "Since neither one of us has the disorder, we won't pass it on."

2. A client has been informed that the result of the pregnancy test indicates she is three weeks pregnant. Which of the following instructions should the nurse give to the client that is most appropriate, given the client's condition?

a. Avoid exercising during pregnancy

b. Stay indoors and avoid going out for the duration of pregnancy

c. Stop using drugs, alcohol, and tobacco

d. Wear comfortable clothes that are not tight or restrictive

3. A nurse is obtaining the genetic history of a pregnant client by questioning family members. Which of the following questions is most appropriate for the nurse to ask?

a. Were there any instances of premature birth in the family?

b. Is there a family history of drinking or drug abuse?

c. What was the cause and age of death for deceased family members?

d. Were there any instances of depression during pregnancy?

4. A nurse is caring for a 37-year-old pregnant client who is expecting twins, both boys. The client used to smoke but has stopped during pregnancy. A cousin of the client has Klinefelter syndrome, and the client wants to find out more about the disorder. Which of the following information will the nurse give the client during genetic counseling?

a. There is a greater risk of Klinefelter syndrome due to the client's age

b. Klinefelter syndrome occurs only in girls, not boys

c. Having twins increases the risk of Klinefelter syndrome

d. The client's previous smoking habit will increase the risk of a genetic disorder

5. A 25-year-old client wants to know if her baby boy is at risk for Down syndrome, because one of her distant relatives was born it. Which of the following will the nurse tell the client while counseling her about Down syndrome?

a. Instances of Down syndrome in the family increase the risk for the baby

b. Children with Down syndrome have 47 chromosomes instead of 46

c. Down syndrome occurs only in females, and there is no risk as the baby is male

d. Children with Down syndrome are intellectually normal

6. A nurse is questioning the family members of a pregnant client to obtain genetic history. While asking questions, which of the following should the nurse keep in mind?

a. Inquire about the socioeconomic status of the family members

b. Avoid questions about race or ethnic background

c. Ask questions regarding physical characteristics of family members

d. Find out if couples are related to each other or have blood ties

7. A pregnant client and her husband have had a session with a genetic specialist. What is the role of the nurse after the client has seen a specialist?

a. Identify the best decision for the client to make

b. Refer client to another specialist for a second opinion

c. Review what has been discussed with the specialist

d. Refer client for further diagnostic and screening tests

8. A nurse is caring for a client who is pregnant with a female baby. The client and her husband are both in their early thirties. They are not directly related by blood but are of Ashkenazi heritage. There has been an instance of Tay-Sachs disease occurring in the family. Which of the following information does the nurse need to give the client regarding Tay-Sachs disease?

a. Tay-Sachs disease affects both male and female babies

b. The age of the client increases the susceptibility of the baby to Tay-Sachs disease

c. There is no risk of Tay-Sachs disease because the parents are not related by blood

d. There is no risk of the baby developing Tay-Sachs disease because both parents are healthy

9. A pregnant client arrives at the community health center for a routine check-up. She informs the nurse that a relative on her mother's side has hemophilia, and she wants to know the chances of her child acquiring hemophilia. Which of the following characteristics of hemophilia should the nurse explain to the client to help the client understand the odds of acquiring the disease? Select all that apply.

a. Affected individuals will have affected parents

b. Affected individuals are usually males

c. Daughters of an affected male are unaffected and are not carriers

d. Female carriers have a 50% chance of transmitting the disorder to their sons

e. Females are affected by the condition if it is a dominant X-linked disorder

10. A nurse is providing genetic counseling to a pregnant client. Which of the following are the nursing responsibilities related to counseling the client? Select all that apply.

a. Explaining basic concepts of probability and disorder susceptibility

b. Ensuring complete informed consent to facilitate decisions about genetic testing

c. Instructing the client on the appropriate decision to be made

d. Knowing basic genetic terminology and inheritance patterns

e. Avoiding explaining ethical or legal issues and concentrating on genetic issues

11. A client has the Huntington disease gene. She is planning to have children and wants to know about the chances of her children inheriting the disease. Which of the following information about Huntington disease should the nurse give to the client?

a. No chances of getting infected if client's husband has a normal matching gene

b. Only male children of parents with the gene are at risk for the disease

c. Presence of the gene mutation means that the individual will eventually have the disease

d. Children of affected parents have a 50% chance of acquiring the disease

12. A nurse is counseling a client who is keen on having a baby about conception. Which of the following should the nurse tell the client about conception? Select all that apply.

a. It occurs around two weeks after the last normal menstrual period

b. It requires only the release of a mature ovum at ovulation

c. It is referred to as the embryonic stage

d. Sperm should be healthy and mobile

e. It takes 12 hours for the sperm to reach the ovum

13. A nurse is caring for a client who has just confirmed her pregnancy. Which of the following hormones is the basis for pregnancy tests?

a. Estrogen

b. Progesterone

c. Human placental lactogen

d. Human chorionic gonadotropin

14. A nurse is counseling a client who is contemplating pregnancy. Which of the following is considered to be the ideal time for genetic counseling?

a. Before conception

b. First week of pregnancy

c. Second trimester

d. Third trimester

15. Given below are the assessments to be performed by a nurse during genetic counseling. Arrange the assessments in the most likely sequence in which they would have occurred.

a. Discover additional details about client's genetic history by questioning family members

b. Obtain a client's genetic history during the initial encounter

c. Provide follow-up counseling support for the family

d. Make referrals to a genetic specialist when appropriate

e. Identify any hereditary conditions from the client's genetic history

CHAPTER 11

Maternal Adaptation During Pregnancy

SECTION I: LEARNING OBJECTIVES

1. Define the key terms utilized in this chapter.

2. Differentiate between subjective (presumptive), objective (probable), and diagnostic (positive) signs of pregnancy.

3. Explain maternal physiologic changes that occur during pregnancy.

4. Summarize the nutritional needs of the pregnant woman and her fetus.

5. Identify the emotional and psychological changes that occur during pregnancy.

SECTION II: ASSESSING YOUR UNDERSTANDING

Activity A *Fill in the blanks.*

1. During the stress of pregnancy, _____, secreted by the adrenal glands, helps keep up the level of glucose in the plasma by breaking down noncarbohydrate sources.

2. _____, or having conflicting feelings at the same time, is an emotion expressed by most women upon learning they are pregnant.

3. _____, released by the posterior pituitary gland, is responsible for milk ejection during breastfeeding.

4. At birth, as soon as the _____ is expelled, and there is a drop in progesterone, lactogenesis can begin.

5. Palmar erythema, a well-delineated pinkish area on the palmar surface of the hands, is caused by elevated _____ levels.

6. The postural changes of pregnancy coupled with the loosening of the _____ joints may result in lower back pain.

7. Constipation, increased venous pressure, and pressure from the gravid uterus can lead to the formation of _____ during pregnancy.

8. During pregnancy, elevated _____ levels cause smooth-muscle relaxation, which results in delayed gastric emptying and decreased peristalsis.

9. _____ is the creamy, yellowish breast fluid that provides nourishment for the newborn during the first few days of life.

10. Most women experience an increase in a whitish vaginal discharge, called _____, during pregnancy.

Activity B *Consider the following figures.*

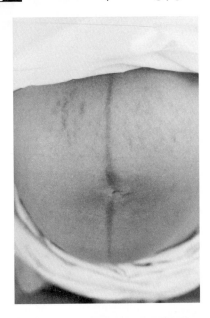

1. Identify the skin change shown in the image.

_____

_____

MyPyramid Plan for Moms

Food Group	1st Trimester	2nd and 3rd Trimesters	What counts as 1 cup or 1 ounce?	Remember to...
	Eat this amount from each group daily.*			
Fruits	2 cups	2 cups	1 cup fruit or juice, ½ cup dried fruit	*Focus on fruits*—Eat a variety of fruit.
Vegetables	2½ cups	3 cups	1 cup raw or cooked vegetables or juice, 2 cups raw leafy vegetables	*Vary your veggies*—Eat more dark green and orange vegetables and cooked dry beans.
Grains	6 ounces	8 ounces	1 slice bread; ½ cup cooked pasta, rice, cereal; 1 ounce ready-to-eat cereal	*Make half your grains whole*—Choose whole instead of refined grains.
Meat and Beans	5½ ounces	6½ ounces	1 ounce lean meat, poultry, fish; 1 egg; ¼ cup cooked dry beans; ½ ounce nuts; 1 tablespoon peanut butter	*Go lean with protein*—Choose low-fat or lean meats and poultry.
Milk	3 cups	3 cups	1 cup milk, 8 ounces yogurt, 1½ ounces cheese, 2 ounces processed cheese	*Get your calcium-rich foods*—Go low-fat or fat-free when you choose milk, yogurt, and cheese.

*These amounts are for an average pregnant woman. You may need more or less than the average. Check with your doctor to make sure you are gaining weight as you should.

2.

    a. What are the good food sources of folic acid?

_____

_____

    b. What foods does the FDA advise pregnant women and nursing mothers to avoid?

_____

_____

Activity C *Match the parts of the female reproductive tract in Column A with the physiologic changes that occur in them during pregnancy, in Column B.*

Column A

_____ **1.** Uterus

_____ **2.** Cervix

_____ **3.** Vagina

_____ **4.** Ovaries

_____ **5.** Ureters

Column B

a. Between weeks 6–8 of gestation, softens due to vasocongestion

b. Elongate, widen, and curve above pelvic rim by tenth gestational week

c. Connective tissue loosens and smooth muscle begins hypertrophy

d. Produce more hormones until weeks 6–7 of gestation

e. Weighs 2 lbs at full term

Activity D *Put the items in correct sequence by writing the letters in the boxes provided below.*

Given below, in random order, are the changes in the uterus as pregnancy progresses. Arrange the changes in sequence.

a. Uterus progressively ascends into the abdomen

b. Fundal height drops as fetus begins to descend and engage into the pelvis

c. Fundus reaches its highest level at the xiphoid process

d. Softening and compressibility of the lower uterine segment are noted

e. Fundus is at the level of the umbilicus and measures 20 cm

☐ → ☐ → ☐ → ☐ → ☐

Activity E *Briefly answer the following.*

1. What are stretch marks?

_____

_____

_____

2. Why does hypertrophy of the heart occur in pregnant women?

_____

_____

_____

3. Why do iron requirements increase during pregnancy?

_____

_____

_____

4. What is pica?

_____

_____

_____

5. What is the role of oxytocin?

_____

_____

_____

6. Why do pregnant women develop varicose veins?

_____

_____

_____

SECTION III: APPLYING YOUR KNOWLEDGE

Activity F *Consider this scenario and answer the questions.*

1. A nurse working in a private doctor's office has been assigned to be the primary nurse for Maggie, 40, who is in her first trimester of pregnancy. Maggie states that she is very nervous about the pregnancy and is concerned because "she is not very excited." She adds that she is also worried about her baby, avoids travel, stays indoors because she feels nauseous most of the time, and has little interaction with the outside world. She asks the nurse if it is normal to feel this way.

a. Describe how the nurse should respond to the client about her lack of excitement.

_____

_____

_____

b. How should the nurse explain to the client how introversion, or focusing on oneself, may be common in early pregnancy?

_____

_____

_____

c. How should the nurse describe to the client how she may feel in the second trimester?

_____

_____

_____

d. How should the nurse reassure Maggie about her mood swings?

_____

_____

_____

SECTION IV: PRACTICING FOR NCLEX

Activity G *Answer the following questions.*

1. A 28-year-old client complains of skipping her menses and suspects she is pregnant. When assessing this client, which of the following would the nurse identify as a presumptive sign of pregnancy?

   a. Positive home pregnancy test
   b. Urinary frequency
   c. Abdominal enlargement
   d. Softening of the cervix

2. A pregnant client complains of an increase in a thick, whitish vaginal discharge. Which of the following information should a nurse provide to this client?

   a. Refrain from any sexual activity
   b. Consult physician for fungal infection
   c. Such discharge is normal during pregnancy
   d. Use local antifungal agents regularly

3. When teaching a client about hormones, which of the following should the nurse identify as responsible in developing the ductal system of the breasts in preparation for lactation during pregnancy?

   a. Estrogen
   b. Prolactin
   c. Progesterone
   d. Oxytocin

4. A 28-year-old client in her first trimester of pregnancy complains of conflicting feelings. She expresses feeling proud and excited about her pregnancy while at the same time feeling fearful and anxious of its implications. Which of the following maternal emotional responses is the client experiencing?

   a. Introversion
   b. Mood swings
   c. Acceptance
   d. Ambivalence

5. A pregnant client arrives at the maternity clinic complaining of constipation. Which of the following factors could be the cause of constipation during pregnancy? Select all that apply.

   a. Decreased activity level
   b. Increase in estrogen levels
   c. Use of iron supplements
   d. Reduced stomach acidity
   e. Intestinal displacement

6. A client in her 10th week of gestation arrives at the maternity clinic complaining of morning sickness. The nurse needs to inform the client about the body system adaptations during pregnancy. Which of the following factors corresponds to the morning sickness period during pregnancy?

   a. Reduced stomach acidity
   b. Elevation of hCG

c. Increase in RBC production

d. Increase in estrogen level

e. Elevation of hPL

7. A pregnant client in her first trimester of pregnancy complains of spontaneous, irregular, painless contractions. What does this indicate?

a. Preterm labor

b. Infection of the GI tract

c. Braxton Hicks contractions

d. Acid indigestion

8. A client in her 29th week of gestation complains of dizziness and clamminess when assuming a supine position. During the assessment, the nurse observes there is a marked decrease in the client's blood pressure. Which of the following interventions should the nurse implement to help alleviate this client's condition?

a. Keep the client's legs slightly elevated

b. Place the client in an orthopneic position

c. Keep the head of the client's bed slightly elevated

d. Place the client in the left lateral position

9. A client in her 20th week of gestation expresses concern about her five-year-old son, who is behaving strangely by not approaching her anymore. He does not seem to be taking the news of a new family member very well. Which of the following strategies can a nurse discuss with the mother to deal with the situation?

a. Provide constant reinforcement of love and care to the child

b. Avoid talking to the child about the new arrival

c. Pay less attention to the child to prepare him for the future

d. Consult a child psychologist about the situation

10. When caring for a newborn, the nurse observes that the neonate has developed white patches on the mucus membranes of the mouth. Which of the following conditions is the newborn most likely to be experiencing?

a. Rubella

b. Thrush

c. Cytomegalovirus infection

d. Toxoplasmosis

11. A client in her 39th week of gestation arrives at the maternity clinic stating that earlier in her pregnancy, she experienced shortness of breath. However, for the past few days, she's been able to breathe easily, but she has also begun to experience increased urinary frequency. A nurse is assigned to perform the physical examination of the client. Which of the following is the nurse most likely to observe?

a. Fundal height has dropped since the last recording

b. Fundal height is at its highest level at the xiphoid process

c. The fundus is at the level of the umbilicus and measures 20 cm

d. The lower uterine segment and cervix have softened

12. A client in her second trimester of pregnancy is anxious about the blotchy, brown pigmentation appearing on her forehead and cheeks. She also complains of increased pigmentation on her breasts and genitalia. When educating the client, which of the following would the nurse identify as the condition experienced by the client?

a. Linea nigra

b. Striae gravidarum

c. Facial melasma

d. Vascular spiders

13. A client in her 39th week of gestation complains of swelling in the legs after standing for long periods of time. The nurse recognizes that these factors increase the client's risk for which of the following conditions?

a. Hemorrhoids

b. Embolism

c. Venous thrombosis

d. Supine hypotension syndrome

14. A nurse is assigned to educate a pregnant client regarding the changes in the structures of the respiratory system taking place during pregnancy. Which of the following conditions are associated with such changes? Select all that apply.

a. Nasal and sinus stuffiness

b. Persistent cough

c. Nosebleed

d. Kussmaul's respirations

e. Thoracic rather than abdominal breathing

15. During a prenatal visit, a client in her second trimester of pregnancy verbalizes positive feelings about the pregnancy and conceptualizes the fetus. Which of the following is the most appropriate nursing intervention when the client expresses such feelings?

    a. Encourage the client to focus on herself, not on the fetus

    b. Inform the primary health care provider about the client's feeling

    c. Inform the client that it is too early to conceptualize the fetus

    d. Offer support and validation about the client's feelings

16. A client in her second trimester of pregnancy complains of discomfort during sexual activity. Which of the following instructions should a nurse provide?

    a. Perform frequent douching, and use lubricants

    b. Modify sexual positions to increase comfort

    c. Restrict contact to alternative, noncoital modes of sexual expression

    d. Perform stress-relieving and relaxing exercises

17. A nurse is educating a client about the various psychological feelings experienced by a woman and her partner during pregnancy. Which of the following is the feeling experienced by the expectant partner during the second trimester of pregnancy?

    a. Ambivalence along with extremes of emotions

    b. Confusion when dealing with the partner's mood swings

    c. Preparation for the new role as a parent and negotiating his or her role during labor

    d. Sympathetic response to the partner's pregnancy

Nursing Management During Pregnancy

SECTION I: LEARNING OBJECTIVES

1. Define the key terms utilized in this chapter.

2. Identify the information typically collected at the initial prenatal visit.

3. Explain the assessments completed at follow-up prenatal visits.

4. Categorize the tests used to assess maternal and fetal well-being, including nursing management for each.

5. Outline appropriate nursing management to promote maternal self-care and minimize the common discomforts of pregnancy.

6. Design the key components of perinatal education.

SECTION II: ASSESSING YOUR UNDERSTANDING

Activity A *Fill in the blanks.*

1. A _____ is a laywoman trained to provide women and their families with encouragement, emotional and physical support, and information through late pregnancy, labor, and birth.

2. A _____ is a woman who has given birth once after a pregnancy of at least 20 weeks.

3. _____ height is the distance (in cm) measured with a tape measure from the top of the pubic bone to the top of the uterus while the client is lying on her back with her knees slightly flexed.

4. In a pregnant woman, darker pigmentation of the nipple and areola develops, along with enlargement of _____ glands in the breast.

5. Bluish coloration of the cervix and vaginal mucosa is known as _____ sign.

6. _____ is the craving for nonfood substances such as clay, cornstarch, laundry detergent, baking soda, soap, paint chips, dirt, ice, or wax.

7. _____ involves a transabdominal perforation of the amniotic sac to obtain a sample of amniotic fluid for analysis.

8. Alpha-fetoprotein (AFP) is a substance produced by the fetal _____ between weeks 13 and 20 of gestation.

9. The basis for the _____ test is that the normal fetus produces characteristic fetal heart rate patterns in response to fetal movements.

10. _____ are varicosities of the rectum which occur as a result of progesterone-induced vasodilation and from pressure of the enlarged uterus on the lower intestine and rectum.

Activity B *Consider the following figures.*

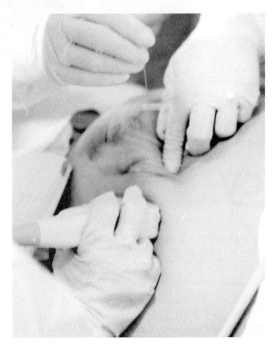

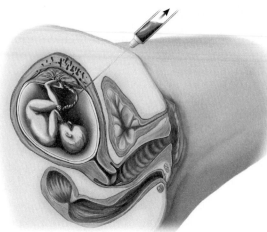

1. a. Identify the technique shown in the figure.

_____

_____

b. What is this technique used for?

_____

_____

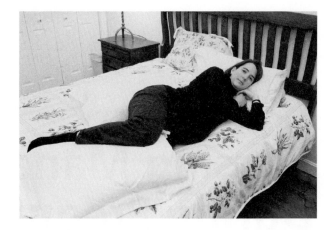

2. a. Identify the figure.

_____

_____

b. Why is this important for the client?

_____

_____

Activity C *Match the different types of assessment tests conducted to determine fetal well-being, in Column A, with their uses in Column B.*

Column A

____ **1.** 1. Ultrasonography

____ **2.** Doppler flow studies

____ **3.** Nuchal translucency screening (ultrasound)

____ **4.** Percutaneous umbilical blood sampling (PUBS)

____ **5.** Contraction stress test (CST)

Column B

a. Allows for earlier detection and diagnosis of some fetal chromosomes and structural abnormalities

b. Permits the collection of a blood specimen directly from the fetal circulation for rapid chromosomal analysis.

c. Determines the fetal heart rate response under stress, such as during contractions.

d. Acts as a guide for the need for invasive intrauterine tests and used to monitor fetal growth and placental location.

e. Help to identify abnormalities in diastolic flow within the umbilical vessels

Activity D *Put the steps in correct sequence by writing the letters in the boxes provided below.*

Given below, in random order, are steps that should be followed by the client who has nosebleeds. Rearrange in the correct sequence.

a. Pinch her nostrils with her thumb and forefinger for 10 to 15 minutes

b. Loosen the clothing around her neck

c. Apply an ice pack to the bridge of her nose

d. Sit with her head tilted forward

$$\square \rightarrow \square \rightarrow \square \rightarrow \square$$

Activity E *Briefly answer the following.*

1. What are the key areas which the nurse should include in preconception care?

_____

_____

_____

2. What is the role of a nurse in preconception care to ensure a positive impact on the pregnancy?

_____

_____

_____

3. What are the assessments the nurse should make during a client's initial prenatal visit?

_____

_____

_____

4. What are the roles of a nurse with regard to providing counseling and education to the client at a prenatal visit?

_____

_____

_____

5. What assessments should a nurse perform when conducting a chest examination for a pregnant client on her first prenatal visit?

_____

_____

_____

6. What assessments should the nurse perform during follow-up visits?

_____

_____

_____

SECTION III: APPLYING YOUR KNOWLEDGE

Activity F *Consider this scenario and answer the questions.*

1. A pregnant client and her husband are preparing for the birth of their first baby. The couple wants to ensure that they are well prepared for the baby's birth and homecoming and seek guidance from the nurse. The pregnant client also wants to know the importance of breastfeeding and wants to prepare for it.

   a. What are the items in the checklist used by the nurse to ensure that the client is well prepared for the newborn's birth and homecoming?

   _____

   _____

   _____

   b. What interventions should the nurse perform in preparing the client for breastfeeding?

   _____

   _____

   _____

c. What advantages of breastfeeding should the nurse educate the pregnant client about?

_____

_____

_____

SECTION IV: PRACTICING FOR NCLEX

Activity G *Answer the following questions.*

1. A 28-year-old client who has just conceived arrives at a health care facility for her first prenatal visit to undergo a physical examination. Which of the following interventions should the nurse perform to prepare the client for the physical examination?
   a. Ensure that the client is lying down
   b. Ensure that the client's family is present
   c. Instruct the client to empty her bladder
   d. Instruct the client to keep taking deep breaths

2. A client in her third month of pregnancy arrives at the health care facility for a regular follow-up visit. The client complains of discomfort due to increased urinary frequency. Which of the following instructions should the nurse offer the client to reduce the client's discomfort?
   a. Avoid consumption of caffeinated drinks
   b. Drink fluids with meals rather than between meals
   c. Avoid an empty stomach at all times
   d. Munch on dry crackers and toast in the early morning

3. A pregnant client has come to a health care provider for her first prenatal visit. The nurse needs to document useful information about the past health history. What is the goal of the nurse in the history-taking process? Select all that apply.
   a. To prepare a plan of care that suits the client's lifestyle
   b. To develop a trusting relationship with the client
   c. To prepare a plan of care for the pregnancy

d. To assess the client's partner's sexual health
e. To urge the client to achieve an optimal body weight

4. A pregnant client has come to a health care facility for a physical examination. Which of the following assessments should a nurse perform when doing a physical examination of the head and neck? Select all that apply.
   a. Assess for previous injuries and sequelae
   b. Check the eye movements
   c. Check for levels of estrogen
   d. Evaluate for limitations in range of motion
   e. Palpate the thyroid gland for enlargement

5. A pregnant client in her 12th week of gestation has come to a health care center for a physical examination of her abdomen. Where should the nurse palpate for the fundus in this client?
   a. At the umbilicus
   b. Below the ensiform cartilage
   c. Midway between the symphysis and umbilicus
   d. At the symphysis pubis

6. A pregnant client has come to a clinic for a pelvic examination. What assessments should a nurse perform when examining external genitalia?
   a. Ensure that the cervix is smooth, long, thick, and closed
   b. Assess for bluish coloration of cervix and vaginal mucosa
   c. Assess for any infection due to hematomas, varicosities, and inflammation
   d. Assess for hemorrhoids, masses, prolapse, and lesions

7. Which of the following nursing interventions should the nurse perform when assessing fetal well-being through abdominal ultrasonography in a client?
   a. Inform the client that she may feel hot initially
   b. Instruct the client to refrain from emptying her bladder
   c. Instruct the client to report the occurrence of fever
   d. Obtain and record vital signs of the client

8. A pregnant client wishes to know if sexual intercourse would be safe during her pregnancy. Which of the following should the nurse confirm before educating the client regarding sexual behavior during pregnancy?

   a. Client does not have an incompetent cervix

   b. Client does not have anxieties and worries

   c. Client does not have anemia

   d. Client does not experience facial and hand edema

9. A client in her second trimester arrives at a health care facility for a follow-up visit. During the exam, the client complains of constipation. Which of the following instructions should the nurse offer to help alleviate constipation?

   a. Ensure adequate hydration and bulk in the diet

   b. Avoid spicy or greasy foods in meals

   c. Practice Kegel exercises

   d. Avoid lying down for two hours after meals

10. A client in the third trimester of pregnancy has to travel a long distance by car. The client is anxious about the effect the travel may have on her pregnancy. Which of the following instructions should the nurse provide to promote easy and safe travel for the client?

    a. Activate the air bag in the car

    b. Use a lap belt that crosses over the uterus

    c. Apply a padded shoulder strap properly

    d. Always wear a three-point seat belt

11. A pregnant client's last menstrual period was March 10. Using Nagele's rule, the nurse knows that which of the following dates should be the client's estimated date of birth (EDB)?

    a. January 7

    b. December 17

    c. February 21

    d. January 30

12. A nurse who has been caring for a pregnant client understands that the client has pica and has been regularly consuming soil. Which of the following conditions should the nurse monitor for in the client as a manifestation of consuming soil?

   a. Iron-deficiency anemia

   b. Constipation

   c. Tooth fracture

   d. Inefficient protein metabolism

13. A client who has just conceived arrives at a health care facility wanting to know of any changes in her eating habits that she should make during her pregnancy. The client informs the nurse that she is a vegetarian. The nurse knows that she has to monitor the client for which of the following risks arising from her vegetarian diet? Select all that apply.

    a. Risk of epistaxis

    b. Iron-deficiency anemia

    c. Decreased mineral absorption

    d. Increased risk of constipation

    e. Low gestational weight gain

14. A nurse is caring for a pregnant client in her second trimester of pregnancy. The nurse educates the client to look for which of the following danger signs of pregnancy needing immediate attention by the physician.

    a. Vaginal bleeding

    b. Painful urination

    c. Severe, persistent vomiting

    d. Lower abdominal and shoulder pain

15. A client in her third trimester of pregnancy wishes to use the method of feeding formula to her infant. Which of the following instructions should the nurse provide to assist the client in feeding her baby?

    a. Mix one scoop of powder with an ounce of water

    b. Feed the infant every 8 hours

    c. Serve the formula at room temperature

    d. Refrigerate any leftover formula

16. A nurse caring for a client in labor has asked her to perform Lamaze breathing techniques to avoid pain. Which of the following should the nurse keep in mind to promote effective Lamaze method breathing?

    a. Ensure deep abdominopelvic breathing

    b. Ensure abdominal breathing during contractions

    c. Ensure client's concentration on pleasurable sensations

    d. Remain quiet during client's period of imagery

17. A nurse is caring for a client in her second trimester of pregnancy. During a regular follow-up visit, the client complains of varicosities of the legs. Which of the following instructions should the nurse provide to help the client alleviate varicosities of the legs?

a. Avoid sitting in one position for long

b. Refrain from crossing legs when sitting for long periods

c. Apply heating pads on the extremities

d. Refrain from wearing any kind of stockings

18. A nurse is assigned to care for a pregnant client as she undergoes a nonstress test. Given below are the steps involved in conducting the nonstress test. Arrange the steps in correct order.

a. Client is handed an event marker

b. Client consumes a meal

c. External electronic fetal monitoring device applied

d. Fetal monitor strip marked for fetal movement

e. Client placed in left lateral recumbent position

Labor and Birth Process

SECTION I: LEARNING OBJECTIVES

1. Outline premonitory signs of labor.

2. Compare and contrast true versus false labor.

3. Categorize the critical factors affecting labor and birth.

4. Analyze the cardinal movements of labor.

5. Identify the maternal and fetal responses to labor and birth.

6. Classify the stages of labor and the critical events in each stage.

7. Explain the normal physiologic/psychological changes occurring during all four stages of labor.

8. Formulate the concept of pain as it relates to the woman in labor.

SECTION II: ASSESSING YOUR UNDERSTANDING

Activity A *Fill in the blanks.*

1. Vaginal birth is most favorable with a _____ type of pelvis because the inlet is round and the outlet is roomy.

2. The thinning out process of the cervix during labor is termed _____.

3. The _____ suture is located between the parietal bones and divides the skull into the right and left halves.

4. _____ station is designated when the presenting part is at the level of the maternal ischial spines.

5. _____ occurs when the fetal presenting part begins to descend into the maternal pelvis.

6. An increase in prostaglandins leads to myometrial _____ and to a reduction in cervical resistance.

7. Oxytocin also aids in stimulating prostaglandin synthesis through receptors in the _____.

8. The birth _____ is the route through which the fetus must travel to be birthed vaginally.

9. A sudden increase in energy on the part of the expectant woman 24 to 48 hours before the onset of labor is sometimes referred to as _____.

10. The elongated shape of the fetal skull at birth as a result of overlapping of the cranial bones is known as _____.

Activity B *Consider the following figures.*

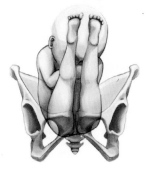

1. a. Identify the figure.

_____

_____

b. In which clients are such cases observed?

_____

_____

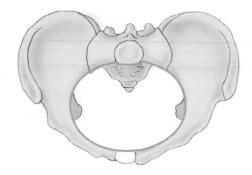

2. a. Identify the figure.

_____

_____

b. What are the possible complications associated with this condition?

_____

_____

Activity C *Match the cardinal movements of labor in Column A with the corresponding fetal movements observed in Column B.*

Column A

_____ **1.** Engagement

_____ **2.** Descent

_____ **3.** Flexion

Column B

a. Occurs when the greatest transverse diameter of the head in vertex passes through the pelvic inlet

_____ **4.** Extension

_____ **5.** External rotation

b. Downward movement of the fetal head until it is within the pelvic inlet

c. Allows the shoulders to rotate internally to fit the maternal pelvis

d. The head emerges through extension under the symphysis pubis, along with the shoulders

e. Occurs as the vertex meets resistance from the cervix, walls of the pelvis, or the pelvic floor

Activity D *Put the items in correct sequence by writing the letters in the boxes provided below.*

Given below, in random order, are the phases of labor. Arrange them in the order of their occurrence.

a. Latent phase

b. Active phase

c. Transition phase

d. Pelvic phase

e. Perineal phase

f. Placental separation

g. Placental expulsion

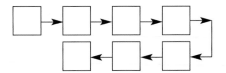

Activity E *Briefly answer the following.*

1. What are the reasons that cause women to adopt back-lying positions during labor?

_____

_____

_____

2. Why should the nurse encourage the pregnant client experiencing contractions to adopt the upright or lateral position?

_____

_____

_____

3. What are the maternal physiologic responses that occur as a woman progresses through childbirth?

_____

_____

_____

4. What are the factors influencing the ability of a woman to cope with labor stress?

_____

_____

_____

5. What are the signs of separation that indicate the placenta is ready to deliver?

_____

_____

_____

6. What are the factors that ensure a positive birth experience for the pregnant client?

_____

_____

_____

SECTION III: APPLYING YOUR KNOWLEDGE

Activity F *Consider this scenario and answer the questions.*

1. Becca is a primigravida at 36 weeks' gestation. During her prenatal visit, she asks the nurse the following questions about labor. Describe how the nurse should respond.

   a. "How will I know I am in labor?"

   _____

   _____

   _____

b. "When should I come to the hospital?"

_____

_____

_____

c. "My sister just had a baby and she told me that the nurse midwife encouraged her to change positions and to walk to help her labor; will this help me in labor?"

_____

_____

_____

d. "How do we determine that it's time to push?"

_____

_____

_____

SECTION IV: PRACTICING FOR NCLEX

Activity G *Answer the following questions.*

1. A client in her third trimester of pregnancy arrives at a health care facility complaining of cramping and low back pain. Physical examination conducted by the nurse indicates that the client has edema of the lower extremities, along with an increase in vaginal discharge. The nurse knows that the client is experiencing which of the following conditions?

   a. Nesting
   b. Lightening
   c. Braxton Hicks contractions
   d. Bloody show

2. A pregnant client who is toward the end of her third trimester presents at a health care facility for a follow-up visit. Assessment of the client reveals that she has increased prostaglandin levels. Which of the following factors should the nurse assess for in the client? Select all that apply.

   a. Reduction in cervical resistance
   b. Myometrial contractions
   c. Boggy appearance of the uterus
   d. Softening and thinning of the cervix
   e. Hypotonic character of the bladder

3. A client experiencing contractions presents at a health care facility. Assessment conducted by the nurse reveals that the client has been experiencing Braxton Hicks contractions. The nurse has to educate the client on the usefulness of Braxton Hicks contractions. Which of the following is the role of Braxton Hicks contractions in aiding labor?

   a. Helps in softening and ripening the cervix

   b. Increases the release of prostaglandins

   c. Increases oxytocin sensitivity

   d. Makes maternal breathing easier

4. A pregnant client wants to know why the labor of a first-time-pregnant woman lasts longer than that of a woman who has already delivered once and is pregnant a second time. What explanation should the nurse offer the client?

   a. Braxton Hicks contractions are not strong enough during first pregnancy

   b. Contractions are stronger during the first pregnancy than the second

   c. The cervix takes around 12 to 16 hours to dilate during first pregnancy

   d. Spontaneous rupture of membranes occurs during first pregnancy

5. A pregnant client is admitted to a maternity clinic for childbirth. The client wishes to adopt the kneeling position during labor. The nurse knows that which of the following is the advantage of adopting a kneeling position during labor?

   a. It helps the woman in labor to save energy

   b. It facilitates vaginal examinations

   c. It facilitates external belt adjustment

   d. It helps to rotate fetus in a posterior position

6. A nurse is caring for a pregnant client who is in labor. Which of the following maternal physiologic responses should the nurse monitor for in the client as the client progresses through childbirth? Select all that apply.

   a. Increase in heart rate

   b. Increase in blood pressure

   c. Increase in respiratory rate

   d. Slight decrease in body temperature

   e. Increase in gastric emptying and pH

7. A nurse is caring for a client in labor who is delivering. Which of the following fetal responses should the nurse monitor for in the client's baby?

   a. Decrease in arterial carbon dioxide pressure

   b. Increase in fetal breathing movements

   c. Increase in fetal oxygen pressure

   d. Decrease in circulation and perfusion to the fetus

8. A client in the third stage of labor has experienced placental separation and expulsion. Why is it necessary for a nurse to massage the woman's uterus briefly until it is firm?

   a. To reduce boggy nature of the uterus

   b. To remove pieces left attached to uterine wall

   c. To constrict the uterine blood vessels

   d. To lessen the chances of conducting an episiotomy

9. A nurse is caring for a pregnant client in labor in a health care facility. The nurse knows that which of the following marks the termination of the first stage of labor in the client?

   a. Diffuse abdominal cramping

   b. Rupturing of fetal membranes

   c. Start of regular contractions

   d. Dilation of cervix diameter to 10 cm

10. A nurse is caring for a client who is in the first stage of labor. The client is experiencing extreme pain due to the labor. The nurse understands that which of the following is causing the extreme pain in the client? Select all that apply.

    a. Lower uterine segment distention

    b. Fetus moving along the birth canal

    c. Stretching and tearing of structures

    d. Spontaneous placental expulsion

    e. Dilation of the cervix

11. A pregnant client in labor has to undergo a sonogram to confirm the fetal position of a shoulder presentation. The nurse has to assess for which of the following conditions associated with shoulder presentation during a vaginal birth?

    a. Uterine abnormalities

    b. Fetal anomalies

    c. Congenital anomalies

    d. Prematurity

12. A nurse is assigned the task of educating a pregnant client about childbirth. Which of the following nursing interventions should the nurse perform as a part of prenatal education for the client to ensure a positive childbirth experience? Select all that apply.

   a. Provide the client clear information on procedures involved

   b. Encourage the client to have a sense of mastery and self-control

   c. Encourage the client to have a positive reaction to pregnancy

   d. Instruct the client to spend some time alone each day

   e. Instruct the client to begin changing the home environment

13. A pregnant client is admitted to a maternity clinic for childbirth. What should the assigned nurse observe to conclude that the client's fetus is in the transverse lie position?

   a. Long axis of fetus is at 60 degrees to that of client

   b. Long axis of fetus is parallel to that of client

   c. Long axis of fetus is perpendicular to that of client

   d. Long axis of fetus is at 45 degrees to that of client

14. A pregnant client is admitted to a maternity clinic after experiencing contractions. The assigned nurse observes that the client experiences pauses between contractions. The nurse knows that which of the following marks the importance of the pauses between contractions during labor?

   a. Effacement and dilation of the cervix

   b. Shortening of the upper uterine segment

   c. Reduction in length of the cervical canal

   d. Restoration of blood flow to uterus and placenta

15. A pregnant client is admitted to a maternity clinic for delivery. Which of the following conditions should the nurse observe in the client during a vaginal birth to identify shoulder presentation?

   a. Multiparity

   b. Uterine abnormalities

   c. Multiple gestation

   d. Congenital anomalies

16. A nurse is caring for a pregnant client during labor. Which of the following methods should the nurse use to provide comfort to the pregnant client? Select all that apply.

   a. Hand holding

   b. Chewing gum

   c. Massaging

   d. Acupressure

   e. Prescribed pain killers

Nursing Management During Labor and Birth

SECTION I: LEARNING OBJECTIVES

1. Define the key terms related to the labor and birth process.

2. Select the measures used to evaluate maternal status during labor and birth.

3. Compare and contrast the advantages and disadvantages of external and internal fetal monitoring, including the appropriate use for each.

4. Choose appropriate nursing interventions to address nonreassuring fetal heart rate patterns.

5. Outline the nurse's role in fetal assessment.

6. Explain the various comfort-promotion and pain-relief strategies used during labor and birth.

7. Summarize the assessment data collected on admission to the perinatal unit.

8. Plan the ongoing assessment involved in each stage of labor and birth.

9. Delineate the nurse's role throughout the labor and birth process.

SECTION II: ASSESSING YOUR UNDERSTANDING

Activity A *Fill in the blanks.*

1. _____ comfort measures are usually simple, safe, effective, and inexpensive to use.

2. If the woman is a diabetic, it is critical to alert the newborn nursery of potential _____ in the newborn.

3. If the nitrazine test is inconclusive, an additional test, called the _____ test, can be used to confirm rupture of membranes.

4. The nurse reviews the prenatal record to identify risk factors that may contribute to a decrease in _____ circulation during pregnancy and/or labor.

5. The _____ spines serve as landmarks for estimating the descent of the fetal presenting part and have been designated as zero station.

6. The primary power of labor is _____ contractions, which are involuntary.

7. The _____ is placed over the uterine fundus in the area of greatest contractility to electronically monitor uterine contractions.

8. _____ describes the irregular variations or absence of FHR due to erroneous causes on the fetal monitor record.

9. Baseline variability represents the interplay between the _____ and sympathetic nervous systems.

10. Fetal _____ are transitory increases in the FHR above the baseline that are associated with sympathetic nervous stimulation.

Activity B *Consider the following figure.*

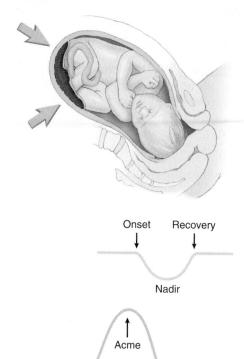

Onset   Recovery

Nadir

Acme

Contraction

1. a. Identify the FHR pattern shown in the image.

_____

_____

b. What causes this FHR pattern?

_____

_____

Activity C *Match the extent of the lacerations in Column A with their depths in Column B.*

Column A

_____ **1.** First-degree laceration

_____ **2.** Second-degree laceration

_____ **3.** Third-degree laceration

_____ **4.** Fourth-degree laceration

Column B

a. Through the anal sphincter muscle

b. Through the muscles of the perineal body

c. Through the skin

d. Through the anterior rectal wall

Activity D *Put the items in correct sequence by writing the letters in the boxes provided below.*

1. Given below, in random order, are nursing interventions during various stages of labor and birth. Arrange them in the correct order.

a. Check the fundus to ensure that it is firm (size and consistency of a grapefruit), located in the midline and below the umbilicus

b. Ascertain whether the woman is in true or false labor

c. Position the woman and cleanse the vulva and perineal areas

d. Check for lengthening of umbilical cord protruding from vagina

e. Check for crowning, low grunting sounds from the woman, and increase in blood-tinged show

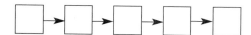

Activity E *Briefly answer the following.*

1. What information should a nurse include when taking the maternal health history?

_____

_____

2. What does the Apgar score assess?

_____

_____

_____

3. What is the purpose of vaginal examination during maternal assessment?

_____

_____

_____

4. What are the advantages and disadvantages of continuous electronic fetal monitoring?

_____

_____

_____

5. What are the typical signs of the second stage of labor?

_____

_____

_____

6. What are the ideal positions for the second stage of labor?

_____

_____

_____

SECTION III: APPLYING YOUR KNOWLEDGE

Activity F   *Consider this scenario and answer the questions.*

1. Susan, a pregnant client, has been admitted to the health care facility because she is in labor. The nurse is prepared to do maternal assessment during labor and delivery. Susan informs the nurse that there is no vaginal bleeding.

a. What nursing intervention should the nurse perform?

_____

_____

_____

b. What is the purpose of vaginal examination during maternal assessment?

_____

_____

_____

c. What is the procedure for conducting vaginal examination?

_____

_____

_____

SECTION IV: PRACTICING FOR NCLEX

Activity G   *Answer the following questions.*

1. It is the nurse's first meeting with a pregnant client. What is the first point that the nurse needs to ascertain as part of the admission assessment to check if the client needs to be admitted?

   a. Whether the client is in true or false labor

   b. Whether the client is pregnant for the first time

   c. Whether the client is addicted to drugs

   d. Whether the client has a history of drug allergy

2. A nurse is assigned to conduct an admission assessment on the phone for a pregnant client. Which of the following information should the nurse obtain from the client? Select all that apply.

   a. Estimated due date

   b. History of drug abuse

   c. Characteristics of contractions

   d. Appearance of vaginal blood

   e. History of drug allergy

3. A nurse is caring for a pregnant client who is in the active phase of labor. At what interval should the nurse monitor the client for maternal vital signs?

   a. Every 15–30 minutes

   b. Every 30 minutes

   c. Every 30–60 minutes

   d. Every 4 hours

4. A nurse is required to obtain the fetal heart rate (FHR) for a pregnant client. If the presentation is cephalic, which maternal site should the nurse monitor to hear the FHR clearly?

   a. Lower quadrant of maternal abdomen

   b. At the level of the maternal umbilicus

   c. Above the level of maternal umbilicus

   d. Just below the maternal umbilicus

5. Which of the following does fetal pulse oximetry help measure?

   a. Weight of the fetus

   b. Fetal blood pH

   c. Fetal oxygen saturation

   d. Fetal position

6. A client in labor is administered lorazepam to help her relax enough so that she can participate effectively during her labor process rather than fighting against it. Which of the following is an adverse effect of the drug that the nurse should monitor for?

   a. Increased sedation

   b. Newborn respiratory depression

   c. Nervous system depression

   d. Decreased alertness

7. A pregnant client with a history of spinal injury is being prepared for a cesarean birth. Which of the following methods of anesthesia is to be administered to the client?

   a. Local infiltration

   b. Epidural block

   c. Regional anesthesia

   d. General anesthesia

8. A pregnant client admitted to a health care center is in the latent phase of labor. How often should the nurse monitor the FHR with the Doppler during the latent phase?

   a. Every 30 minutes

   b. Every hour

   c. Every 15–30 minutes

   d. Continuously

9. During an admission assessment of a client in labor, the nurse observes that there is no vaginal bleeding yet. What nursing intervention is appropriate in the absence of vaginal bleeding when the client is in the early stage of labor?

   a. Monitor vital signs

   b. Assess amount of cervical dilation

   c. Obtain urine specimen for urinalysis

   d. Monitor hydration status

10. A pregnant client is admitted with vaginal bleeding. The nurse performs a nitrazine test to confirm that the membranes have ruptured. The nitrazine tape remains yellow to olive green, with pH between 5 and 6. What does this indicate?

   a. Membranes have ruptured

   b. Presence of amniotic fluid

   c. Presence of vaginal fluid

   d. Presence of excess blood

11. A nurse assisting a pregnant client during pregnancy is to monitor uterine contractions. Which of the following factors should the nurse assess to monitor uterine contraction? Select all that apply.

   a. Uterine resting tone

   b. Frequency of contractions

   c. Change in temperature

   d. Change in blood pressure

   e. Intensity of contractions

12. The nurse performing Leopold's maneuvers for a pregnant client explains to the client the purpose of the maneuvers. Which of the following is the purpose of Leopold's maneuvers? Select all that apply.

   a. Determining the presentation of the fetus

   b. Determining the position of the fetus

   c. Determining the lie of the fetus

   d. Determining the weight of the fetus

   e. Determining the size of the fetus

13. A nurse caring for a pregnant client in labor observes that the FHR is below 110. Which of the following interventions should the nurse perform? Select all that apply.

   a. Turn the client on her left side

   b. Reduce IV fluid rate

   c. Administer oxygen by mask

   d. Assess client for underlying causes

   e. Ignore questions from the client

14. The nurse caring for a client in preterm labor observes nonreassuring FHR patterns. Which of the following nursing interventions should the nurse perform?

   a. Application of vibroacoustic stimulation

   b. Tactile stimulation

   c. Administration of oxygen by mask

   d. Fetal scalp stimulation

15. A nurse is caring for a client administered an epidural block. Which of the following symptoms must the nurse monitor the client for?

    a. Respiratory depression
    b. Accidental intrathecal blockade
    c. Inadequate or failed block
    d. Postdural puncture headache

16. A client administered combined spinal-epidural analgesia is showing signs of hypotension and associated FHR changes. What interventions should the nurse perform to manage the changes?

    a. Assist client to a supine position
    b. Provide supplemental oxygen
    c. Discontinue IV fluid
    d. Turn client to her left side

17. A nurse is caring for a client administered general anesthesia for an emergency cesarean birth. What complications associated with general anesthesia should the nurse monitor for?

    a. Pruritus
    b. Uterine relaxation
    c. Inadequate or failed block
    d. Maternal hypotension

18. A pregnant client has opted for hydrotherapy for pain management during labor. Which of the following should the nurse consider when assisting the client during the birthing process?

    a. Initiate the technique only when the client is in active labor
    b. Do not allow the client to stay in the bath for long
    c. Ensure that the water temperature exceeds body temperature
    d. Allow the client into the water only if her membranes have ruptured

19. A nurse is teaching a couple about patterned breathing during their childbirth education. Which of the following techniques should the nurse suggest for slow-paced breathing?

    a. Inhale and exhale through the mouth at a rate of 4 breaths every 5 seconds
    b. Inhale slowly through nose and exhale through pursed lips
    c. Punctuated breathing by a forceful exhalation through pursed lips every few breaths
    d. Hold breath for 5 seconds after every three breaths

20. A pregnant client requires administration of an epidural block for management of pain during labor. Which of the following conditions should the nurse check for in the client before administering the epidural block? Select all that apply.

    a. Spinal abnormality
    b. Hypovolemia
    c. Varicose veins
    d. Coagulation defects
    e. Skin rashes or bruises

CHAPTER 15

Postpartum Adaptations

SECTION I: LEARNING OBJECTIVES

1. Define the key terms bolded in this chapter.

2. Explain the systemic physiologic changes occurring in the woman after childbirth.

3. Identify the phases of maternal role adjustment as described by Reva Rubin.

4. Analyze the psychological adaptations occurring in the mother's partner after childbirth.

SECTION II: ASSESSING YOUR UNDERSTANDING

Activity A *Fill in the blanks.*

1. Within 10 days of birth, the fundus of the uterus usually cannot be palpated because it has descended into the true _____.

2. If retrogressive changes do not occur as a result of retained placental fragments or infection, _____ results.

3. _____ are the painful uterine contractions some women experience during the early postpartum period.

4. Increased prolactin levels and abundant milk supply, combined with inadequate emptying of the breast, may cause breast _____.

5. During pregnancy, stretching of the abdominal wall muscles occurs to accommodate the enlarging _____.

6. _____ acts so that milk can be ejected from the alveoli to the nipple.

7. For _____ women, menstruation usually resumes 7 to 9 weeks after giving birth.

8. _____ is the secretion of milk by the breasts.

9. _____ from the anterior pituitary gland, secreted in increasing levels throughout pregnancy, triggers synthesis and secretion of milk after giving birth.

10. The profuse _____ that is common during the early postpartum period is one of the most noticeable adaptations in the integumentary system and is a way of eliminating excess body fluids retained during pregnancy.

Activity B *Match the terms in Column A with their descriptions in Column B.*

Column A

____ 1. Engrossment

____ 2. Involution

____ 3. Lochia

____ 4. Puerperium

____ 5. Uterine atony

Column B

a. The discharge that occurs after birth

b. Encompasses the time after delivery as the woman's body begins to return to the prepregnant state

c. Allows excessive bleeding

d. The father's developing a bond with his newborn, which is a time of intense absorption, preoccupation, and interest

e. Involves three retro-gressive processes, which are contraction of muscle fibers, catabolism, and regeneration of uterine epithelium

Activity C *Put the items in correct sequence by writing the letters in the boxes provided below.*

1. Lochia refers to the discharge that occurs after birth. Given below, in random order, are the three stages of lochia. Choose the correct sequence in which they appear after birth.

   a. Lochia alba

   b. Lochia rubra

   c. Lochia serosa

   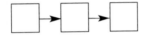

2. Given below, in random order, are the three stages a woman goes through immediately after she gives birth to a child. Choose the correct sequence in which they occur.

   a. Letting-go phase

   b. Taking-hold phase

   c. Taking-in phase

   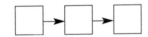

Activity D *Briefly answer the following.*

1. Explain why breastfeeding is not a reliable method of contraception.

   _____

   _____

   _____

2. Why are afterpains more acute in multiparous women?

   _____

   _____

   _____

3. What are the factors that facilitate uterine involution?

   _____

   _____

   _____

4. What are the factors that inhibit involution?

   _____

   _____

   _____

5. Why do women who have had cesarean births tend to have less flow of lochial discharge?

   _____

   _____

   _____

6. Why are afterpains usually stronger during breastfeeding? What can be done to reduce this discomfort?

   _____

   _____

   _____

SECTION III: APPLYING YOUR KNOWLEDGE

Activity E *Consider this scenario and answer the questions.*

1. A nurse is caring for two clients, one who is breastfeeding and has developed breast engorgement, and another who is not breastfeeding and has developed breast engorgement.

   a. What relief measures should the nurse suggest to resolve engorgement in the client who is breastfeeding?

   _____

   _____

   _____

   b. What relief measures should a nurse suggest for non-breastfeeding engorgement?

   _____

   _____

   _____

SECTION IV: PRACTICING FOR NCLEX

Activity F *Answer the following questions.*

1. A nurse is caring for a client in the postpartum period. Which of the following processes should the nurse identify as retrogressive processes involved in involution? Select all that apply.
   a. Contraction of muscle fibers
   b. Return of breasts to their prepregnancy size
   c. Catabolism, which reduces individual myometrial cells
   d. Regeneration of uterine epithelium
   e. Retention of urine

2. A client who gave birth about 12 hours ago informs the nurse that she has been voiding small amounts of urine frequently. The nurse examines the client and notes the displacement of the uterus from the midline to the right. What intervention should the nurse suggest or perform?
   a. Warm shower
   b. Good body mechanics
   c. Warm compress
   d. Catheterization

3. A client who has given birth a week ago complains to the nurse of discomfort when defecating and ambulating. The birth involved an episiotomy. Which of the following should the nurse suggest to the client to provide local comfort? Select all that apply.
   a. Maintain correct posture
   b. Use of warm sitz baths
   c. Use of anesthetic sprays
   d. Use of witch hazel pads
   e. Use good body mechanics

4. A nurse is caring for a client who has had a vaginal birth. The nurse understands that pelvic relaxation can occur in any woman experiencing a vaginal birth. Which of the following should the nurse recommend to the client to improve pelvic floor tone?
   a. Kegel exercises
   b. Witch hazel pads
   c. Good body mechanics
   d. Sitz baths

5. The nurse is caring for a client who had been administered an anesthetic block during labor. Which of the following are risks that the nurse should watch for in the client? Select all that apply.
   a. Incomplete emptying of bladder
   b. Bladder distention
   c. Ambulation difficulty
   d. Urinary retention
   e. Perineal laceration

6. A client who delivered a baby 36 hours ago informs the nurse that she has been passing unusually large volumes of urine very often. How should the nurse explain this to the client?
   a. Bruising and swelling of the perineum
   b. Swelling of tissues surrounding the urinary meatus
   c. Retention of extra fluids during pregnancy
   d. Decreased bladder tone due to anesthesia

7. A client complains to the nurse of pain in the lower back, hips, and joints 10 days after the birth of her baby. What instruction should the nurse give the client after birth to prevent low back pain and injury to the joints?
   a. Use anesthetic sprays
   b. Maintain correct position
   c. Practice Kegel exercises
   d. Apply ice

8. A concerned client tells the nurse that her husband, who was so excited about the baby before its birth, is apparently happy but seems to be afraid of caring for the baby. What suggestions should the nurse give to the client's husband to resolve the issue?
   a. Hold the newborn
   b. Speak to his friends
   c. Read up on parental care
   d. Speak to the physician

9. A client who gave birth five days ago complains to the nurse of profuse sweating during the night. What should the nurse recommend to the client in this regard?
   a. Use good body mechanics
   b. Use sitz baths
   c. Change her gown
   d. Practice Kegel exercises

10. A client is undergoing a routine check-up two months after the birth of her child. The nurse understands that the client is not practicing Kegel exercises. Which of the following should the nurse tell the client is caused by poor perineal muscular tone?

    a. Pain in the joints

    b. Pain in the lower back

    c. Urinary incontinence

    d. Postpartum diuresis

11. A breastfeeding client informs the nurse that she is unable to maintain her milk supply. What instructions should the nurse give to the client to improve milk supply?

    a. Take cold baths

    b. Apply ice to the breasts

    c. Empty the breasts frequently

    d. Perform Kegel exercises

12. A nurse is examining a client who underwent a vaginal birth 24 hours ago. The client tells the nurse that she is bleeding profusely. What explanation should the nurse give the client about lochia rubra?

    a. Discharge consists of mucus, tissue debris, and blood

    b. Discharge consists of leukocytes, decidual tissue, RBCs, and serous fluid

    c. Discharge consists of RBCs and leukocytes

    d. Discharge consists of leukocytes and decidual tissue

13. A nurse is caring for a client who gave birth a week ago. The client informs the nurse that she experiences painful uterine contractions when breastfeeding the baby. What should the nurse explain is the cause for such afterpains?

    a. Relaxin

    b. Progesterone

    c. Prolactin

    d. Oxytocin

CHAPTER 16

Nursing Management During the Postpartum Period

SECTION I: LEARNING OBJECTIVES

1. Define the key terms that are bolded throughout the chapter.

2. Categorize the parameters requiring assessment during the postpartum period.

3. Compare the bonding and attachment process.

4. Identify behaviors that enhance or inhibit the attachment process.

5. Outline nursing management for the woman and her family during the postpartum period.

6. Design the role of the nurse in promoting successful breastfeeding.

7. Plan areas of health education needed for discharge planning, home care, and follow-up.

SECTION II: ASSESSING YOUR UNDERSTANDING

Activity A *Fill in the blanks.*

1. The _____ is a plastic squeeze bottle filled with warm tap water that is sprayed over the perineal area after each voiding and before applying a new perineal pad.

2. Palpate the breasts for any nodules, masses, or areas of warmth, which may indicate a plugged duct that may progress to _____ if not treated promptly.

3. Elevations in blood pressure from the woman's baseline might suggest pregnancy-induced _____.

4. _____ is considered the fifth vital sign.

5. _____ hypotension can occur when the woman changes rapidly from a lying or sitting position to a standing one.

6. The top portion of the uterus, known as the _____, is assessed to determine uterine involution.

7. Women who experience _____ births will have less lochia discharge than those having a vaginal birth.

8. _____ is the process by which the infant's capabilities and behavioral characteristics elicit parental response.

9. _____ refers to the enduring nature of the attachment relationship.

10. Any discharge from the nipple should be described and documented if it is not _____, or foremilk.

Activity B *Match the terms in Column A with their descriptions in Column B.*

Column A

___ **1.** Bonding

___ **2.** Proximity

___ **3.** Process of attachment

___ **4.** Postpartum blues

Column B

a. Physical and psychological experience of the parents being close to their infant

b. Transient emotional disturbances

c. Development of a close emotional attachment to a newborn by the parents during the first 30 to 60 minutes after birth

d. Development of strong affectional ties between an infant and a significant other (e.g., mother, father, sibling, caretaker)

Activity C *Briefly answer the following.*

1. What does the postpartum assessment of the mother include?

_____

_____

_____

2. What nutritional recommendations can a nurse provide to a client during the postpartum period?

_____

_____

_____

3. What are the causes of postpartum stress?

_____

_____

_____

4. What are the postpartum danger signs?

_____

_____

_____

5. Discuss ways a nurse can model behavior to facilitate parental role adaptation and attachment during the postpartum period.

_____

_____

_____

6. What suggestions can a nurse provide to the parents to minimize sibling rivalry during the postpartum period?

_____

_____

_____

SECTION III: APPLYING YOUR KNOWLEDGE

Activity D *Consider this scenario and answer the questions.*

1. A nurse is caring for a client who has just delivered a healthy baby girl. The client is aware of the benefits of breastfeeding. She expresses her desire to breastfeed her newborn.

a. What assessments should the nurse perform in this regard?

_____

_____

b. How often should the client breastfeed her infant during the postpartum period?

_____

_____

_____

SECTION IV: PRACTICING FOR NCLEX

Activity E *Answer the following questions.*

1. A nurse has been assigned to the care of a client who has just given birth. How frequently should the nurse perform the assessments during the first hour after delivery?
   a. Every 30 minutes
   b. Every 15 minutes
   c. After 60 minutes
   d. After 45 minutes

2. A nurse, assigned to check the pulse, discerns tachycardia in a postpartum client. Which of the following does it suggest?
   a. Pulmonary edema
   b. Atelectasis
   c. Excessive blood loss
   d. Pulmonary embolism

3. A client complains of uterine complications. Which of the following signs should the nurse look for while monitoring the uterus for uterine atony?
   a. Fundus feels firm
   b. Foul-smelling urine
   c. Purulent drainage
   d. Boggy or relaxed uterus

4. The nurse observes a two-inch lochia stain on the perineal pad of a postpartum client. Which of the following terms should the nurse use to describe the amount of lochia present?
   a. Light
   b. Scant
   c. Moderate
   d. Large

5. A nurse is caring for a client who has just had an episiotomy. The nurse observes that the laceration extends through the perineal area and continues through the anterior rectal wall. Which of the following classifications will the nurse use to describe the laceration?
   a. First-degree laceration
   b. Second-degree laceration
   c. Third-degree laceration
   d. Fourth-degree laceration

6. A nurse is required to apply ice packs to a client who has had a vaginal delivery. Which of the following interventions should the nurse perform to ensure that the client gets the optimum benefits of the procedure?
   a. Apply ice packs directly to the perineal area
   b. Apply ice packs for 40 minutes continuously
   c. Ensure ice pack is changed frequently
   d. Use ice packs for a week after delivery

7. Which of the following exercises should a nurse suggest to the client during the first day of postpartum?
   a. Abdominal exercises
   b. Buttock exercises
   c. Thigh-toning exercises
   d. Kegel exercises

8. A first-time mother is nervous about breastfeeding. Which of the following interventions should the nurse perform to reduce maternal anxiety about breastfeeding?
   a. Reassure the mother that some newborns "latch on and catch on" right away, and some newborns take more time and patience
   b. Explain that breastfeeding comes naturally to all mothers
   c. Tell her that breastfeeding is a mechanical procedure that involves burping once in a while and that she should try finishing it quickly
   d. Ensure that the mother breastfeeds the infant using the cradle method only

9. A client who has a breastfeeding infant complains of sore nipples. Which of the following interventions can the nurse do to alleviate the client's condition?
   a. Recommend a moisturizing soap to clean the nipples
   b. Encourage use of breast pads with plastic liners
   c. Offer suggestions based on observation to correct positioning or latching
   d. Fasten nursing bra flaps immediately after feeding

10. A client who has given birth is being discharged from the health care facility. She wants to know how safe it would be for her to have intercourse. Which of the following instructions should the nurse provide to the client regarding intercourse after childbirth?

    a. Avoid use of water-based gel lubricants

    b. Resume intercourse if bright-red bleeding stops

    c. Avoid performing pelvic floor exercises

    d. Use oral contraceptives for contraception

11. A client has been discharged from the maternity clinic after a cesarean delivery. Which of the following is the most appropriate time for scheduling a follow-up appointment for the client?

    a. Within 3 weeks of hospital discharge

    b. Between 4 and 6 weeks after hospital discharge

    c. Within 2 weeks of hospital discharge

    d. Within 1 week of hospital discharge

12. A client is Rh-negative and has given birth to an infant who is Rh-positive. Within how many hours should Rh immunoglobulin be injected in the mother?

    a. 72

    b. 75

    c. 78

    d. 80

13. A nurse is to care for a client during the postpartum period. The client complains of pain and discomfort in her breasts. What signs should a nurse look for to find out if the client has engorged breasts? Select all that apply.

    a. Breasts are hard

    b. Breasts are tender

    c. Nipples are fissured

    d. Nipples are cracked

    e. Breasts are taut

14. A nurse is assessing a client during the postpartum period. Which of the following indicate normal postpartum adjustment? Select all that apply.

    a. Abdominal pain

    b. Active bowel sounds

    c. Tender abdomen

    d. Passing gas

    e. Nondistended abdomen

15. Which of the following interventions should the nurse perform to ensure that the nutritional requirements of newborn infants are met? Select all that apply.

    a. Give infants water and other foods to balance nutritional needs

    b. Show mothers how to initiate breastfeeding within 30 minutes of birth

    c. Encourage breastfeeding of the newborn infant on demand

    d. Provide breastfeeding infants with pacifiers

    e. Place baby in uninterrupted skin-to-skin contact with the mother

CHAPTER 17

Newborn Adaptation

SECTION I: LEARNING OBJECTIVES

1. Define the key terms.

2. Identify the major changes in body systems that occur as the newborn adapts to extrauterine life.

3. Enumerate the primary challenges faced by the newborn during the adaptation to extrauterine life.

4. Explain the three behavioral patterns of newborn behavioral adaptation.

5. Distinguish the five typical behavioral responses of the newborn.

SECTION II: ASSESSING YOUR UNDERSTANDING

Activity A *Fill in the blanks.*

1. _____ is the newborn's ability to process and respond to visual and auditory stimuli.

2. A _____ is an involuntary muscular response to a sensory stimulus.

3. The immune system's responses may be natural or _____.

4. _____ is the first stool passed by the newborn, which is composed of amniotic fluid, shed mucosal cells, intestinal secretions, and blood.

5. Human milk provides a passive mechanism to protect the newborn against the dangers of a deficient _____ defense system.

6. At birth, the pH of the stomach contents is mildly acidic, reflecting the pH of the _____ fluid.

7. _____ refers to the yellowing of the skin, sclera, and mucous membranes as a result of increased bilirubin blood levels.

8. The source of bilirubin in the newborn is the _____ of erythrocytes.

9. Newborn iron stores are determined by total body _____ content and length of gestation.

10. The primary body temperature regulators are located in the _____ and the central nervous system.

Activity B *Match the blood-supplying structures in Column A with their corresponding functions in Column B.*

Column A

____ 1. Umbilical vein

____ 2. Ductus venosus

____ 3. Foramen ovale

____ 4. Ductus arteriosus

Column B

a. Allows majority of the umbilical vein blood to bypass liver and merge with blood moving through the vena cava, bringing it to the heart sooner

b. Connects pulmonary artery to the aorta, which allows bypassing of the pulmonary circuit

c. Allows more than half the blood entering the right atrium to cross immediately to the left atrium

d. Carries oxygenated blood from placenta to

Activity C *Briefly answer the following.*

1. What is a newborn's response to auditory and visual stimuli?

_____

_____

_____

2. What are the expected neurobehavioral responses of the newborn?

_____

_____

_____

3. What events must occur before a newborn's lungs can maintain respiratory function?

_____

_____

_____

4. How is the amniotic fluid removed from the lungs of a newborn?

_____

_____

_____

5. What signs of abnormality should a nurse observe in a newborn's respiration?

_____

_____

_____

6. What are the nursing interventions that may help minimize regurgitation?

_____

_____

_____

SECTION III: APPLYING YOUR KNOWLEDGE

Activity D *Consider this scenario and answer the questions.*

1. A newborn is under the observation of a nurse in a health care facility. The child is crying and its heartbeat has increased. Usually, heartbeats are highest after birth and reach a plateau within a week after birth. During the first few minutes after birth, a newborn's heart rate is approximately 120 to 180 bpm. Thereafter, the heart rate begins to decrease to somewhere between 120 and 130 bpm.

   a. What are the factors that increase the heart rate and blood pressure in a newborn?

   _____

   _____

   _____

   b. What are the factors that affect the hematologic values of a newborn?

   _____

   _____

   _____

   c. What are the benefits of delayed cord clamping after birth?

   _____

   _____

   _____

SECTION IV: PRACTICING FOR NCLEX

Activity E *Answer the following questions.*

1. A client delivers a newborn in a local health care facility. What guidance should the nurse give to the client before discharge regarding care of the newborn at home?

   a. Ensure cool air is circulating over the newborn to ward off the heat

   b. Keep the newborn wrapped in a blanket, with a cap on its head

c. Hold the newborn close to the body after taking a shower

d. Refrain from using clothing and blankets in the crib

2. A nurse is explaining the benefits of breast-feeding to a client who has just delivered. Which of the following immunoglobulins does breast milk contain that boost a new-born's immune system as opposed to for-mula?

a. IgA

b. IgD

c. IgE

d. IgM

3. Which of the following are factors that in-crease the risk of overheating in a newborn? Select all that apply.

a. Limited sweating ability

b. Underdeveloped lungs

c. Too-warm crib

d. Limited insulation

e. Lack of brown fat

4. A two-month-old infant is admitted to a local health care facility after experiencing heat loss. Which of the following manifestations should the nurse observe in the infant in order to confirm the occurrence of cold stress?

a. Change in color of the urine

b. Increase in the body temperature

c. Lethargy and hypotonia

d. Change in the color of the skin

5. Which of the following is a risk factor for the development of jaundice in a newborn?

a. Formula feeding

b. Oxytocin dosage

c. Female gender

d. Hepatitis A vaccine

6. Which of the following possibilities should a nurse keep in mind while administering IV therapy to a newborn?

a. Heart rate increase

b. Lower blood pressure

c. Decrease in alertness

d. Fluid overload

7. A client is worried that her newborn's stools are greenish, with an unpleasant odor. The newborn is being formula-fed. What instruc-tion should the nurse give this client?

a. Switch to breast milk

b. Greenish stools with an unpleasant odor are normal

c. Increase newborn's fluid intake

d. Administer vitamin K supplements

8. A mother wants to know the caloric intake for her two-week-old newborn. Which of the following should the nurse suggest as the ideal caloric intake for a term newborn to re-gain lost weight?

a. 80 kcal/kg/day

b. 108 kcal/kg/day

c. 150 kcal/kg/day

d. 200 kcal/kg/day

9. Which of the following newborns are at a greater risk for cold stress?

a. Preterm newborns

b. Newborns being fed formula

c. Post-term newborns

d. Larger–than-average newborns

10. A client delivers a baby in the maternity unit of a local health care facility. Which of the following behaviors of the newborn should the nurse identify as the self-quieting ability of a newborn?

a. Hand-to-mouth movements

b. Movement of head and eyes

c. Hyperactivity

d. Movements of the legs

11. A nurse needs to check the blood glucose lev-els of a newborn under observation at a health care facility. When should the nurse check the newborn's initial glucose level?

a. After the newborn has been fed

b. 24 hours after admission to the nursery

c. On admission to the nursery

d. 5 hours after admission to the nursery

12. Which of the following interventions can a nurse perform to maintain a neutral thermal environment?

    a. Promote early breastfeeding
    b. Avoid skin-to-skin contact with the mother
    c. Keep the infant transporter cool
    d. Avoid bathing the newborn

13. A nurse is required to assess the temperature of a newborn, using a skin temperature probe. Which of the following points should the nurse keep in mind while taking the newborn's temperature?

    a. Ensure that the newborn is lying on his or her abdomen
    b. Place the temperature probe on the forehead
    c. Place the temperature probe over the liver
    d. Place the temperature probe on the buttocks

14. A nurse is assigned to care for an infant with high bilirubin levels. Which of the following symptoms of jaundice should the nurse monitor?

    a. Yellow mucous membranes
    b. Pinkish appearance of tongue
    c. Heart rate of 120 bpm
    d. Bluish skin discoloration

15. Which of the following is a characteristic of the stools of a breastfed newborn?

    a. Formed in consistency
    b. Completely odorless
    c. Firm in shape
    d. Yellowish gold color

CHAPTER 18

Nursing Management of the Newborn

SECTION I: LEARNING OBJECTIVES

1. Define the key terms bolded throughout the chapter.

2. Differentiate the assessments performed during the immediate newborn period.

3. Select the interventions appropriate to meet the immediate needs of the term newborn.

4. Distinguish the components of a typical physical examination of a newborn.

5. Identify common variations that can be noted during a newborn's physical examination.

6. Categorize common concerns regarding the newborn and appropriate interventions.

7. Compare the importance of the newborn screening tests.

8. Explain the common interventions appropriate during the early newborn period.

9. Delineate the nurse's role in meeting the newborn's nutritional needs.

10. Outline discharge planning content and education needed for the family with a newborn.

SECTION II: ASSESSING YOUR UNDERSTANDING

Activity A *Fill in the blanks.*

1. The _____ score is used to evaluate newborns at 1 minute and 5 minutes after birth.

2. _____ refers to the soft, downy hair on the newborn's body.

3. _____ babies are babies with placental aging who are born after 42 weeks.

4. Babies weighing more than the 90th percentile on standard growth charts are referred to as _____ for gestational age.

5. Vitamin K, a fat-soluble vitamin, promotes blood clotting by increasing the synthesis of _____ by the liver.

6. Persistent cyanosis of fingers, hands, toes, and feet with mottled blue or red discoloration and coldness is called _____.

7. _____ are unopened sebaceous glands frequently found on a newborn's nose.

8. _____ sign refers to the dilation of blood vessels on only one side of the body, giving the newborn the appearance of paleness on one side of the body and ruddiness on the other.

9. The _____ fontanel of the baby is diamond shaped and closes by age 18 to 24 months.

10. _____ is a localized effusion of blood beneath the periosteum of the skull of the newborn.

Activity B *Consider the following figures.*

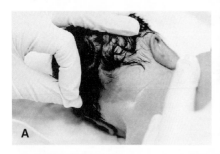

A

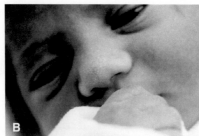

B

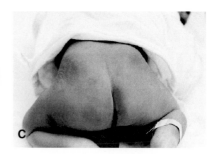

C

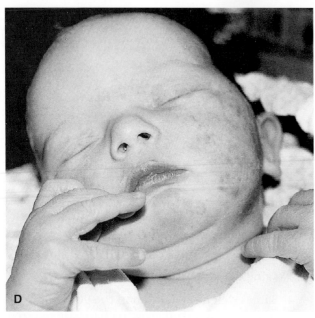

D

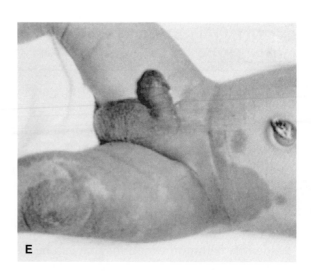

E

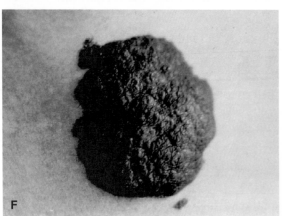

F

1. Identify the conditions in the figures.

_____

_____

2. What does the figure depict?

_____

_____

Activity C *Match the following anthropometric measurements of a term newborn in Column A with their appropriate value in Column B.*

Column A

_____ **1.** Head circumference

_____ **2.** Chest circumference

_____ **3.** Weight

_____ **4.** Length

Column B

a. 30–33 cm

b. 33–37 cm

c. 2500–4000 g

d. 45–55 cm

Activity D *Put the terms in correct sequence by writing the letters in the boxes provided below.*

1. Arrange the following reflexes in the correct order of their disappearance into adulthood.

a. Stepping

b. Babinski sign

c. Grasp

d. Rooting

e. Gag reflex

☐→☐→☐→☐→☐

Activity E *Briefly answer the following.*

1. How can a mother achieve the football hold position for breastfeeding?

_____

_____

_____

2. What is colostrum?

_____

_____

_____

3. What is the use of fiber optic pads in treatment of physiologic jaundice?

_____

_____

_____

4. How can a nurse test Moro's reflex?

_____

_____

_____

5. What is caput succedaneum?

_____

_____

_____

6. What is erythema toxicum?

_____

_____

_____

SECTION III: APPLYING YOUR KNOWLEDGE

Activity F *Consider this scenario and answer the questions.*

1. Karen, a first-time mother, is worried that her baby does not sleep properly and wakes up every two hours. Karen informs the nurse that she often brings the baby to her bed to nurse and falls asleep with the baby in her bed.

   a. What information should the nurse offer regarding the sleeping habits of newborns?

   _____

   _____

   _____

   b. What safety precautions should the mother take when putting the baby to sleep?

   _____

   _____

   _____

   c. What education should the nurse impart to Karen to discourage bed-sharing?

   _____

   _____

   _____

SECTION IV: PRACTICING FOR NCLEX

Activity G *Answer the following questions.*

1. The nurse caring for a newborn has to perform assessment at various intervals. When should the nurse complete the second assessment for the newborn?

   a. Immediately after birth, in the birthing area

   b. Within the first 2 to 4 hours, when newborn is in the nursery

   c. Before the newborn is discharged

   d. The day after the newborn's birth

2. A nurse is caring for a five-hour-old newborn. The physician has asked the nurse to maintain the newborn's temperature between 97.7° and 99.5°F (between 36.5° and 37.5°C). What nursing intervention should the nurse perform to maintain the temperature within the recommended range?

   a. Avoid measuring the weight of the infant, as scales may be cold

   b. Use the stethoscope over the baby's garment

   c. Place the newborn close to the outer wall in the room

   d. Place the newborn skin-to-skin with the mother

3. As a part of the newborn assessment, the nurse determines the skin turgor. Which of the following nursing interventions is relevant when observing the turgor of the newborn's skin?

   a. Pinch skin and note return to original position

   b. Examine for stork bites or salmon patches

   c. Check for unopened sebaceous glands

   d. Inspect for blue or purple splotches on buttocks

4. Which of the following information should the nurse give to a client who is breastfeeding her newborn regarding the nutritional requirements of newborns, as per the recommendations of AAP?

   a. Feed the infant at least 10 mL/kg of water daily

   b. Give iron supplements to the infant daily

   c. Give daily Vitamin D supplements for the first 2 months

   d. Ensure adequate fluoride supplementation

5. A first-time mother informs the nurse that she is unable to breastfeed her baby through the day, as she is usually away at work. She adds that she wants to express her breast milk and store it for her baby. What instruction should the nurse offer the woman to ensure the safety of frozen expressed breast milk?

   a. Use sealed and chilled milk within 24 hours

   b. Use frozen milk within 6 months of obtaining it

   c. Use microwave ovens to warm chilled milk

   d. Refreeze the used milk for later use

6. A nurse is educating the mother of a newborn about feeding and burping. Which of the following strategies should the nurse offer to the mother regarding burping?

   a. Hold the baby upright with the baby's head on her mother's shoulder

   b. Lay the baby on her back on her mother's lap

   c. Gently rub the baby's abdomen while the baby is in a sitting position

   d. Lay the baby on her mother's lap and give her frequent sips of warm water

7. The mother of a seven-month-old baby wishes to start the weaning process. What information should the nurse offer the client regarding introduction of solid foods?

   a. Introduce fruits after vegetables and eggs are introduced

   b. Introduce just one new single-ingredient food at a time to watch for allergies

   c. Coax the infant to eat if he or she is not willing to eat

   d. Avoid using a variety of solid foods in the diet

8. A nurse, while examining a newborn, observes salmon patches on the nape of the neck and on the eyelids. Which of the following is the most likely cause of the salmon patches?

   a. Concentration of pigmented cells

   b. Eosinophils reacting to environment

   c. Immature autoregulation of blood flow

   d. Concentration of immature blood vessels

9. A nurse is required to obtain the temperature of a healthy newborn who is placed in an ordinary crib. Which of the following is the most appropriate method for measuring a newborn's temperature?

   a. Tape electronic thermistor probe to the abdominal skin

   b. Obtain temperature orally

   c. Place electronic temperature probe in the midaxillary area

   d. Obtain temperature rectally

10. A nurse observes that a newborn has a 1-minute Apgar score of 5 points. What should the nurse conclude from the observed Apgar score?

    a. Severe distress in adjusting to extrauterine life

    b. Better condition of the newborn

    c. Moderate difficulty in adjusting to extrauterine life

    d. Abnormal central nervous system status

11. The mother of a newborn observes a diaper rash on her baby's skin. Which of the following should the nurse instruct the parent to prevent diaper rash?

    a. Expose the newborn's bottom to air several times a day

    b. Use plastic pants while bathing the infant

    c. Use products such as powder and items with fragrance

    d. Place the newborn's buttocks in warm water often

12. A nurse is caring for a newborn with transient tachypnea. What nursing interventions should the nurse perform while providing supportive care to the newborn? Select all that apply.

    a. Provide warm water to drink

    b. Provide oxygen supplement

    c. Massage the infant's back

    d. Ensure the newborn's warmth

    e. Observe respiratory status frequently

13. A nurse is caring for a newborn with hypoglycemia. What symptoms of hypoglycemia should the nurse monitor the newborn for? Select all that apply.

    a. Lethargy

    b. Low-pitched cry

    c. Cyanosis

    d. Skin rashes

    e. Jitteriness

14. A mother who is four days postpartum expresses to the nurse that her breast seems to be tender and engorged. What education should the nurse give to the mother to relieve breast engorgement? Select all that apply.

   a. Take warm-to-hot showers to encourage milk release
   b. Feed the newborn in the sitting position only
   c. Express some milk manually before breast-feeding
   d. Massage the breasts from the nipple toward the axillary area
   e. Apply warm compresses to the breasts prior to nursing

15. A nurse is performing detailed newborn assessment of a female baby. Which of the following observations indicate a normal finding? Select all that apply.

   a. Mongolian spots
   b. Enlarged fontanelles
   c. Swollen genitals
   d. Low-set ears
   e. Short, creased neck

CHAPTER 19

Nursing Management of Pregnancy at Risk: Pregnancy-Related Complications

SECTION I: LEARNING OBJECTIVES

1. Define the term *high-risk pregnancy*.

2. Explain common factors that might put a pregnancy at high risk.

3. Identify the causes of vaginal bleeding during early and late pregnancy.

4. Outline nursing assessment and management for the pregnant woman experiencing vaginal bleeding.

5. Develop a plan of care for the woman experiencing preeclampsia, eclampsia, and HELLP syndrome.

6. Explain the pathophysiology of polyhydramnios and subsequent management.

7. Select factors in a woman's prenatal history that place her at risk for premature rupture of membranes (PROM).

8. Formulate a teaching plan for maintaining the health of pregnant women experiencing a high-risk pregnancy.

SECTION II: ASSESSING YOUR UNDERSTANDING

Activity A *Fill in the blanks.*

1. _____ is a decreased amount of amniotic fluid (<500 mL) between 32 and 36 weeks' gestation.

2. _____ is the presence of rhythmic involuntary contractions, most often at the foot or ankle.

3. The time interval from rupture of membranes to the onset of regular contractions is termed the _____ period.

4. Brisk reflexes, or _____, are a common presenting symptom of preeclampsia and are the result of an irritable cortex.

5. Rh _____ is a condition that develops when a woman with Rh-negative blood type is exposed to Rh-positive blood cells and subsequently develops circulating titers of Rh antibodies.

6. _____ twins develop when a single, fertilized ovum splits during the first 2 weeks after conception.

7. A foul odor of amniotic fluid indicates

   _____.

8. A _____ abortion refers to the loss of a fetus resulting from natural causes—that is, not elective or therapeutically induced by a procedure.

9. The most common cause for _____ trimester abortions is fetal genetic abnormalities, usually unrelated to the mother.

10. _____ hypertension is characterized by hypertension without proteinuria after 20 weeks of gestation and a return of the blood pressure to normal postpartum.

Activity B *Consider the following figures.*

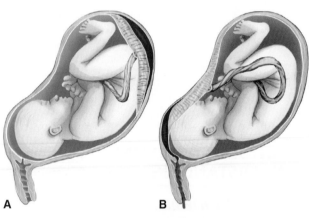

A   B

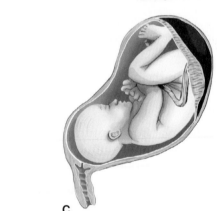

C

1. Identify the classifications of abruption placenta shown in the images.

   _____

   _____

Activity C *Match the following conditions commonly associated with pregnancy-related complications in Column A with their definitions in Column B.*

Column A

____ **1.** Spontaneous abortion

____ **2.** Ectopic pregnancy

____ **3.** Gestational trophoblastic disease

____ **4.** Cervical insufficiency

____ **5.** Placenta previa

Column B

a. Spectrum of neoplastic disorders that originate in the human placenta

b. Weak, structurally defective cervix that spontaneously dilates in the absence of contractions in the second trimester, resulting in the loss of the pregnancy

c. Loss of an early pregnancy, usually before the 20th week of gestation

d. Painless bleeding condition that occurs in the last two trimesters of pregnancy

e. Pregnancy in which the fertilized ovum implants outside the uterine cavity

Activity D *Put the terms in correct sequence by writing the letters in the boxes provided below.*

1. Given below, in random order, are the steps for assessing the patellar reflex. Write the correct sequence.

   a. Using a reflex hammer or the side of the hand, strike the area of the patellar tendon firmly and quickly

   b. Have the woman flex her knee slightly

   c. Place the woman in the supine position

   d. Repeat the procedure on the opposite leg

   e. Note the movement of the leg and foot

   f. Place a hand under the knee to support the leg and locate the patellar tendon

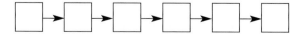

Activity E *Briefly answer the following.*

1. What are some possible complications of hyperemesis gravidarum?

2. What are the conditions associated with early bleeding during pregnancy?

3. What are the causes of ectopic pregnancies?

4. What are the risk factors for hyperemesis gravidarum?

5. What should a nurse include in prevention education for ectopic pregnancies?

6. What is the Kleihauer–Betke test?

SECTION III: APPLYING YOUR KNOWLEDGE

Activity F *Consider this scenario and answer the questions.*

1. The Labor and Birth triage nurse is admitting Jenna. By completing Jenna's history, the nurse learns that she is a single, 17-year-old African-American, G-3 P-0020, who registered for prenatal care at the local clinic at 16 weeks. Her prenatal course has been unremarkable except for a urinary tract infection at 22 weeks that was treated with antibiotics. She did not return to the clinic for a follow-up urine culture following treatment. She is presenting at the hospital now, at 26 weeks, complaining of lower backache, cramping, and malaise. She reports to the nurse that she feels normal fetal movement and denies vaginal bleeding or discharge. She states that she feels her uterus "balling up" every 5–10 minutes. This has been going on all day, even after she came home from school and rested. The external fetal monitor, tocodynamometer, and ultrasound are applied to Jenna. The nurse's initial assessment indicates Jenna having contractions every 4–5 minutes that last 30–40 seconds, and the nurse palpates the contractions as mild.

   a. Name the symptoms that indicate preterm labor and birth.

   b. The nurse caring for Jenna must ensure that she receives basic information about preterm labor, including information about harmful lifestyles, the signs of genitourinary infections, and preterm labor. What information should the nurse provide to Jenna to help better educate her in prevention strategies?

SECTION IV: PRACTICING FOR NCLEX

Activity G *Answer the following questions.*

1. A pregnant client with hyperemesis gravidarum needs advice on how to minimize nausea and vomiting. Which of the following instructions should a nurse give this client?

   a. Lie down or recline for at least two hours after eating

   b. Avoid dry crackers, toast and soda

   c. Eat small, frequent meals throughout the day

   d. Decrease intake of carbonated beverages

2. When caring for a client with premature rupture of membranes (PROM), the nurse observes an increase in the client's pulse. What does this increase in pulse indicate?

   a. Infection

   b. Preterm labor

   c. Cord compression

   d. Respiratory distress syndrome

3. A nurse is caring for a client who has just undergone delivery. What is the best method for the nurse to assess this client for postpartum hemorrhage?

   a. By assessing skin turgor

   b. By assessing blood pressure

   c. By frequently assessing uterine involution

   d. By monitoring hCG titers

4. A nurse is monitoring a client with premature rupture of membranes (PROM) who is in labor and observes meconium in the amniotic fluid. What does this indicate?

   a. Cord compression

   b. Fetal distress related to hypoxia

   c. Infection

   d. CNS involvement

5. The nurse is caring for a pregnant client with severe preeclampsia. Which of the following nursing interventions should a nurse perform to institute and maintain seizure precautions in this client?

   a. Provide a well-lit room

   b. Keep head of bed slightly elevated

   c. Place the client in a supine position

   d. Keep the suction equipment readily available

6. A client with preeclampsia is receiving magnesium sulfate to suppress or control seizures. Which of the following nursing interventions should a nurse perform to determine the effectiveness of therapy?

   a. Assess deep tendon reflexes

   b. Monitor intake and output

   c. Assess client's mucous membrane

   d. Assess client's skin turgor

7. A nurse is assessing pregnant clients for the risk of placenta previa. Which of the following clients faces the greatest risk for this condition?

   a. A 23-year-old client

   b. A client with a history of alcohol ingestion

   c. A client with a structurally defective cervix

   d. A client who had undergone a myomectomy to remove fibroids

8. A client is seeking advice for his pregnant wife, who is experiencing mild elevations in blood pressure. In which of the following positions should a nurse recommend the pregnant client rest?

   a. Supine position

   b. Lateral recumbent position

   c. Left lateral lying position

   d. Head of the bed slightly elevated

9. A nurse is caring for a client with hyperemesis gravidarum. Which of the following should be the first choice for fluid replacement for this client?

   a. Total parenteral nutrition

   b. IV fluids and antiemetics

   c. Percutaneous endoscopic gastrostomy

   d. 5% dextrose in lactated Ringer's solution with vitamins and electrolytes

10. A nurse has been assigned to assess a pregnant client for abruptio placenta. Which of the following is a classic manifestation of this condition that the nurse should assess for?

    a. Painless bright red vaginal bleeding

    b. Increased fetal movement

    c. "Knife-like" abdominal pain with vaginal bleeding

    d. Generalized vasospasm

11. A nurse is caring for a client undergoing treatment for ectopic pregnancy. Which of the following symptoms is observed in a client if rupture or hemorrhaging occurs before successfully treating the ectopic pregnancy?

    a. Phrenic nerve irritation

    b. Painless bright red vaginal bleeding

    c. Fetal distress

    d. Tetanic contractions

12. The nurse is required to assess a pregnant client who is complaining of vaginal bleeding. Which of the following assessments should be considered as a priority by the nurse?
   a. Monitoring uterine contractility
   b. Assessing signs of shock
   c. Determining the amount of funneling
   d. Assessing the amount and color of the bleeding

13. The nurse is required to monitor a pregnant client with fallopian tube rupture. Which of the following interventions should a nurse perform to identify development of hypovolemic shock in this client?
   a. Monitor the client's beta-hCG level
   b. Monitor the mass with transvaginal ultrasound
   c. Monitor the client's vital signs, bleeding
   d. Monitor the fetal heart rate

14. Which of the following instructions should a nurse give an Rh-negative nonimmunized client in her early weeks of pregnancy to prevent complications of blood incompatibility?
   a. Obtain RhoGAM at 28 weeks' gestation
   b. Consume a well-balanced, nutritional diet
   c. Avoid sexual activity until after 28 weeks
   d. Undergo periodic transvaginal ultrasound

15. A nurse is caring for a pregnant client with eclamptic seizure. Which of the following should the nurse know as a characteristic of eclampsia?
   a. Muscle rigidity is followed by facial twitching
   b. Respirations are rapid during the seizure
   c. Coma occurs after seizure
   d. Respiration fails after the seizure

16. A nurse is assessing a pregnant client with preeclampsia for suspected dependent edema. Which of the following is a characteristic of dependent edema?
   a. Dependent edema leaves a small depression or pit after finger pressure is applied to a swollen area
   b. Dependent edema occurs only in clients on bed rest
   c. Dependent edema can be measured when pressure is applied
   d. Dependent edema may be seen in the sacral area if the client is on bed rest

17. The nurse is assessing a client who is in her 24th week of pregnancy. The nurse knows that which of the client's presenting symptoms should be further assessed as a possible sign of preterm labor? Select all that apply.
   a. Increase in vaginal discharge
   b. Phrenic nerve irritation
   c. Rupture of membranes
   d. Uterine contractions
   e. Hypovolemic shock

18. A pregnant client is brought to the health care facility with signs of PROM (premature rupture of membranes). Which of the following are the associated conditions and complications of premature rupture of the membranes? Select all that apply.
   a. Prolapsed cord
   b. Abruptio placenta
   c. Spontaneous abortion
   d. Placenta previa
   e. Preterm labor

19. The nurse is required to assess a client for HELLP syndrome. Which of the following are the signs and symptoms of this condition? Select all that apply.
   a. Blood pressure higher than 160/110
   b. Epigastric pain
   c. Oliguria
   d. Upper right quadrant pain
   e. Hyperbilirubinemia

20. A nurse is monitoring a client with spontaneous abortion who has been prescribed misoprostol. The nurse knows that which of the following symptoms are common adverse effects associated with misoprostol? Select all that apply.
   a. Constipation
   b. Dyspepsia
   c. Headache
   d. Hypotension
   e. Tachycardia

Nursing Management of the Pregnancy at Risk: Selected Health Conditions and Vulnerable Populations

SECTION I: LEARNING OBJECTIVES

1. Identify at least two conditions present before pregnancy that can have a negative effect on a pregnancy.

2. Explain how a condition present before pregnancy can impact the woman physiologically and psychologically when she becomes pregnant.

3. Differentiate the nursing assessment and management for a pregnant woman with diabetes from that of a pregnant woman without diabetes.

4. Explore how congenital and acquired heart conditions can affect a woman's pregnancy.

5. Describe the nursing assessment and management of a pregnant woman with cardiovascular disorders and respiratory conditions.

6. Differentiate among the types of anemia affecting pregnant women in terms of prevention and management.

7. Describe the most common infections that can jeopardize a pregnancy and propose possible preventive strategies.

8. Explain the nurse's role in the prevention and management of adolescent pregnancy.

9. Identify the impact of pregnancy for a woman over the age of 35.

10. Develop a plan of care for the pregnant woman who is HIV-positive.

11. Examine the effects of substance abuse during pregnancy.

SECTION II: ASSESSING YOUR UNDERSTANDING

Activity A *Fill in the blanks.*

1. Human placental lactogen and growth hormone _____ increase in direct correlation with the growth of placental tissue, causing insulin resistance.

2. _____ diabetes of any severity increases the risk of fetal macrosomia.

3. Asthma is known as reactive _____ disease.

4. The _____ is the major site of involvement in the client with tuberculosis.

5. _____ results in reduced capacity of the blood to carry oxygen to the vital organs of the mother and fetus as a result of reduced quantities of RBCs or hemoglobin.

6. Vaginal and rectal specimens are cultured for the presence of a _____.

7. _____ is a widespread parasitic infection caused by a one-celled protozoan.

8. _____ spans the time frame from the onset of puberty to the cessation of physical growth, roughly from 11 to 19 years of age.

9. _____ found in cigarettes causes vasoconstriction, transfers across the placenta, and reduces blood flow to the fetus, contributing to fetal hypoxia.

10. _____ is a psychoactive drug derived from the leaves of the coca plant, which grows in the Andes Mountains of Peru, Ecuador, and Bolivia.

Activity B *Consider the following figure.*

1. a. Identify the disorder shown in the image.

_____

_____

b. What are the characteristics of this disorder?

_____

_____

Activity C *Match the substances in Column A with their effect on pregnancy in Column B.*

Column A

____ **1.** Alcohol

____ **2.** Caffeine

____ **3.** Nicotine

____ **4.** Cocaine

____ **5.** Narcotics

____ **6.** Sedatives

Column B

a. Respiratory problems, feeding difficulties, disturbed sleep

b. Neonatal abstinence syndrome, preterm labor, IUGR, and preeclampsia

c. Vasoconstriction, tachycardia, hypertension, abruptio placenta, abortion, prune belly syndrome, IUGR

d. Reduced uteroplacental blood flow, decreased birth weight, abortion, prematurity, abruptio placenta

e. Decreased iron absorption; increased risk of anemia

f. Growth deficiencies, facial abnormalities, CNS impairment, behavioral disorders, and abnormal intellectual development

Activity D *Briefly answer the following.*

1. What are the complications in a pregnant client with hypertension?

_____

_____

_____

2. What elements should be included during the physical examination of pregnant clients with asthma?

_____

_____

_____

3. What are the factors the nurse should include in the teaching plan for a pregnant client with asthma?

_____

_____

_____

4. What is the procedure involved in the assessment of tuberculosis in pregnant clients?

_____

_____

_____

5. What are the developmental tasks associated with adolescent behavior?

_____

_____

_____

6. What are the effects of abuse of sedatives by the mother on her infant?

_____

_____

_____

SECTION III: APPLYING YOUR KNOWLEDGE

Activity E *Consider this scenario and answer the questions.*

1. A nurse is caring for a pregnant client with asthma. During pregnancy, the respiratory system of the client is affected by hormonal changes, mechanical changes, and prior respiratory conditions.

    a. When is a pregnant client likely to suffer an increase in asthma attacks?

    _____

    _____

    _____

    b. What does successful management of asthma in pregnancy involve?

    _____

    _____

    _____

c. What are the nursing interventions involved for a client with asthma during labor?

_____

_____

_____

SECTION IV: PRACTICING FOR NCLEX

Activity F *Answer the following questions.*

1. A nurse is caring for a pregnant client. The nurse learns from the report that the client is diabetic. Which of the following should the nurse identify as the effect of insulin resistance in the client?

    a. Hypertension

    b. Postprandial hyperglycemia

    c. Hypercholesterolemia

    d. Myocardial infarction

2. A nurse is caring for a pregnant client. During assessment, the nurse learns that the client has cardiovascular disease. Which of the following should the nurse identify as a major risk that can be faced by the offspring of the client?

    a. Respiratory distress syndrome

    b. Congenital varicella syndrome

    c. Sudden infant death syndrome

    d. Prune belly syndrome

3. What is the role of the nurse during the preconception counseling of a pregnant client with chronic hypertension?

    a. Stressing the avoidance of dairy products

    b. Stressing the positive benefits of a healthy lifestyle

    c. Stressing the increased use of vitamin D supplements

    d. Stressing regular walks and exercise

4. Which of the following should the nurse recognize as a symptom of cardiac decompensation?

    a. Swelling of the face

    b. Dry, rasping cough

    c. Slow, labored respiration

    d. Elevated temperature

5. A nurse is caring for a pregnant client with heart disease in a labor unit. Which of the following is the most important intervention for this client in the first 48 hours postpartum?

   a. Limiting sodium intake

   b. Inspecting the extremities for edema

   c. Ensuring that the client consumes a high-fiber diet

   d. Assessing for cardiac decompensation

6. A nurse is caring for a pregnant client with asthma. Which of the following interventions should the nurse include during physical examination of this client?

   a. Monitoring temperature frequently

   b. Assessing for signs of fatigue

   c. Monitoring frequency of headache

   d. Assessing for feeling nauseated

7. What important instruction should the nurse give a pregnant client with tuberculosis?

   a. Maintain adequate hydration

   b. Avoid direct sunlight

   c. Avoid red meat

   d. Wear light, cotton clothes

8. Which of the following should the nurse identify as a risk associated with anemia during pregnancy?

   a. Newborn with heart problems

   b. Fetal asphyxia

   c. Preterm birth

   d. Newborn with an enlarged liver

9. A nurse is caring for a client with cardiovascular disease who has just delivered. What nursing intervention should the nurse perform when caring for this client?

   a. Assess for shortness of breath

   b. Assess for possible fluid overload

   c. Assess for edema and note any pitting

   d. Auscultate heart sounds for abnormalities

10. A nurse is caring for a pregnant client who works at a daycare center and is in regular contact with children. What instructions should the nurse give this client in order to minimize risk of transmission of cytomegalovirus (CMV) to the fetus?

    a. Ensure thorough handwashing

    b. Seek consultation for antibiotics

    c. Avoid interacting with children

    d. Drink plenty of fluids

11. A nurse is caring for a pregnant adolescent client admitted to the maternity unit of a health care center. Which of the following is an important area that the nurse should address during assessment of the client?

    a. Sexual development of the client

    b. Whether sex was consensual

    c. Stress level of the client

    d. Knowledge of child development

12. A nurse is caring for a 40-year-old pregnant client. About which of the following should the nurse inform this client?

    a. Risk for coronary artery disease

    b. Avoid excessive exposure to sunlight

    c. Avoid consumption of poultry products

    d. Perform aerobic exercises daily

13. A nurse is caring for a pregnant client who is HIV-positive. Which of the following is the most important issue that the nurse should discuss with the client?

    a. Relationship with the spouse

    b. Physical contact with infant

    c. Visiting crowded places

    d. Avoidance of breastfeeding

14. A nurse is caring for a pregnant client who admits to occasional substance abuse. Which risk factor associated with substance abuse during pregnancy should the nurse caution the client about?

    a. Post-term birth

    b. High levels of anxiety

    c. Stillbirth

    d. Transient tachypnea of the newborn

15. A nurse is caring for a pregnant client. The initial interview reveals that the client is accustomed to drinking coffee at regular intervals. What possible effect of maternal coffee consumption during pregnancy should the nurse make the client aware of?

    a. Increased risk of heart disease

    b. Increased risk of anemia

    c. Increased risk of rickets

    d. Increased risk of scurvy

16. The nurse is caring for a pregnant client whose Kardex indicates that she is fond of meat, works with children, and has a pet cat. Which of the following instructions should the nurse give this client to prevent toxoplasmosis? Select all that apply.

    a. Eat meat cooked to 160°F

    b. Avoid cleaning the cat's litter box

    c. Keep the cat outdoors at all times

    d. Feed the cat only uncooked meat

    e. Avoid outdoor activities such as gardening

17. A pregnant client has been diagnosed with gestational diabetes. Which of the following are risk factors for developing gestational diabetes? Select all that apply.

    a. Maternal age less than 18 years

    b. Genitourinary tract abnormalities

    c. Obesity

    d. Hypertension

    e. Previous LGA infant

18. A nurse is caring for a pregnant client with sickle cell anemia. What should the nursing care for the client include? Select all that apply.

    a. Teach the client meticulous handwashing

    b. Assess serum electrolyte levels of the client at each visit

    c. Instruct client to consume protein-rich food

    d. Assess hydration status of the client at each visit

    e. Urge the client to drink 8 to 10 glasses of fluid daily

19. A nurse is caring for a newborn with fetal alcohol spectrum disorder. What characteristic of the fetal alcohol spectrum disorder should the nurse assess for in the newborn?

    a. Small head circumference

    b. Decreased blood glucose level

    c. Poor breathing pattern

    d. Wide eyes

20. A nurse is documenting a dietary plan for a pregnant client with pregestational diabetes. What instructions should the nurse include in the dietary plan for this client?

    a. Include more dairy products in the diet

    b. Include complex carbohydrates in the diet

    c. Eat only two meals per day

    d. Eat at least one egg per day

CHAPTER 21

Nursing Management of Labor and Birth at Risk

SECTION I: LEARNING OBJECTIVES

1. Define dystocia.

2. Identify the four major abnormalities or problems associated with dysfunctional labor patterns, giving examples of each problem.

3. Describe the nursing management for the woman with dysfunctional labor experiencing a problem with the powers, passenger, passageway, and psyche.

4. Develop a plan of care for the woman experiencing preterm labor.

5. Discuss the nursing assessment and management of the woman experiencing a post-term pregnancy.

6. Explain four obstetric emergencies that can complicate labor and birth, including appropriate management for each.

7. Compare and contrast the nursing management for the woman undergoing labor induction or augmentation versus forceps and vacuum–assisted birth.

8. Summarize the plan of care for a woman who is to undergo a cesarean birth.

9. Discuss the key areas to be addressed when caring for a woman who is to undergo vaginal birth after cesarean (VBAC).

SECTION II: ASSESSING YOUR UNDERSTANDING

Activity A *Fill in the blanks.*

1. Abnormal or difficult labor is known as _____.

2. _____ presentation is frequently associated with multifetal pregnancies and grand multiparity.

3. _____ maneuver is used to identify deviations in fetal presentation or position.

4. _____ drugs promote uterine relaxation by interfering with uterine contraction.

5. _____ are given to enhance fetal lung maturity between 24 weeks and 34 weeks of gestation.

6. Fetal _____, a glycoprotein produced by the chorion, is found at the junction of the chorion and deciduas.

7. _____ score helps to identify women who would be most likely to achieve a successful induction.

8. _____ dilators absorb endocervical and local tissue fluids; as they enlarge they expand the endocervix and provide controlled mechanical pressure.

9. An _____ involves inserting a cervical hook through the cervical os to artificially rupture the membranes.

10. _____ is produced naturally by the posterior pituitary gland and stimulates contractions of the uterus.

Activity B *Consider the following figures.*

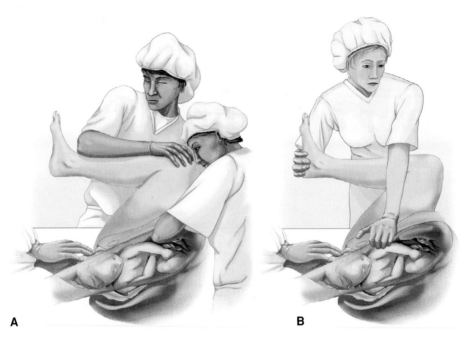

A   B

1. What do the figures depict?

_____

_____

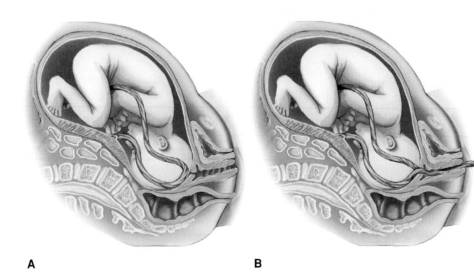

A   B

2. Identify the figures.

_____

_____

Activity C *Match the tests in Column A with their purposes in Column B.*

Column A

___ **1.** Ultrasound

___ **2.** Pelvimetry

___ **3.** Nonstress test

___ **4.** Phosphatidyl-glycerol (PG) level

___ **5.** Nitrazine paper and/or fern test

Column B

a. To rule out fetopelvic disproportion

b. To assess fetal lung maturity

c. To evaluate fetal size, position, and gestational age and to locate the placenta

d. To confirm ruptured membranes

e. To evaluate fetal well-being

Activity D *Put the terms in correct sequence by writing the letters in the boxes provided below.*

1. Given below, in random order, are steps for administering oxytocin. Choose the correct sequence.

a. Use an infusion pump on a secondary line connected to the primary infusion.

b. Prepare the oxytocin infusion by diluting 10 units of oxytocin in 1,000 mL of lactated Ringer's solution.

c. Perform or assist with periodic vaginal examinations to determine cervical dilation and fetal descent.

d. Start the oxytocin infusion in mU/min or mL/hour as ordered.

e. Monitor the characteristics of the FHR, including baseline rate, baseline variability, and decelerations.

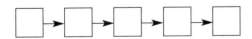

Activity E *Briefly answer the following.*

1. What are symptoms of preterm labor?

_____

_____

_____

2. What is cervical ripeness?

_____

_____

_____

3. What is uterine rupture?

_____

_____

_____

4. What are the indications and contraindications of amnioinfusion?

_____

_____

_____

5. What care should the nurse take when assessing the client for risk of cord prolapse?

_____

_____

_____

6. What are maternal and fetal complications in shoulder dystocia?

_____

_____

_____

SECTION III: APPLYING YOUR KNOWLEDGE

Activity F *Consider this scenario and answer the questions.*

1. Amnioinfusion is a technique in which a volume of warmed, sterile, normal saline or Ringer's lactate solution is introduced into the uterus through an intrauterine pressure catheter to increase the volume of fluid when oligohydramnios is present. It is used to change the relationship of the uterus, placenta, cord, and fetus to improve placental and fetal oxygenation. A nurse is caring for an antenatal mother who is advised to undergo amnioinfusion due to oligohydramnios. The nurse prepares the client for the procedure. What nursing interventions should the nurse follow when caring for the client to prevent maternal and fetal complications?

_____

_____

_____

SECTION IV: PRACTICING FOR NCLEX

Activity G *Answer the following questions.*

1. A nurse is assigned to care for a client who has to undergo a forceps and vacuum–assisted birth. The nurse understands that which of the following factors has contributed to a forceps and vacuum–assisted birth?

   a. A prolonged second stage of labor
   b. Oligohydramnios due to placental insufficiency
   c. Preterm labor with premature rupture of membranes
   d. Rupture of uterus

2. A nurse is assigned to care for a client who has been diagnosed with placental abruption. The nurse knows that which of the following could have led to placental abruption in the client?

   a. Obesity or excess weight gain
   b. Cardiovascular disease
   c. Gestational diabetes
   d. Gestational hypertension

3. A nurse is caring for a client who is experiencing acute onset of dyspnea and hypotension. The physician suspects the client has amniotic fluid embolism. Which of the following symptoms should a nurse monitor to verify the presence of this condition in the client?

   a. Cyanosis
   b. Arrhythmia
   c. Hyperglycemia
   d. Hematuria

4. A nurse is caring for obstetric clients. The nurse should be aware of which of the following as an indication for labor induction?

   a. Chorioamnionitis
   b. Complete placenta previa
   c. Abruptio placenta
   d. Transverse fetal lie

5. A nurse is caring for a client who is undergoing amnioinfusion. Which of the following should the nurse ensure to confirm that amnioinfusion is not contraindicated in this client?

   a. Client does not have uterine hypertonicity
   b. Client does not have an active genital herpes infection
   c. There are no signs of abruptio placentae
   d. Client does not have invasive cervical cancer

6. A client is experiencing shoulder dystocia during delivery. Which of the following should the nurse identify as risks to the fetus in such a condition?

   a. Extensive lacerations
   b. Bladder injury
   c. Infection
   d. Nerve damage

7. A full-term pregnant client is being assessed for induction of labor. Her Bishop score is less than six. Which of the following does it indicate?

   a. Cervical ripening method should be used
   b. A cesarean may be required
   c. Vaginal birth will be successful
   d. Labor will occur spontaneously

8. Which of the following postoperative interventions should a nurse perform when caring for a client who has undergone a cesarean section?

   a. Assess uterine tone to determine fundal firmness
   b. Delay breastfeeding the newborn for a day
   c. Ensure that the client does not cough or breathe deeply
   d. Avoid early ambulation to prevent respiratory problems

9. A client with full-term pregnancy who is not in active labor has been ordered oxytocin intravenously. Which of the following is a contraindication for oxytocin administration?

   a. Dysfunctional labor pattern

   b. Post-term status

   c. Prolonged ruptured membranes

   d. Overdistended uterus

10. A client who is in labor presents with shoulder dystocia of the fetus. Which of the following is an important nursing intervention?

    a. Assist with positioning the woman in squatting position

    b. Assess for complaints of intense back pain in first stage of labor

    c. Anticipate possible use of forceps to rotate to anterior position at birth

    d. Assess for prolonged second stage of labor with arrest of descent

11. A nurse is assessing the cause of multiple gestations in clients. Which of the following factors should the nurse assess as contributors to increased probability of multiple gestations?

    a. Infertility treatment

    b. Medications

    c. Advanced maternal age

    d. Adolescent pregnancies

12. A client is admitted to the health care facility with a gestational age of 42 weeks. The client is to undergo a cesarean section. Which of the following would be the fetal risk associated with post-term pregnancy?

    a. Underdeveloped suck reflex

    b. Congenital heart defects

    c. Intraventricular hemorrhage

    d. Cephalopelvic disproportion

13. A nurse is caring for a client who has been diagnosed with precipitous labor. For which of the following potential fetal complications should the nurse monitor as a result of precipitous labor?

    a. Facial nerve injury

    b. Cephalhematoma

    c. Intracranial hemorrhage

    d. Facial lacerations

14. A nurse is newly posted to the obstetric unit of the health care facility. Which of the following are the causes of intrauterine fetal demise in late pregnancy that the nurse should be aware of?

    a. Hydramnios

    b. Multifetal gestation

    c. Prolonged pregnancy

    d. Malpresentation

15. A nurse is caring for an antenatal mother diagnosed with umbilical cord prolapse. Which of the following should the nurse monitor for in a fetus in cases of umbilical cord prolapse?

    a. Fetal hypoxia

    b. Preeclampsia

    c. Coagulation defects

    d. Placental pathology

CHAPTER 25

Growth and Development of the Newborn and Infant

SECTION I: LEARNING OBJECTIVES

1. Identify normal developmental changes occurring in the newborn and infant.

2. Identify the gross and fine motor milestones of the newborn and infant.

3. Express an understanding of language development in the first year of life.

4. Describe nutritional requirements of the newborn and infant.

5. Develop a nutritional plan for the first year of life.

6. Identify common issues related to growth and development in infancy.

7. Demonstrate knowledge of appropriate anticipatory guidance for common developmental issues.

SECTION II: ASSESSING YOUR UNDERSTANDING

Activity A *Fill in the blanks.*

1. _____ is defined as inconsolable crying that lasts 3 hours or longer per day without any physical cause.

2. The education of parents about what to expect in the next phase of development is referred to as _____ guidance.

3. When playing with toys, the infant usually engages in _____ play.

4. _____ is the sequential process by which infants and children gain various skills and functions.

5. _____ refers to an increase in functionality of various body systems or developmental skills.

6. _____, or blueness of the hands and feet, is normal in the newborn; it decreases over the first few days of life.

7. The ability to fuse two ocular images into one cerebral picture is called _____.

8. _____ anxiety is an indicator that the infant is recognizing himself or herself as separate from others.

9. _____ is an individual's nature; it is referred to as the "how" of behavior.

10. Sudden infant death syndrome (SIDS) has been associated with _____ positioning of newborns and infants, so the infant should be placed to sleep on the back.

Activity B *Consider the following figure.*

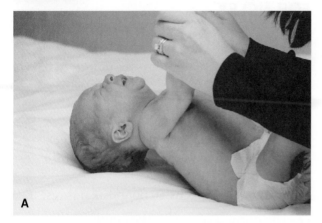

A

1. a. Identify the figure.

_____

_____

b. How do the gross motor skills develop in the infant?

cephalocaudal- head to tail

Activity C *Match the age of the infant in Column A with the proper motor skill in Column B.*

Column A

 1. One month old

 2. Two months old

_c_ **3.** Three months old

_a_ **4.** Four months old

_d_ **5.** Five months old

 6. Six months old

Column B

a. Rolls from prone to supine

b. Raises head and chest

c. Holds open hand to face

d. Grasps rattle or toy

e. Lifts head while prone

f. Sits in tripod fashion

Activity D *Put the terms in correct sequence by writing the letters in the boxes provided below.*

1. Given here, in random order, is the development of fine motor skills in infancy. Choose the correct sequence in which they occur.

a. Bangs objects together

b. Pokes with index finger

c. Involuntary hand movements with fists mostly clenched

d. Offers objects to others and releases them

e. Releases objects in hand to take another

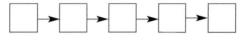

2. Given below, in random order, is the development of gross motor skills in infancy. Choose the correct sequence in which they occur.

a. Lifts head and looks around, rolls from prone to supine

b. Sits alone with some use of hands for support

c. Sits from standing position, walks independently

d. Crawls with abdomen off the floor

e. Raises head and chest and holds position, improving head control

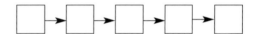

Activity E *Briefly answer the following.*

1. What are the nursing interventions that will help achieve the Healthy People 2010 objective of increasing the proportion of mothers who breastfeed?

_____

_____

_____

2. What causes the infant to spit up? What can be done to control spitting up?

_____

_____

_____

3. How can nurses help parents determine what type of temperament their infant has so that they can most effectively interact with their child?

_____

_____

_____

4. What are the different states of consciousness that a normal newborn will move through?

_____

_____

_____

5. What are the anatomic differences in an infant's respiratory system as compared to an adult's respiratory system?

_____

_____

_____

6. What is the sequence and average age of tooth eruption in infants?

_____

_____

_____

SECTION III: APPLYING YOUR KNOWLEDGE

Activity F *Consider this scenario and answer the questions.*

1. Eight-month-old Carla Jan is brought to the clinic by her parents for her eight-month well-child check-up. As new parents, Carla's parents have many questions and concerns.

   a. Carla's parents are worried about her breaking into sudden "crying spells" on seeing visitors. How should the nurse address Carla's parents' concerns?

   _____

   _____

   _____

   b. Carla's mother had been feeding her iron-fortified rice cereal with formula. She wanted to know if she can feed her any other foods. Considering Carla is normal and healthy, what suggestions can the nurse provide to the mother?

   _____

   _____

   _____

SECTION IV: PRACTICING FOR NCLEX

Activity G *Answer the following questions.*

1. The nurse is examining a six-month-old girl who was born eight weeks early. Which of the following findings is cause for concern?

   a. The child measures 21 inches in length

   b. The child exhibits palmar grasp reflex

   c. Head size has increased 5 inches since birth

   d. The child weighs 10 pounds 2 ounces

2. The nurse is caring for the family of a two-month-old boy with colic. Which of the following interventions would provide the most help in the short term?

   a. Urging the parents to get time away from the child

   b. Educating the parents about when colic stops

   c. Assessing the parents' care and feeding skills

   d. Watching how the parents respond to the child

3. The nurse is providing anticipatory guidance to the parents of a one-year-old girl. Which of the following is the most accurate guidance for disciplining the child as she grows?

   a. Establishing the coffee table as off limits

   b. Telling the child that she will be punished for bad behavior

   c. Keeping her in a child-safe room

   d. Saying "no" in appropriate instances

4. The nurse is teaching the parents of a six-month-old boy about proper child dental care. Which of the following actions will the nurse indicate as the most likely to cause dental caries?

   a. Not cleaning the boy's gums when he has finished eating

   b. Putting the child to bed with a bottle of milk or juice

   c. Using a cloth instead of a brush for cleaning teeth

   d. Failing to clean the teeth with fluoridated toothpaste

5. The nurse is assessing the sleeping practices of the parents of a four-month-old girl who wakes repeatedly during the night. Which of the following parent comments might reveal a cause for the night waking?

   a. They sing to her before she goes to sleep

   b. They put her to bed when she falls asleep

   c. If she is safe, they lay her down and leave

   d. The child has a regular, scheduled bedtime

6. The nurse is educating the mother of a six-month-old boy about the symptoms of teething. Which of the following symptoms would the nurse identify?

   a. The child may run a mild fever or vomit

   b. The child avoids hard foods in favor of soft ones

   c. The child increases biting and sucking

   d. The child has frequent loose stools

7. The nurse is teaching healthy eating habits to the parents of a seven-month-old girl. Which of the following recommendations is the most valuable teaching?

   a. Let the child eat only the foods she prefers

   b. Actively urge the child to eat new foods

   c. Provide small portions that must be eaten

   d. Keep serving a new food 20 times or more

8. The nurse is providing helpful tips on breast-feeding to the mother of a two-week-old boy. Which of the following recommendations will best help the child feed effectively?

   a. Maintaining a feed-on-demand approach

   b. Applying warm compresses to the breast

   c. Encouraging the infant to latch on properly

   d. Maintaining adequate diet and fluid intake

9. The nurse is providing anticipatory guidance to the mother of a one-week-old girl. Which of the following is a reason for the mother to contact her care provider?

   a. The dried umbilical cord stump falls off

   b. Rectal temperature is greater than 100.4°F

   c. The child is eating but still losing weight

   d. The child wets her diaper eight times per day

10. The nurse is observing a six-month-old boy for developmental progress. Which of the following milestones would be typical for him?

   a. Shifts a toy to his left hand and reaches for another

   b. Picks up an object using his thumb and fingertips

   c. Puts down a little ball to pick up a stuffed toy

   d. Enjoys hitting a plastic bowl with a large spoon

11. A nurse is observing primitive reflexes in an infant. The infant fans and hyperextends his toes when the nurse strokes along the lateral aspect of the sole and across the plantar surface. Which of the following reflexes is the infant exhibiting?

   a. Babinski

   b. Step

   c. Moro

   d. Plantar grasp

12. A nurse is educating the parents regarding the consistency of their infant's stools. Which of the following is of concern and should be reported to the primary care provider?

   a. Dark green to black color

   b. Yellowish or tan color

   c. Loose and seedy texture

   d. Mucus-like or frothy

13. A nurse is assessing the development of a three-month-old girl. Which of the following is a warning sign of possible problems with social or emotional development in the infant?

   a. Does not make sounds

   b. Does not laugh or squeal

   c. Does not smile at people

   d. Does not babble

14. A nurse is educating the mother of a six-month-old girl regarding the preparation and storage of bottles and formula. About which of the following should the nurse inform the mother?

   a. Microwave formula and transfer to bottle

   b. Avoid sweetening formula with honey

   c. Add cereal to the formula in the bottle

   d. Reheat unused portion for the next feed

CHAPTER 26

Growth and Development of the Toddler

SECTION I: LEARNING OBJECTIVES

1. Explain normal physiologic, psychosocial, and cognitive changes occurring in the toddler.

2. Identify the gross and fine motor milestones of the toddler.

3. Demonstrate an understanding of language development in the toddler years.

4. Discuss sensory development of the toddler.

5. Demonstrate an understanding of emotional/social development and moral/spiritual development during toddlerhood.

6. Implement a nursing care plan to address common issues related to growth and development in toddlerhood.

7. Encourage growth and learning through play.

8. Develop a teaching plan for safety promotion in the toddler period.

9. Demonstrate an understanding of toddler needs related to sleep and rest, as well as dental health.

10. Develop a nutritional plan for the toddler based on average nutritional requirements.

11. Provide appropriate anticipatory guidance for common developmental issues that arise in the toddler period.

12. Demonstrate an understanding of appropriate methods of discipline for use during the toddler years.

13. Identify the role of the parent in the toddler's life and determine ways to support, encourage, and educate the parents about toddler growth, development, and concerns during this period.

SECTION II: ASSESSING YOUR UNDERSTANDING

Activity A *Fill in the blanks.*

1. _____ results in improved coordination and equilibrium as well as the ability to exercise sphincter control.

2. By 30 months of age, the toddler should have a full set of _____ (baby) teeth.

3. _____ language development is the ability to understand what is being said or asked.

4. The _____ remains short in both male and female toddlers, making them more susceptible than adults to urinary tract infections.

5. The abdominal musculature is _____ in early toddlerhood, resulting in a pot-bellied appearance.

6. _____ defines the toddler period as a time of autonomy versus shame and doubt.

7. Toddlers typically play alongside another child rather than cooperatively; this is known as _____ play.

8. The ability to self-soothe is a function of _____ and is viewed as a sign of a nurturing environment.

9. Adequate _____ intake and appropriate exercise lay the foundation for proper bone mineralization in the toddler.

10. _____ involves systematic ignoring of the undesired behavior.

Activity B *Match the terms related to development in the toddler in Column A with their definitions in Column B.*

Column A

_____ **1.** Animism

_____ **2.** Parachute reflex

_____ **3.** Echolalia

_____ **4.** Individuation

_____ **5.** Food jag

Column B

a. Repeating words and phrases without understanding

b. Forming a sense of self and learning to exert control over one's environment

c. Attributing human feelings to objects

d. Using outstretched arms to catch oneself when falling

e. Preferring one particular food for several days, then not wanting it for weeks

Activity C *Put the terms in correct sequence by writing the letters in the boxes provided below.*

1. Given below in random order are descriptions of expressive language. Arrange them in the order in which the toddler will display them.

a. Uses descriptive words such as "hungry" and "hot"

b. Talks about something that happened in the past

c. Uses a finger to point to things

d. Babbles in what sounds like sentences

☐ → ☐ → ☐ → ☐

2. Given below in random order are descriptions of receptive language. Arrange them in the order the toddler will display them.

a. Points to pictures in books

b. Follows a one-step command accompanied by a gesture

c. Participates in short conversations

d. Understands the word "no"

e. Follows a series of two independent commands

☐ → ☐ → ☐ → ☐ → ☐

Activity D *Briefly answer the following.*

1. Why do toddlers have temper tantrums?

_____

_____

_____

2. What is "toddler gait"?

_____

_____

_____

3. What is telegraphic speech?

_____

_____

_____

4. What are the play habits of toddlers?

_____

_____

_____

5. What should the parent look for when choosing a preschool?

_____

_____

_____

6. What can parents do to prevent caries in toddlers?

_____

_____

_____

SECTION III: APPLYING YOUR KNOWLEDGE

Activity E *Consider this scenario and answer the questions.*

1. Alena Wimund is a two-year-old girl brought to the clinic by her parents for her two-year-old check-up.

   a. Alena's parents state, "We speak to Alena in German at home and are working to make her bilingual." What should the nurse consider when assessing language development in Alena?

   _____

   _____

   _____

   b. Alena's mother asks what they can do to encourage Alena's language development.

   _____

   _____

   _____

   c. Alena's father states that Alena's favorite word is "no." He asks if this is normal at this age. How should the nurse respond to this case? (Include a discussion on Erikson's stage of development and suggestions for dealing with this.)

_____

_____

_____

   d. What are the specific developmental warnings that the nurse should assess Alena for?

   _____

   _____

   _____

SECTION IV: PRACTICING FOR NCLEX

Activity F *Answer the following questions.*

1. The parents of an overweight two-year-old boy admit that their child is a bit chunky but argue that he is a picky eater who will eat only junk food. Which is the best response by the nurse to facilitate a healthier diet?

   a. "You may have to serve a new food 10 or more times."

   b. "Serve only healthy foods. He'll eat when he's hungry."

   c. "Give him healthier choices with less junk food available."

   d. "Calorie requirements for toddlers are less than infants."

2. The nurse is assessing a 36-month-old boy during a well-child visit. Which motor skill has he most recently acquired?

   a. Able to undress himself

   b. Can push a toy lawnmower

   c. Can kick a ball

   d. Pull a toy while walking

3. The nurse is providing anticipatory guidance to the parents of an 18-month-old girl. Which recommendation will be most helpful to the parents?

   a. Giving the child time out for 90 seconds

   b. Ignoring bad behavior and praising good behavior

   c. Slapping her hand using one or two fingers

   d. Describing proper behavior when she misbehaves

4. The nurse is teaching a first-time mother with a 14-month-old boy about child safety. Which is the most effective overall safety information to provide guidance for the mother?

a. "Place a gate at the top of stairways."

b. "Never let him out of your sight."

c. "Keep chemicals in a locked cabinet."

d. "Don't smoke in the house or car."

5. The parents of a two-year-old girl are concerned with her behavior. For which behavior would the nurse share their concern?

a. The child refuses to share her toys with her sister.

b. She frequently babbles to herself when playing.

c. The child likes to change toys frequently.

d. She plays by herself even when other children are present

6. The nurse is discussing sensory development with the mother of a two-year-old boy. Which parental comment suggests that the child may have a sensory problem?

a. "He wasn't bothered by the paint smell."

b. "He was licking up the dishwashing soap."

c. "He doesn't respond if I wave to him."

d. "I dropped a pan behind him and he cried."

7. The nurse is assessing the language development of a three-year-old girl. Which finding would suggest a problem?

a. The child speaks in two- to three-word sentences

b. The child can make simple conversation

c. She tells the nurse she saw Na-Na today

d. She can tell the nurse what her name is

8. The nurse is observing a three-year-old boy in a daycare center. Which behavior might suggest an emotional problem?

a. The child has persistent separation anxiety

b. He goes from calm to tantrum suddenly

c. The child sucks his thumb periodically

d. He is unable to share toys with others

9. The nurse is teaching a mother of a one-year-old girl about weaning her from the bottle and breast. Which recommendation would be part of the nurse's plan?

a. Wean from breast at 18 months of age

b. Switch the child to a no-spill sippy cup

c. Wean from the bottle at 15 months of age

d. Give the child an iron-fortified cereal

10. When performing a regular assessment for an 18-month-old boy, the nurse observes that the boy uses a pacifier. About which of the following should the nurse inform the parents regarding the use of a pacifier? Select all that apply.

a. Use only one-piece pacifiers

b. Replace worn pacifiers with new ones

c. Tie the pacifier around the toddler's neck

d. Avoid pacifier use until permanent teeth erupt

e. Limit pacifier use to stressful situations

11. A young couple with a toddler is expecting their second child. The parents are concerned that the toddler may exhibit sibling rivalry. About which of the following should the nurse inform the parents to help minimize issues with sibling rivalry?

a. Modify toddler's routine to suit the baby's schedule

b. Spend more time with the toddler than with the baby

c. Involve the toddler in the care of the baby

d. Treat the toddler like a baby

12. The parents of a two-year-old girl are concerned about the child's nutritional needs. Which of the following should the nurse tell the parents regarding nutrition for the toddler? Select all that apply.

a. Provide high fat, high-sugar, processed food

b. Limit milk intake to 16 to 24 ounces per day

c. Limit juice intake to 10 to 20 ounces per day

d. Provide foods rich in iron and Vitamin C

e. Offer three full meals and two snacks daily

13. The nurse is assessing a twenty-month-old boy who has started eating solid foods. What teaching should the nurse provide to the parents to prevent the child from choking?

a. Cut nuts and raw carrots into bite-sized pieces

b. Supervise the toddler when he is eating

c. Use a child-sized spoon and fork with dull tines

d. Cut grapes and hot dogs into halves

CHAPTER 27

Growth and Development of the Preschooler

SECTION I: LEARNING OBJECTIVES

1. Identify normal physiologic, cognitive, and psychosocial changes occurring in the preschool-aged child.

2. Express an understanding of language development in the preschool years.

3. Implement a nursing care plan that addresses common concerns or delays in the preschooler's development.

4. Integrate knowledge of preschool growth and development with nursing care and health promotion of the preschool-aged child.

5. Develop a nutrition plan for the preschool-aged child.

6. Identify common issues related to growth and development during the preschool years.

7. Demonstrate knowledge of appropriate anticipatory guidance for common developmental issues that arise in the preschool period.

SECTION II: ASSESSING YOUR UNDERSTANDING

Activity A *Fill in the blanks.*

1. Overconsumption of cow's milk may result in a deficiency of _____ due to calcium blocking its absorption.

2. Communication in preschool children is _____ in nature, because they are not yet capable of abstract thought.

3. Preschool children are more susceptible to bladder infections than are adults because of the length of the _____.

4. _____ development is focused on the accomplishment of initiative.

5. Through _____ thinking, preschool children satisfy their curiosity about differences in the world around them.

6. The preschooler extrapolates from a particular situation to another, even though the events may be unrelated; in other words, he or she uses _____ when reasoning.

7. As the preschooler's _____ system continues to mature, existing motor skills become refined and new ones develop.

8. If a three-year-old is using short sentences that contain only the essential information, he or she is using _____ speech.

9. Parents should encourage _____ activity in the preschooler to stimulate the development of his or her gross motor skills.

10. Daily brushing and flossing help prevent dental _____.

Activity B *Match the age and ability in Column A with the demonstrated behavior in Column B.*

Column A

_____ **1.** Age 4 gross motor

_____ **2.** Age 4 fine motor

_____ **3.** Age 4 communication

_____ **4.** Age 5 gross motor

_____ **5.** Age 5 fine motor

Column B

a. Somersaults

b. Kicks ball forward

c. 75% of speech understood by those outside the family

d. Draws circles and squares

e. Prints some letters

Activity C *Put the terms in correct sequence by writing the letters in the boxes provided below.*

1. Given below, in random order, are motor skills acquired by a child. Choose the correct sequence in which they are acquired.

    a. Dresses or undresses without assistance

    b. Throws ball overhand

    c. Swings and climbs well

    d. Copies circles and traces squares

    ☐→☐→☐→☐

Activity D *Briefly answer the following.*

1. Describe the cognitive abilities of a child in the intuitive phase.

    _____

    _____

    _____

2. Give a few suggestions that parents of preschoolers can use to prevent accidental poisoning.

    _____

    _____

    _____

3. Name three ways to promote healthy teeth and gums in preschoolers.

    _____

    _____

    _____

4. Justify protecting preschoolers from second-hand tobacco smoke.

    _____

    _____

    _____

5. What are the nutritional needs of a typical three- to five-year-old?

    _____

    _____

    _____

6. What are the gross motor skills you can expect of a typical preschooler? ?

    _____

    _____

    _____

SECTION III: APPLYING YOUR KNOWLEDGE

Activity E *Consider this scenario and answer the questions.*

1. Sonia Maule is a four-year-old girl brought to the clinic by her parents for her school check-up.

    a. Sonia's mother states, "Sonia loves to play make-believe. She is constantly playing in a fantasy world. I am not sure if this is healthy behavior." How should the nurse address Mrs. Maule's concerns?

    _____

    _____

    _____

b. Sonia's parents express concerns about the transition to kindergarten. What guidance should the nurse give them regarding this?

_____

_____

_____

c. During assessment, Sonia's mother asks what findings would be of concern to the nurse. Discuss specific developmental warning signs that the nurse should assess Sonia for.

_____

_____

_____

SECTION IV: PRACTICING FOR NCLEX

Activity F *Answer the following questions.*

1. The nurse is conducting a well-child assessment of a four-year-old. Which of the following assessment findings would warrant further investigation?
   a. Presence of 20 deciduous teeth
   b. Presence of 10 deciduous teeth
   c. Absence of dental caries
   d. Presence of 19 deciduous teeth

2. The nurse is conducting a health screening of a five-year-old boy as required for kindergarten. The mother informs the nurse that the boy is fearful about going to a new school. Which of the following is the best response by the nurse?
   a. "Kindergarten is a big step for a child. Be patient with him."
   b. "Remind him that kindergarten will be a lot of fun and he'll make new friends."
   c. "Be aware that he may have difficulty adjusting being away from home five days a week."
   d. "Talk to your son's new teacher and schedule a tour with him."

3. The nurse is assessing the height of a four-year-old during a well-child examination. The nurse would expect that the child's height would have increased by which of the following since the previous year's examination?
   a. One-half to 1 inch
   b. 1 to 2 inches
   c. 2.5 to 3 inches
   d. 3.5 to 4 inches

4. A nurse is performing a routine wellness examination for a five-year-old boy. Which of the following responses by the parents indicates a need for an additional referral or follow-up?
   a. "We often have to translate his speech to others."
   b. "He can count to 30 but gets confused after that."
   c. "He is always talking and telling detailed stories."
   d. "He knows his name and address."

5. The parents of a four-year-old girl tell the nurse that their daughter is having frequent nightmares. Which of the following statements would indicate that the girl is having night terrors instead of nightmares?
   a. "She comes and wakes us up after she awakens."
   b. "She is scared after she wakes up."
   c. "She screams and thrashes when we try to touch her."
   d. "She has a hard time going back to sleep."

6. The nurse is teaching bike safety to the mother of a four-year-old girl. Which of the following statements by the mother indicates a need for further teaching?
   a. "The balls of her feet should reach both pedals while sitting."
   b. "Pedal-back brakes are better for her age group."
   c. "She should always ride on the sidewalk."
   d. "She can ride on the street if I am riding with her."

7. The nurse is conducting a health screening for a three-year-old boy as required by his preschool. Which of the following statements by the parents would warrant further discussion and intervention?

a. "The school has a looser environment, which is a good match for his temperament."

b. "The food they serve at the school is primarily organic, with little processing."

c. "The school is quite structured and advocates corporal punishment."

d. "There is a very low student-to-teacher ratio and they do a lot of hands-on projects."

8. A nurse is caring for a four-year-old girl. The parents state that their daughter often reports that objects in the house are her friends. They are concerned because the girl says that the grandfather clock in the hallway smiles and sings to her. How should the nurse respond?

a. "Your daughter is demonstrating animism, which is common."

b. "Attributing life-like qualities to inanimate objects is quite normal at this age."

c. "Do you think your daughter is hallucinating?"

d. "Is there a family history of mental illness?"

9. The nurse is teaching safety measures to the parents of a four-year-old girl. Which of the following statements by the parents would indicate a need for further teaching?

a. "She should use a helmet only when riding her bike."

b. "She still needs a booster seat in the car."

c. "We need to know the basics of CPR and first aid."

d. "We need to continually remind her about safety rules."

10. The nurse is teaching proper dental care to the parents of a five-year-old girl. Which of the following responses indicates a need for further teaching?

a. "Too much fluoride can contribute to fluorosis."

b. "She needs to floss her teeth before brushing."

c. "She should see a dentist every 6 months."

d. "We should use only a pea-sized amount of toothpaste."

11. A nurse is performing a routine wellness examination for a four-year-old girl. Which of the following responses by the parents indicates a need for an additional referral or follow-up?

a. "She sleeps about eight hours every day."

b. "She is afraid of the dark and cannot sleep unless we put on the nightlight."

c. "She refuses to sleep unless she has her favorite doll by her side."

d. "She takes a nap during the day, too."

12. A nurse is discussing the development of a five-year-old girl with her parents. Which of the following responses by the parents indicates the need for an intervention?

a. "We are planning to enroll her in swimming class."

b. "We generally do not keep tabs on what television she watches."

c. "We never coax her to try new foods."

d. "We do not spank to discipline her."

13. The nurse assessing a preschooler observes that the child uses a no-spill sippy cup. Why should the nurse discourage the preschooler from using no-spill sippy cups?

a. They contribute to dental caries

b. They limit the intake of fluids

c. They increase appetite for solid foods

d. The preschooler must use a glass

14. A nurse is performing a routine wellness examination for a preschooler. Which of the following responses by the parents indicates the need for an intervention?

a. "She eats only certain foods over a several-day period."

b. "She pilots an imaginary airplane."

c. "She watches television 4 hours a day."

d. "She stutters while talking."

15. The nurse is conducting a health screening for a three-year-old boy as required by his preschool. Which of the following statements by the parents would call for further discussion?

a. "He is afraid of loud noises made by firecrackers."

b. "He tends to lie a lot."

c. "He does not drink more than 10 ounces of milk a day."

d. "He is not able to stand on one foot."

CHAPTER 28

Growth and Development of the School-Age Child

SECTION I: LEARNING OBJECTIVES

1. Identify normal physiologic, cognitive, and moral changes occurring in the school-age child.

2. Describe the role of peers and schools in the development and socialization of the school-age child.

3. Identify the developmental milestones of the school-age child.

4. Identify the role of the nurse in promoting safety for the school-age child.

5. Demonstrate knowledge of the nutritional requirements of the school-age child.

6. Identify common developmental concerns regarding the school-age child.

7. Demonstrate knowledge of the appropriate nursing guidance for common developmental concerns.

SECTION II: ASSESSING YOUR UNDERSTANDING

Activity A *Fill in the blanks.*

1. _____ is the period that typically occurs in the two years before the beginning of puberty.

2. Teeth grinding during sleep is known as _____.

3. Malalignment of the eyes is known as _____.

4. Children who are home alone without adult supervision, with both parents in the workforce, are known as _____ kids.

5. The principle of _____ states that matter does not change when its form changes.

6. During the school-age years, all 20 primary _____ teeth are lost.

7. School-age children develop the ability to think about language and comment on its properties, known as _____ awareness.

8. Continuous _____ relationships provide the most important social interaction for school-age children.

9. Compared with the earlier years, caloric needs of the school-age child are _____.

10. The number of hours of sleep required for growth and development _____ with age.

Activity B *Match the theorists listed in Column A with their theories for the school-age child, in Column B.*

Column A

___ 1. Kohlberg

___ 2. Freud

___ 3. Piaget

___ 4. Erikson

Column B

a. Conventional: "good child, bad child"

b. Industry vs. Inferiority

c. Latency

d. Concrete operational

Activity C *Put the terms in correct sequence by writing the letters in the boxes provided below.*

1. Given below, in random order, are developmental milestones in a school-age child. Choose the correct order.

a. Brain growth is complete

b. Fine motor skills develop

c. Development of frontal sinuses is complete

d. Gross motor skills develop

e. Lymphatic tissue growth is complete

☐ → ☐ → ☐ → ☐ → ☐

Activity D *Briefly answer the following.*

1. Describe the development of children's gross motor skills as they correspond to age groups.

_____

_____

_____

2. Describe the child who is labeled "slow to warm."

_____

_____

_____

3. Detail the sleep requirements for school-age children.

_____

_____

_____

4. What is the meaning of school phobia?

_____

_____

_____

5. What are the characteristics of latchkey kids?

_____

_____

_____

6. How can sense of smell and touch be tested in the school-age child?

_____

_____

_____

SECTION III: APPLYING YOUR KNOWLEDGE

Activity E *Consider this scenario and answer the questions.*

1. Olivia Anderson, 9 years old, is brought to the clinic by her mother for her annual check-up.

a. During your assessment, you note the interaction between the mother and the daughter. When you ask Olivia about her friends at school, the mother responds, "Olivia does not have many friends. I have told her that if she would just care more about her appearance, other children will want to spend time with her." How would you respond to the mother?

_____

_____

_____

b. Olivia's mother expresses concerns regarding discipline and how best to approach this. How would you respond?

_____

_____

_____

c. During your assessment, you discover that Olivia spends most of her time watching television and playing video games. What guidance can you give to Olivia and her mother regarding this?

_____

_____

_____

SECTION IV: PRACTICING FOR NCLEX

Activity F *Answer the following questions.*

1. The nurse is about to see a nine-year-old girl for a well-child checkup. Knowing that the child is in Piaget's period of concrete operational thought, which of the following characteristics will the child display?

   a. The child classifies or groups objects by their common elements
   b. The child does not understand the reason behind rules
   c. The child develops social skills in relating to same-sex friends
   d. The child develops feelings of inferiority with failures and lack of support

2. The nurse is educating the parents of a six-year-old boy about how to manage the child's transition to elementary school. The child has an easy temperament. Which of the following would the nurse most likely suggest?

   a. Comforting the child when he is frustrated
   b. Helping the child deal with minor stresses
   c. Visiting the school before classes start
   d. Being firm with moodiness and irritability

3. The mother of a seven-year-old girl is asking the nurse's advice about getting her daughter a two-wheel bike. Which of the following responses should the nurse make?

   a. "Teach her to try to land on the grass if she falls"
   b. "Be sure to get the proper size bike"
   c. "She won't need a helmet if she has training wheels"
   d. "Learning to ride the bike will improve her coordination"

4. The school nurse is assessing the nutritional status of an overweight 12-year-old girl. Which of the following questions would be appropriate for the nurse to ask the girl?

   a. "Does your family have rules about foods and how they are prepared?"
   b. "What does your family do for exercise?"
   c. "How often does everyone in your family eat together?"
   d. "Have you gained weight recently?"

5. The nurse has taken a health history and performed a physical exam for a 12-year-old boy. Which of the following findings was probably made?

   a. The child's body fat has decreased since last year
   b. The child's food preferences are different from those of his parents
   c. The child has a leaner body mass than a girl at this age.
   d. The child describes a somewhat reduced appetite

6. The nurse is teaching the parents of an 11-year-old girl how to deal with the issues of tobacco and alcohol use. Which of the following suggestions provides the best course of action for the parents?

   a. Avoid smoking in the house or in front of the child
   b. Hide alcoholic beverages out of the child's reach
   c. Forbid the child to have friends who smoke or drink
   d. Discuss tobacco and alcohol use with the child

7. The nurse is assessing the nutritional needs of an eight-year-old girl who weighs 65 pounds. Which of the following would be the proper daily caloric intake for this child?

   a. 1,895 calories per day

   b. 2,065 calories per day

   c. 2,245 calories per day

   d. 2,385 calories per day

8. The nurse is talking with the parents of an eight-year-old boy who has been cheating at school. Which of the following comments should be the primary message for the nurse to present?

   a. "Be firm with your punishment to show how serious you are."

   b. "Make sure that your behavior around your son is exemplary."

   c. "Resolve this by providing an opportunity for him to cheat and then dealing with it."

   d. "You may be putting too much pressure on him to succeed."

9. A nine-year-old boy has arrived for a health maintenance visit. Which of the following milestones of physical growth would the nurse expect to observe?

   a. Brain growth is complete and the head is longer

   b. Lymphatic tissue growth is complete, providing greater resistance to infections

   c. Frontal sinuses are developed; tonsils have decreased in size

   d. All deciduous teeth are replaced by 32 permanent teeth

10. A nurse is talking to the parents of a ten-year-old boy with complaints from teachers about his frequent absences from school. The boy says he feels scared to attend school and makes excuses to stay at home. Which of the following should the nurse suggest to the parents?

    a. Tell the child that he will be harshly punished by his teacher

    b. Tell the child that his fears are baseless and force him to attend school

    c. Have the child spend part of the day in the counselor's office

    d. Ask the teachers if they have been harsh with the child

11. A working mother of an 11-year-old girl tells the nurse that she is constantly worried about her daughter, who is home alone for long hours. Which of the following should the nurse suggest to the parent?

    a. Ask the child to have friends in the house when her parents are not home

    b. Ask the child to play with friends outside as much as possible

    c. Ensure that the child knows the name, address, and phone number of a neighbor

    d. Instruct the child to tell anyone who visits or phones that Mom is not home

12. A nurse is counseling the parents of a six-year-old girl, who has recently developed a habit of lying and telling tall tales to them. To which of the following reasons could the nurse attribute the child's problem?

    a. Fear of being punished

    b. Unmet family expectations

    c. Urge to impress others

    d. Low self-esteem

13. A nurse is counseling a mother on discipline for her nine-year-old child. Which of the following traits in nine-year-olds should the nurse explain to the parent?

    a. They realize the consequences of their behaviors

    b. They express emotions with violence

    c. They are beginning to understand the effects of behaviors on others

    d. They learn only from the natural consequences of their actions

14. A parent wants to know about safety techniques while driving a car with his seven-year-old son. Which of the following techniques should the nurse suggest to the parent?

    a. Place the child in the front seat only if the vehicle has an airbag

    b. Place the child in the rear seat, using a three-point restraint system

    c. Place the child in a booster seat without belts

    d. Place the child in the front seat without a restraint system

CHAPTER 29

Growth and Development of the Adolescent

SECTION I: LEARNING OBJECTIVES

1. Identify normal physiologic changes, including puberty, occurring in the adolescent.

2. Discuss psychosocial, cognitive, and moral changes occurring in the adolescent.

3. Identify changes in relationships with peers, family, teachers, and community during adolescence.

4. Describe interventions to promote safety during adolescence.

5. Demonstrate knowledge of the nutritional requirements of the adolescent.

6. Demonstrate knowledge of the development of sexuality and its influence on dating during adolescence.

7. Identify common developmental concerns of the adolescent.

8. Demonstrate knowledge of the appropriate nursing guidance for common developmental concerns.

SECTION II: ASSESSING YOUR UNDERSTANDING

Activity A *Fill in the blanks.*

1. The _____ of the skeletal system is completed earlier in girls than in boys.

2. _____ glands are all over the body, and they produce sweat that helps to eliminate body heat through evaporation.

3. _____ occurs in approximately 50% of adolescents, resulting from facial and mandibular bone growth.

4. Biological changes that occur during adolescence are known as _____.

5. Tanning can cause _____ cancer later in life.

6. The liver, spleen, kidneys, and digestive tract enlarge during the growth spurt but do not change in _____.

7. The prevalence of obesity is highest in _____ and African-American teens between the ages of 12 and 19.

8. According to Erikson, it is during adolescence that teenagers achieve a sense of _____.

9. _____ groups play an essential role in the identity of the adolescent.

10. Second only to growth during _____, adolescence involves the most rapid and dramatic changes in size and proportions.

Activity B *Match the nutrient in Column A with the daily requirement for teenagers in Column B.*

Column A

____ **1.** Calcium (boys and girls)

____ **2.** Iron (boys)

____ **3.** Iron (girls)

____ **4.** Protein (boys)

____ **5.** Protein (girls)

Column B

a. 45 to 59 g/day

b. 12 mg/day

c. 15 mg/day

d. 46 g/day

e. 1,200 to 1,500 mg/day

Activity C *Put the terms in correct sequence by writing the letters in the boxes provided below.*

1. Given below, in random order, are the changes that occur in adolescent females. Choose the correct sequence in which they occur.

   a. First menstrual period

   b. Pubic hair begins to curl and spread over mons pubis

   c. Breast bud and areola continue to enlarge

   d. Areola and papilla separate from the contour of the breast to form a secondary mound

Activity D *Briefly answer the following.*

1. Explain how the school experience is an integral component of the adolescent's preparation for the future.

   _____

   _____

   _____

2. How can a nurse promote appropriate physical growth in terms of appropriate weight gain in an adolescent?

   _____

   _____

   _____

3. What safety measures should a nurse suggest to an adolescent who is eager to learn to drive?

   _____

   _____

   _____

4. What practices can prevent and control obesity?

   _____

   _____

   _____

5. What are the long-term effects and consequences of drug and alcohol use?

   _____

   _____

   _____

6. What are the effects of smoking on health?

   _____

   _____

   _____

SECTION III: APPLYING YOUR KNOWLEDGE

Activity E *Consider this scenario and answer the questions.*

1. Pamela, a 15-year-old, is brought to the clinic by her mother for her annual school checkup.

   a. During your assessment, Pamela states she wants to get her belly button pierced but her parents refuse. She states, "They just don't understand that there is really no risk. I have at least 10 friends who have one, and none of them have had any problems." How should the nurse address this?

   _____

   _____

   _____

b. During your assessment, she confides to the nurse that she always feels inadequate in front of her peers and nervous when with parents. She also feels that she is being pulled by her friends and parents in opposite directions. How should the nurse address her dilemma?

_____

_____

_____

c. After the exam, Pamela's mother expresses concerns about communicating with her daughter. How would you respond?

_____

_____

_____

SECTION IV: PRACTICING FOR NCLEX

Activity F _Answer the following questions._

1. The nurse knows that the 13-year-old girl in the exam room is in the process of developing her own set of values. Which of the following will this child be experiencing, according to Erikson's psychosocial theory?

a. Wishing her parents were more understanding

b. Assuming everyone is interested in her favorite pop star

c. Wondering about the meaning of life

d. Taking more responsibility for her behaviors

2. The school nurse is providing nutritional guidance during a ninth-grade health class. Which of the following foods would be recommended as a good source of calcium?

a. Strawberries, watermelon, and raisins

b. Beans, poultry, and fish

c. Peanut butter, tomato juice, and whole grain bread

d. Cheese, yogurt, and white beans

3. The school nurse is assessing a 16-year-old girl. She appears drowsy and has constricted pupils. Which of the following drugs might she be using?

a. Opiates

b. Barbiturates

c. Amphetamines

d. Marijuana

4. The nurse is providing anticipatory guidance for violence prevention to a group of parents with adolescent children. Which of the following actions would be most effective in preventing suicide?

a. Checking for signs of depression or lack of friends

b. Becoming acquainted with the teen's friends

c. Watching for aggressive behavior or racist remarks

d. Monitoring video games, TV shows, and music

5. A 16-year-old girl has arrived for her sports physical with a new piercing in her navel. What is the best approach for the nurse to use?

a. "I hope for your sake the needle was clean."

b. "Be sure to clean the navel several times a day."

c. "This is a risk for hepatitis, tetanus, and AIDS."

d. "This is a wound and can become infected."

6. Throughout a health surveillance visit, a 12-year-old boy complains to the nurse about his parents intruding into his personal space, but then says he is looking forward to the family vacation. Which of the following characteristics also suggests the boy has entered adolescence?

a. Understands that actions have consequences

b. Feels secure with his body image

c. Growing interest in attracting girls' attention

d. Experiences frequent mood changes

7. A nurse is assessing a 14-year-old boy whose front tooth got knocked out while playing soccer. Which of the following is one of the first steps the nurse should attempt to do?

   a. Ask the child to gargle with cold milk

   b. Instruct him to not play outdoor games in future

   c. Help him clean his mouth and then discard the knocked-out tooth

   d. Try reinserting the tooth into its socket if possible

8. A 16-year-old boy is brought to the clinic by his parents, who are afraid that their son is using drugs. Which of the following symptoms shown by the boy would indicate the use of drugs? Select all that apply.

   a. Pressured speech

   b. Considerable weight loss in the past two months

   c. Discoloration of teeth

   d. Euphoria

   e. Bleeding gums

9. During a health checkup, a 17-year-old boy confides to a nurse that, sometimes, he happens to ejaculate when he is sleeping. Which of the following would be the best approach for the nurse?

   a. "You need immediate treatment."

   b. "You should improve your diet."

   c. "Emissions are hereditary."

   d. "Emissions are normal occurrences."

10. A nurse is providing a routine wellness examination for a 14-year-old girl. Which of the following statements by the parents needs intervention and further discussion?

    a. "We always compliment her."

    b. "We ensure that we always get enough time to discuss things."

    c. "We believe in setting fair rules and limits."

    d. "We trust her enough to not know anything about her friends."

11. A nurse is conducting a health screening of a 13-year-old boy. Which of the following statements by the boy needs intervention and further discussion?

    a. "I wash my face three times a day."

    b. "I don't like to scrub my face vigorously, as it irritates the skin."

    c. "I always squeeze out the acne so that it doesn't increase."

    d. "I apply sunscreen lotion on my face."

12. A nurse is conducting a health screening of a 17-year-old boy, who is engaged in a part-time job that requires being out in the sun for long hours. Which of the following would be the best instruction for the nurse to give the client?

    a. "Apply and keep reapplying sunscreen or sunblock when out in the sun."

    b. "You may have skin cancer because you have been out in the sun."

    c. "You can cut down your exercise time each day because work would compensate for that."

    d. "Scrub the face well to keep away the effects of tanning."

13. A 15-year-old boy has arrived for his health screening with a new tattoo on his shoulder. What is the best approach for the nurse to use?

    a. "You should have known that a tattoo is an open wound predisposed to infection."

    b. "You could have had some allergy to the dyes used in the tattoo process."

    c. "Is this a mark of some gang membership?"

    d. "Cleanse the tattoo with an antibacterial soap and water several times a day."

CHAPTER 30

Health Supervision

SECTION I: LEARNING OBJECTIVES

1. Describe the principles of health supervision.

2. List the three components of a health supervision visit.

3. Utilize instruments appropriately for developmental and functional testing of children.

4. Demonstrate knowledge of the principles of immunization.

5. Identify barriers to immunization.

6. Identify challenges to health supervision for children with chronic illnesses.

SECTION II: ASSESSING YOUR UNDERSTANDING

Activity A *Fill in the blanks.*

1. _____ screenings are brief assessment procedures that identify those children who warrant more intensive assessment and testing.

2. A _____ home is any primary health care provider with a long-term and comprehensive relationship with the family.

3. Disease _____ is defined as interventions performed to protect clients from a disease or identify it at an early stage and lessen its consequences.

4. _____ tests are procedures or laboratory analyses intended to identify those who may have a treatable condition.

5. _____ polio vaccine (IPV) is the only polio vaccine currently recommended in the United States.

6. Foreign materials in the body are called _____.

7. When an antigen is recognized by the immune system, the immune system responds by producing _____.

8. Newborns with ocular structural abnormalities are at high risk for _____ impairment.

9. Toxoid vaccines contain protein products produced by bacteria called _____.

10. Human papilloma virus causes genital warts and is responsible for the development of _____ cancer.

Activity B *Consider the following figure.*

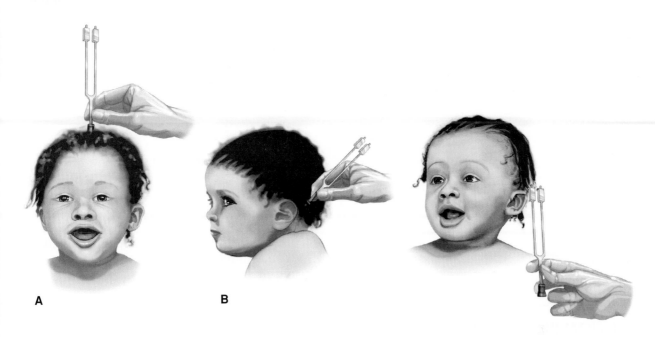

A   B

1. Identify the tests shown in the figure.

_____

_____

Activity C *Match the age and developmental warning sign listed in Column A with the developmental concern in Column B.*

Column A

_____ 1. Primitive reflex persistence at 6 months

_____ 2. Persistent head lag after 4 months

_____ 3. Repetitive speech at 24 months

_____ 4. Rolls over before 3 months

Column B

a. Autism spectrum disorders

b. Hypotonia

c. Hypertonia

d. Neurologic dysfunction

Activity D *Put the items in correct sequence by writing the letters in the boxes provided below.*

Given here, in random order, are steps followed while using a screening vision chart for children. Arrange the steps in order.

a. Align the child's heels on the mark.

b. The child reads each line with both eyes.

c. The child reads each line with one eye covered and then with the other eye covered.

d. Place a mark on the floor 20 feet from the chart.

e. Place the chart at the child's eye level.

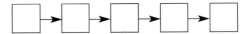

Activity E *Briefly answer the following.*

1. What are the different types of vaccines?

_____

_____

_____

2. What are the elements of proper documentation in the child's permanent record of immunization?

_____

_____

_____

3. What is rotavirus vaccine?

_____

_____

_____

4. What are the psychosocial assessment issues in comprehensive health supervision?

_____

_____

_____

5. What are the components of developmental surveillance?

_____

_____

_____

6. What are the types of immunity?

_____

_____

_____

SECTION III: APPLYING YOUR KNOWLEDGE

Activity F *Consider this scenario and answer the questions.*

1. Jasmine Chase, a 15-year-old girl, is seen in the clinic for her annual exam. During this health supervision visit, Jasmine expresses concerns about her weight. She states she has been attempting to diet and has started skipping breakfast. She also decided to give up meat, fish, and poultry, and eats mostly salads for lunch and dinner.

   a. During the health interview and exam, what information should the nurse elicit?

   _____

   _____

   _____

   b. What screening test may be warranted for Jasmine, and why?

   _____

   _____

   _____

c. During the examination, the nurse determines that Jasmine's height is 5 feet and her weight is 150 pounds. What can the nurse do to help promote a healthy weight for Jasmine?

_____

_____

_____

_____

SECTION IV: PRACTICING FOR NCLEX

Activity G *Answer the following questions.*

1. A three-year-old child has been diagnosed with asthma. For which of the following community factors should the nurse assess as a contributing factor to asthma?
   a. Loss of support systems
   b. Violence and abuse
   c. Breakdown of family relationships
   d. Substandard housing

2. A school health nurse is conducting a comprehensive health supervision of the school-children. Which of the following is an additional component of health supervision in children, not found in adult health supervision?
   a. Developmental screening
   b. Disease prevention
   c. Health promotion
   d. Immunization

3. The nurse is performing a vision screening for a five-month-old child. Which of the following should the nurse use when performing vision screening?
   a. The "tumbling E" chart
   b. The traditional Snellen chart
   c. The Allen figures
   d. Objects with black and white patterns

4. It is important to administer vaccines by the correct route. Which of the following vaccines are administered subcutaneously?
   a. Influenza
   b. Hepatitis A
   c. Varicella
   d. Pneumococcal

5. A nurse is caring for a client diagnosed with phenylketonuria. Which of the following functions of the body is compromised?

a. Amino acid metabolism

b. Organic acid metabolism

c. Fatty acid oxidation

d. Hemoglobin

6. A primary health nurse is assigned to hold a vaccination camp. The nurse reviews the types of vaccines and their functions. Which of the following is a characteristic of conjugate vaccines?

a. Use modified living organisms that are weakened

b. Contain protein products produced by bacteria

c. Increase the immune response dramatically

d. Use genetically engineered organisms

7. A community health nurse is assigned to take care of an immunization program which is held at the community level. The nurse, prior to the administration of any immunization, should be aware of the temporary and permanent contraindications of vaccination. Which of the following is a permanent contraindication of the pertussis vaccination?

a. Encephalopathy

b. Immunosuppression

c. Recent blood transfusion

d. Severe illness with a high fever

8. A nurse is conducting a hearing screening of a six-month-old child through Auditory Brainstem Response. Which of the following is an important nursing intervention?

a. Allow the child to sit on the parent's lap

b. Offer two presentations of stimulus to ensure reliability

c. Sedate the child if the child is not quiet

d. Administer conditioning trials

9. The primary health nurse is assigned to administer *Haemophilus influenzae* type B vaccine to four-year-old children. Which of the following infections can be prevented by the vaccine?

a. Septic arthritis

b. Measles

c. Mumps

d. Rubella

10. During the physical assessment of a six-year-old child, the nurse observes that the child has lost a tooth, and the nurse uses the opportunity to promote oral health care. Which of the following comments should be the focus of this discussion?

a. "Oral health can affect general health."

b. "Fluoridated water has significantly reduced cavities."

c. "Try to keep the child's hands out of the mouth."

d. "Limit the amount of soft drinks in the child's diet."

11. The nurse is promoting healthy weight to an overweight 12-year-old child and her parents. Which of the following approaches is best?

a. Showing the family the appropriate weight for the child

b. Asking what activities she enjoys, such as dance or sports

c. Suggesting that the child join a softball team

d. Pointing out fattening foods and excesses in their diet

12. A nurse plans to perform a screening test for a ten-month-old child. Which of the following developmental screening tools should the nurse use?

a. Battelle Developmental Inventory Screening Test

b. Denver Articulation Screening

c. Goodenough-Harris Drawing Test

d. Denver II

13. On a home visit, the nurse finds that the two-year-old child has developed a sunburn. Which of the following interventions should the nurse teach the family members to prevent sunburns? Select all that apply.

   a. Apply sunscreen lotions

   b. Avoid peak sun hours

   c. Wear proper clothing

   d. Encourage hand-washing

   e. Pursue exercise activity

14. A nurse is vaccinating a child against the Hepatitis A virus. Which of the following factors predispose young children to Hepatitis A infection? Select all that apply.

   a. Functional asplenia

   b. Close contact with other children

   c. Inadequate hygiene practices

   d. Immunosuppression

   e. Tendency to place everything in their mouth

15. A nurse is administering pneumococcal vaccines to a two-year-old child who is at high risk of developing pneumococcal sepsis. Which of the following are the conditions that place a child at high risk for pneumococcal sepsis and warrant the vaccine against *Streptococcus pneumoniae*? Select all that apply.

   a. Meningitis

   b. Epiglottitis

   c. Sickle-cell disease

   d. Immunosuppression

   e. Diabetes mellitus

Health Assessment of Children

SECTION I: LEARNING OBJECTIVES

1. Demonstrate an understanding of the appropriate health history to obtain from the child and the parent or primary caregiver.

2. Individualize elements of the health history depending upon the age of the child.

3. Discuss important concepts related to health assessment in children.

4. Describe the appropriate sequence of the physical examination in the context of the child's developmental stage.

5. Perform a health assessment using approaches that relate to the age and developmental stage of the child.

6. Distinguish normal variations in the physical examination from differences that may indicate serious alterations in health status.

7. Determine the sexual maturity of females and males on the basis of evaluation of the secondary sex characteristics.

SECTION II: ASSESSING YOUR UNDERSTANDING

Activity A *Fill in the blanks.*

1. A _____ is used to measure the height of children capable of standing independently.

2. The physical examination of children begins with a systematic _____.

3. All infants display some degree of _____, which is soft, downy hair on the body.

4. When assessing the thorax and lungs, an inspiratory high-pitched sound is referred to as audible _____.

5. Transient blueness of the hands and feet of a few-days-old baby is called _____.

6. A _____ response causes mottling of the skin over the trunk and extremities.

7. Lack of color in skin, hair, and eyes is related to _____.

8. A _____ is used to assess the mobility of the eardrum.

9. Pulse _____ determines the oxygen saturation (SaO_2) in blood.

10. _____ is a waxy substance normally found lubricating and protecting the external ear canal.

Activity B *Consider the following figures.*

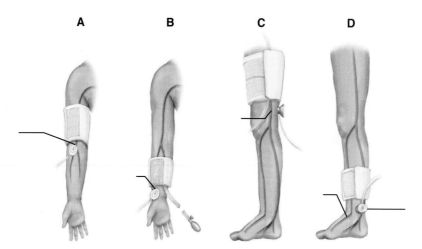

A   B   C   D

1. Label the following arteries shown in the images:
   - Brachial artery
   - Dorsalis pedis artery
   - Popliteal artery
   - Radial artery

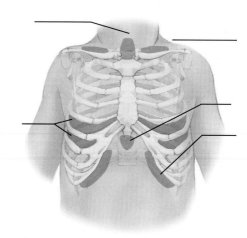

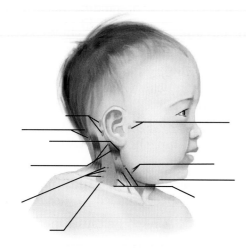

3. Label the following locations for retractions shown in the image:
   - Clavicular
   - Subcostal
   - Substernal
   - Suprasternal

2. Label the following lymph nodes shown in the image:
   - Preauricular
   - Occipital
   - Superficial cervical
   - Deep cervical chain

Activity C *Match the heart sounds in Column A with their descriptions in Column B.*

Column A	Column B
____ **1.** S1	**a.** Usually most intense at the aortic and pulmonic areas
____ **2.** S2	**b.** Usually loudest at the mitral and tricuspid areas
____ **3.** S3	**c.** May indicate congestive heart failure
____ **4.** S4	**d.** Most often occurs with cardiac disease

Activity D *Put the items in correct sequence by writing the letters in the boxes provided below.*

1. Given below, in random order, are questions in the health interview of an adolescent. Choose the correct sequence in which they should be asked.

   a. Are you sexually active?

   b. What is your name?

   c. What can I help you with today?

   d. Do you have any allergies?

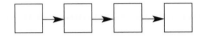

Activity E *Briefly answer the following.*

1. Write a short note on BMI.

   _____

   _____

   _____

2. Why is inspecting the skin important?

   _____

   _____

   _____

3. What are the most important factors included in a complete physical examination?

   _____

   _____

   _____

4. What are the points a nurse should bear in mind while assessing the respiratory rate of an infant or a young child?

   _____

   _____

   _____

5. Differentiate between primitive and protective reflexes.

   _____

   _____

   _____

6. Write a note about PMI (Point of Maximum Intensity).

   _____

   _____

   _____

SECTION III: APPLYING YOUR KNOWLEDGE

Activity F *Consider this scenario and answer the questions.*

1. a. A three-day-old infant is brought to the clinic by his parents for an examination. The mother states, "Though my baby is kept well-fed and warm, his hands and feet appear blue. I am not sure if this is healthy." How should the nurse address the mother's concerns?

   _____

   _____

   _____

   b. How can the nurse check if the infant is dehydrated?

   _____

   _____

   _____

   c. The father states that he is very glad about the few teeth that have erupted in the baby's mouth. What response should the nurse give the parents regarding this?

   _____

   _____

   _____

SECTION IV: PRACTICING FOR NCLEX

Activity G *Answer the following questions.*

1. The nurse is preparing to see a 14-month-old child and needs to establish the chief complaint or purpose of the visit. Which of the following would be the best way to approach the parent or guardian?
   a. "What is your chief complaint?"
   b. "What can I help you with today?"
   c. "Is your child feeling sick?"
   d. "Has your child been exposed to infectious agents?"

2. A nurse is conducting a physical examination of an uncooperative preschooler. What could the nurse say to encourage deep breathing during lung auscultation?
   a. "Do you want your mother to listen to your lungs?"
   b. "Do you think you can blow out the light bulb on this pen?"
   c. "You may not leave until I listen to your breathing."
   d. "You must breathe deeply so I can hear your lungs."

3. The nurse is examining the genitals of a healthy newborn girl. The nurse would expect to observe which of the following normal findings?
   a. Swollen labia minora
   b. Lesions on the external genitalia
   c. Labial adhesions
   d. Swollen labia majora

4. The nurse is caring for a 13-year-old girl. As part of a routine health assessment, the nurse needs to address areas relating to sexuality and substance abuse. Which of the following should the nurse say first to encourage communication?
   a. "Do you smoke cigarettes or marijuana?"
   b. "I promise not to tell your mother any of your responses."
   c. "Tell me about some of your current activities at school."
   d. "Are you considering sexual activity?"

5. A nurse is caring for a very shy three-year-old girl. During the well-child assessment the nurse must take the girl's blood pressure. Which of the following is the best approach?
   a. "Help me take your doll's blood pressure."
   b. "Your sister did a great job when I took hers."
   c. "May I take your blood pressure?"
   d. "Will you let me put this cuff on your arm?"

6. The nurse is conducting a physical examination of a healthy six-year-old. Which of the following would the nurse do first?
   a. Auscultate the heart, lungs, and abdomen
   b. Tap the knee with a reflex hammer to check for deep tendon reflexes
   c. Palpate the skin for texture and hydration
   d. Observe the skin for its overall color and characteristics

7. A nurse is assessing an infant's reflexes. The nurse places his or her thumb to the ball of the infant's foot to elicit which reflex?
   a. Palmar grasp
   b. Plantar grasp
   c. Parachute
   d. Babinski

8. A nurse is inspecting the skin of a dark-skinned three-month-old baby. Which of the following observations needs a follow-up?
   a. Lanugo
   b. Hyperpigmented nevi
   c. Mottling of the skin over the trunk
   d. Rashes

9. A nurse is inspecting the abdomen of a two-week old baby. Which of the following observations will need immediate intervention and follow-up?
   a. Absence of granulation at umbilical site
   b. Visible peristaltic waves
   c. Dry, black, and hard umbilical stump
   d. Protrusion of umbilical hernia

10. A nurse is required to take the temperature of a neurologically impaired child. Assuming that equipment for each of the methods are available to her, which of the following will be the best method for the task?

    a. Oral

    b. Axillary

    c. Temporal

    d. Rectal

11. The nurse is conducting a physical examination of a five-year-old girl. The nurse asks the girl to stand still with her eyes closed and arms down by her side. The girl immediately begins to lean. What does this response tell the nurse?

    a. The child has average coordination and balance.

    b. The child has a negative Romberg test; no further testing is necessary.

    c. The child warrants further testing for cerebellar dysfunction.

    d. The child has a possible inner ear infection.

12. A nurse is inspecting a two-year-old baby. Which of the following observations is normal?

    a. Anterior fontanels cannot be felt

    b. Drainage from ear canals

    c. Hair is extremely coarse and dry

    d. Nails are dry and brittle

13. A nurse is inspecting a four-month-old baby. Which of the following observations will require immediate intervention?

    a. Teeth have not erupted.

    b. Ear canal is pink and has tiny hairs.

    c. Tympanic membrane appears gray.

    d. The fontanels are sunken.

14. A nurse is inspecting a newborn. Which of the following observations would indicate a serious health problem?

    a. Milia on the cheeks

    b. Greasy, scaly plaque on the scalp

    c. Low-set ears

    d. Pink nasal mucosa

15. A nurse is testing the eyes of a four-year-old child to check if they demonstrate accommodation. Which of the following reactions will be expected for the given purpose?

    a. The pupil should constrict as the object moves closer

    b. The pupils should not react to the approaching object

    c. The eyes should not blink

    d. The eyes should exhibit strabismus

CHAPTER 32

Nursing Care of Children During Illness and Hospitalization

SECTION I: LEARNING OBJECTIVES

1. Identify the major impact and stressors of illness and hospitalization for children in the various developmental stages.

2. Identify the reactions and responses of children and their families during illness and hospitalization.

3. Explain the factors that influence the reactions and responses of children and their families during illness and hospitalization.

4. Describe the nursing care that minimizes the stressors of children who are ill or hospitalized.

5. Examine the major components of admission of children to the hospital.

6. Outline the nursing interventions required for children in the specific units or situations in the hospital.

7. Use appropriate safety measures when caring for children of all ages.

8. Describe basic care procedures for children in various health care settings.

9. Review the major components and nursing responsibilities related to patient education and discharge from the hospital.

SECTION II: ASSESSING YOUR UNDERSTANDING

Activity A *Fill in the blanks.*

1. Therapeutic _____ is the use of a holding position that promotes close physical contact between the child and a parent or caregiver.

2. Restraints should be checked every fifteen minutes following initial placement and then every _____ for proper placement.

3. A good time to assess the skin is during _____ time.

4. Forcing a child to eat can exacerbate any nausea or vomiting and can lead to an _____ to food that extends past the hospital stay.

5. Emotional outlet play or _____ play allows a child to act out or dramatize real-life stressors.

6. _____ units are used to keep hospital stays short and decrease the cost of hospitalization.

7. The first phase of separation anxiety, _____, occurs when the child is separated from his or her parents or primary caretaker.

8. Preschooler thinking is _____; they believe that some personal deed or thought has caused their illness, which can lead to guilt and shame.

9. When the child's _____ activity is restricted, anger and hyperactivity may result.

10. All techniques used to prepare the child for hospitalization should emphasize the philosophy of _____ care.

Activity B *Consider the following figures.*

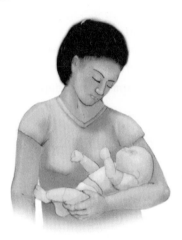

1. Identify the method used to carry the infant.

_____

_____

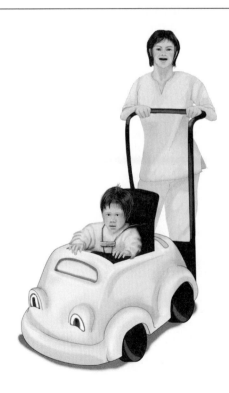

2. Identify the equipment in the figure.

_____

_____

Activity C *Match the terms in Column A with their definitions in Column B.*

Column A

_____ 1. Denial

_____ 2. Regression

_____ 3. Sensory overload

_____ 4. Separation anxiety

_____ 5. Magical thinking

Column B

a. The child returns to a previous stage of development

b. The child experiences increased stimulation

c. The type of thinking that allows for fantasies and creativity

d. The distress related to removal from family and familiar surroundings

e. The child forms coping mechanisms to protect self from further emotional pain

Activity D *Put the terms in correct sequence by writing the letters in the boxes provided below.*

1. Given below, in random order, are the stages of separation anxiety. Choose the correct sequence.

a. Denial

b. Protest

c. Despair

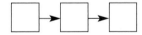

Activity E *Briefly answer the following.*

1. How can the nurse address and minimize a hospitalized child's separation anxiety?

_____

_____

_____

2. Why does discharge planning begin upon admission?

_____

_____

_____

3. What are the fears and anxieties experienced by children during hospitalization?

_____

_____

_____

4. What are the factors affecting a child's response to illness and hospitalization?

_____

_____

_____

5. What are the general reactions of the parents of the hospitalized child?

_____

_____

_____

6. What are the factors that influence the reactions of the family of the hospitalized child?

_____

_____

_____

SECTION III: APPLYING YOUR KNOWLEDGE

Activity F _Consider this scenario and answer the questions._

1. Leslie Lucas, a six-month-old girl with a club foot repair, is hospitalized after surgery. She has been irritable and difficult to console.

   a. Identify the interventions and rationale for Leslie.

_____

_____

_____

SECTION IV: PRACTICING FOR NCLEX

Activity G _Answer the following questions._

1. The nurse is caring for an 18-month-old boy hospitalized with a gastrointestinal disorder. The nurse knows that the child is at risk for separation anxiety. Which of the following behaviors would indicate the first phase of separation anxiety?

   a. Displaying hopelessness by withdrawing from others

   b. Rejecting others who attempt to comfort him

   c. Lack of interest in play and food

   d. Exhibiting apathy and depression

2. The nurse is caring for a preschooler who is hospitalized with a suspected blood disorder. The nurse needs to draw some blood and knows to use which of the following approaches?

   a. "I need to take some blood."

   b. "We need to put a little hole in your arm."

   c. "I need to remove a little blood."

   d. "Why don't you sit on your mom's lap?"

3. The nurse is caring for a child hospitalized with complications from asthma. Which of the following statements by the parents indicates a need for careful observation of the child's anxiety level?

   a. "My mother passed away here after surgery."

   b. "Our twins were born here 18 months ago."

   c. "My son was born at this hospital."

   d. "We attended a living-with-asthma class here."

4. A nurse is caring for a six-year-old boy hospitalized due to an infection. The child needs intravenous antibiotic therapy. His motor activity is restricted and he is acting out—yelling, kicking, and screaming. Which of the following responses by the nurse would help promote positive coping?

    a. "This medicine is the only way you will get better."

    b. "Let me explain why you need to sit still."

    c. "Would you like to read or play video games?"

    d. "Do I need to call your parents?"

5. A nurse is telling the parents how to help their ten-year-old daughter deal with an extended hospital stay due to surgery followed by traction. Which of the following responses indicates a need for further teaching?

    a. "I should not tell her how long she will be here."

    b. "She will watch our reactions carefully."

    c. "We must prepare her in advance."

    d. "She will be sensitive to our concerns."

6. A nurse is preparing to admit a child for a tonsillectomy. How should the nurse establish rapport?

    a. "Let's take a look at your tonsils."

    b. "Do you understand why you are here?"

    c. "Are you scared about having your tonsils out?"

    d. "Tell me about the cute stuffed dog you have."

7. The nurse is preparing to admit a four-year-old girl who will be having tympanostomy tubes placed in both ears. Which of the following strategies would most likely reduce the child's fears of the procedure?

    a. "The physician is going to insert tympanostomy tubes in your ears."

    b. "Don't worry; you will be asleep the whole time."

    c. "Let me show you how tiny these tubes are."

    d. "Let me show you the operating room."

8. A nurse is developing a preoperative plan of care for a two-year-old. To which of the following age-related fears should the nurse pay particular attention?

    a. Separation from friends

    b. Separation from parents

    c. Loss of control

    d. Loss of independence

9. The nurse is teaching the parents of a seven-year-old boy about preparing him for scheduled surgery. Which of the following statements by the parents indicates a need for further teaching?

    a. "We should talk about going to the hospital and what it will be like coming home."

    b. "We should visit the hospital and go through the pre-admission tour in advance."

    c. "It's best to wait and let him bring up the surgery or any questions he has."

    d. "It is a good idea to read stories about experiences with hospital or surgery."

10. The nurse is caring for a seven-year-old boy in a body cast. He is shy and seems fearful of the numerous personnel who are in and out of his room. How can the nurse help reduce his fear?

    a. Remind the boy he will be going home soon

    b. Encourage the boy's parents to stay with him at all times

    c. Write the name of his nurse on a board and identify all staff on each shift, every day

    d. Tell him not to worry; explain that everyone is here to care for him

11. A nurse is assigned to care for a child with typhoid. The child is to be admitted to the health care facility. Which of the following techniques will help to reduce the child's fears and increase his or her ability to cope with the hospital experience?

    a. Talk to the child and parents in medical terms

    b. Allow the child to practice nursing care on dolls

    c. Ask the child to avoid touching the equipment

    d. Introduce the child to the health care personnel

Activity B *Match the developmental stages in Column A with the corresponding effects of chronic illness on the child in Column B.*

Column A

____ **1.** Infants

____ **2.** Toddlers

____ **3.** Preschoolers

____ **4.** School-age children

____ **5.** Adolescents

Column B

a. May fail to develop a sense of trust or attach appropriately with the parents

b. May experience difficulty developing autonomy because of increased dependence on the parent

c. May have difficulty in developing a sense of initiative because of limited opportunities

d. May feel as though they are different from their peers because of their lack of skills or abilities

e. May have limited opportunities to achieve a sense of industry because of school absence

Activity C *Briefly answer the following.*

1. What is Vulnerable Child Syndrome?

_____

_____

_____

2. What are the inorganic causes of failure to thrive (FTT)?

_____

_____

_____

3. What are the advantages of home care for children with special care needs?

_____

_____

_____

4. How is the growth and development of the premature infant assessed?

_____

_____

_____

5. What are the principles of palliative care?

_____

_____

_____

6. What is hippotherapy?

_____

_____

_____

SECTION III: APPLYING YOUR KNOWLEDGE

Activity D *Consider this scenario and answer the questions.*

1. Georgia Lansing, a seven-year-old girl, has been diagnosed with lymphoma. She recently had a relapse and has not responded to treatment. The family has decided on palliative care. Georgia understands that she is going to die and becomes very anxious when alone in a room or if any procedures are done on her. The family is grieving about the anticipated loss.

   a. How can the nurse alleviate Georgia's anxiety and fear?

   _____

   _____

   _____

   b. What can the nurse do to support Georgia's family?

   _____

   _____

   _____

SECTION IV: PRACTICING FOR NCLEX

Activity E *Answer the following questions.*

1. A nurse is preparing a baby for discharge from the NICU. Which of the following parental teaching is important for effective home care of the baby?

   a. Developmentally appropriate skills

   b. Cues and behavior of the child

   c. Emphasize positive qualities

   d. Provide consistent caregivers

2. A 14-year-old boy is terminally ill and is aware of this fact. Which action would best meet his need for self-esteem and sense of worth?

   a. Listening to his fears and concerns about dying

   b. Giving direct, honest answers to his questions

   c. Helping to establish sense of control in daily activities

   d. Providing full participation in decision-making

3. The nurse is caring for a child who requires long-term rehabilitation. Which intervention is most important to the parents?

   a. Evaluating the emotional strength of the parents

   b. Educating the parents about the course of treatment

   c. Preparing a list of supplies the family will need

   d. Assessing the adequacy of the home environment

4. The nurse at a hospice is caring for a 12-year-old girl. Which intervention best meets the needs of this child?

   a. Helping to establish a sense of control

   b. Encouraging her to help make decisions

   c. Urging her to invite her friends to visit

   d. Explaining her condition to her in detail

5. A 15-year-old boy with special needs is attending high school. Which nursing intervention will be most beneficial to his education?

   a. Serving on his individualized education plan committee

   b. Collaborating with the school nurse about his care

   c. Discussing future plans like vocation and college

   d. Assessing how attending school will affect his health

6. A nurse is caring for a seven-year-old child with special needs. Which of the following interventions should the nurse implement to promote the child's growth and development?

   a. Begin developmentally appropriate discipline

   b. Reinforce that illness is not punishment

   c. Encourage mastery of self-help skills

   d. Educate the child about course of treatment

7. A six-month-old girl is significantly underweight. Which nursing action will point to an inorganic cause?

   a. Observe the infant to see if the infant refuses nipple

   b. Observe the mother and child for eye contact

   c. Ask the mother if the birth was premature

   d. Check the health history for risk factors

8. The nurse learns that a 15-year-old boy admitted with cystic fibrosis does not disclose his illness to his friends and gives false explanations regarding his hospitalization. The nurse is aware that adolescents may ignore their health care needs to fit into their peer groups. Which intervention will help avert the child's neglect of his health needs?

   a. Monitoring compliance with treatment

   b. Assessing for signs of depression

   c. Encouraging participation in activities

   d. Urging him to join a support group

9. A nurse is caring for a two-year-old medically fragile child. Which of the following developmental milestones would be affected?

   a. Sense of trust

   b. Sense of autonomy

   c. Sense of initiative

   d. Sense of industry

10. A nurse is planning the discharge for a former premature infant. The baby was managed in the neonatal care unit because of the inability to maintain his vital functions of respiration and circulation. Which of the following medical problems may arise after discharge?

    a. Attention-deficit disorder

    b. Cerebral palsy

    c. Apnea of prematurity

    d. Cognitive delay

11. A nurse is caring for a 12-year-old child who is terminally ill. Which of the following is an appropriate intervention for helping the family with end-of-life decision-making?

    a. Provide the family with honest information

    b. Make judgments on their behalf

    c. Ask for clarifications on decisions

    d. Discourage vacillations in decision-making

12. A nurse is caring for a 16-year-old girl with special needs. Which of the following interventions should the nurse adopt to help the adolescent in making the transition to adulthood?

    a. Help in getting Supplemental Security Income (SSI) assistance

    b. Inform about available Internet resources

    c. Determine the eligibility for insurance

    d. Ensure that transition plan is initiated

13. A nurse is preparing a discharge plan for a ten-year-old girl who is technologically dependent. Which of the following nursing interventions is required before the client is discharged?

    a. Encourage high level of parental participation

    b. Modify the office routine to promote child comfort

    c. Promote liaison with community resources

    d. Develop written health plans for the child's care

14. A nurse is caring for a child who is underweight and experiencing failure to thrive (FTT). Which of the following is an inorganic cause for failure to thrive?

    a. Poor feeding techniques

    b. Alterations in metabolism

    c. Inability to swallow correctly

    d. Malabsorption

15. A nurse is caring for a ten-year-old girl who is nearing death. Which of the following interventions should the nurse follow to minimize the child's discomfort?

    a. Involve the child in decision-making

    b. Answer the child's questions honestly

    c. Change the child's position frequently

    d. Explain all aspects of care to the child

CHAPTER 34

Medication Administration, Intravenous Therapy, and Nutritional Support

SECTION I: LEARNING OBJECTIVES

1. Describe atraumatic methods for preparing children for procedures.

2. Describe the "eight rights" of pediatric medication administration.

3. Explain the physiologic differences in children affecting a medication's pharmacodynamic and pharmacokinetic properties.

4. Accurately determine recommended pediatric medication doses.

5. Demonstrate the proper technique for administering medication to children via the oral, rectal, ophthalmic, otic, intravenous, intramuscular, and subcutaneous routes.

6. Integrate the concepts of atraumatic care in medication administration for children.

7. Identify the preferred sites for peripheral and central intravenous medication administration.

8. Describe nursing management related to maintenance of intravenous infusions in children, as well as prevention of complications.

9. Explain nursing care related to enteral tube feedings.

10. Describe nursing management of the child receiving total parenteral nutrition.

SECTION II: ASSESSING YOUR UNDERSTANDING

Activity A *Fill in the blanks.*

1. An Infus-A-Port is a type of _____ port used in the administration of medications, fluids, and nutrition in children.

2. _____ is the behavior of a medication at the cellular level.

3. Encouraging the child to count aloud or asking a child to blow bubbles during a medical procedure is a means of creating a _____.

4. When it is necessary to insert a rectal suppository for a child under the age of 3, the nurse should use the _____ finger.

5. Total parenteral nutrition (TPN) has a high concentration of sugar. _____ typically occurs with too-rapid cessation of TPN.

6. Movement of drugs throughout the body via absorption, distribution, metabolism, and excretion is called _____ .

7. _____ , or the alteration of chemical structures from their original form, which allows for the eventual excretion of the substance, is different in children than in adults because of differences in hepatic enzyme production and metabolic rate.

8. The amount of gastric contents remaining in the stomach, or the gastric _____ , indicates gastric emptying time.

9. Intermittent enteral feedings are commonly called _____ feedings.

10. Most children are very active, even when they are ill. When selecting an IV site in an extremity, always choose the most _____ site.

Activity B *Consider the following figures.*

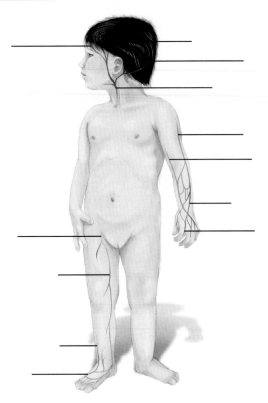

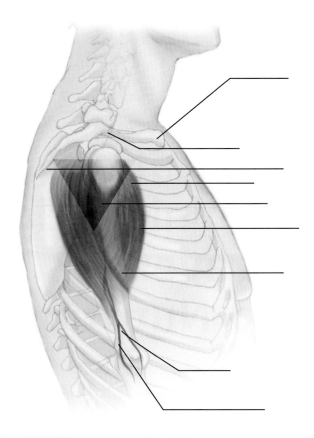

2. Label the following parts shown in the image.
- Clavicle
- Radial nerve
- Humerus
- Acromion process

Activity C *Match the terms in Column A with their definitions in Column B.*

Column A

_____ **1.** Gavage feeding

_____ **2.** Enteral nutrition

_____ **3.** Intermittent feeding

_____ **4.** Parenteral nutrition

Column B

a. Administration of a specified feeding solution at specific intervals, usually over a short period of time

b. Nutrition delivered directly into the intestinal tract

c. Feeding administered via a tube into the stomach or intestines

d. Intravenous delivery of nutritional substances

1. Label the following preferred peripheral sites for IV insertion shown in the image.
- Cephalic
- Digital
- Great saphenous
- External jugular

Activity D *Put the items in correct sequence by writing the letters in the boxes provided below.*

1. Given below, in random order, are some of the steps for administering medication through a syringe pump. Arrange them in the sequence in which they should be undertaken.

   a. Purge the air from the tubing

   b. Attach the syringe pump tubing to the medication syringe

   c. Set the infusion rate

   d. Verify the medication order

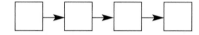

2. Given below, in random order, are some of the steps for inserting a gavage feeding tube. Arrange them in the sequence in which they should be undertaken.

   a. Lubricate the tube with a generous amount of sterile water/water-soluble lubricant

   b. Determine the tubing length for insertion

   c. Inspect the child's nose and mouth

   d. Advance the tube slowly to the designated length

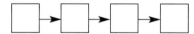

Activity E *Briefly answer the following.*

1. How can the nurse ensure that the medication is being administered to the right patient?

_____

_____

_____

2. What are the physiologic factors affecting distribution of medication in children?

_____

_____

_____

3. Describe the procedure of administering nose drops.

_____

_____

_____

4. State a few measures that the nurse can take to ensure proper enteral feeding and avoid complications during the process.

_____

_____

_____

5. What method should be used to stabilize a gastronomy tube if there is skin breakdown or irritation at the insertion site?

_____

_____

_____

6. What are the differences between peripheral parenteral nutrition (PPN) and total parenteral nutrition (TPN) with respect to the use, the route, and the child's status?

_____

_____

_____

SECTION III: APPLYING YOUR KNOWLEDGE

Activity F *Consider this scenario and answer the questions.*

1. Jennifer Michels, a seven-month-old, has a rectal temperature of 102.5°F. The nurse caring for her is preparing to administer oral acetaminophen per the physician's order. Jennifer's weight is 15 lbs.

   a. Discuss the steps the nurse will take for administering a PRN dose of oral acetaminophen to Jennifer.

   _____

   _____

   _____

b. The physician ordered 70 mg PO q4h for fever or discomfort. Calculate the correct dose for Jennifer's weight. Is the physician's order a safe and therapeutic dose?

_____

_____

_____

c. How much should be drawn up of an 80 mg/0.8 mL concentration of Tylenol infant drops?

_____

_____

_____

SECTION IV: PRACTICING FOR NCLEX

Activity G *Answer the following questions.*

1. The nurse is caring for a four-year-old who requires a venipuncture. Which of the following explanations is most appropriate to prepare the child for the procedure?
   a. "The doctor will look at your blood to see why you are sick."
   b. "The doctor wants to see if you have strep throat."
   c. "The doctor needs to take your blood to see why you are sick."
   d. "The doctor needs to culture your blood to see if you have strep."

2. The nurse is caring for a child with an intravenous device in his hand. Which of the following signs would alert the nurse that infiltration is occurring?
   a. Warmth, redness
   b. Tender skin
   c. Induration
   d. Cool, puffy skin

3. The nurse is preparing to administer a medication via a syringe pump as ordered for a two-month-old girl. What is the priority nursing action?
   a. Gather the medication
   b. Verify the medication order
   c. Gather the necessary equipment and supplies
   d. Wash hands and put on gloves

4. A nurse is teaching the parents of a five-year-old boy how to administer oral medication. The child has been ordered daily oral medication. Which of the following responses indicates a need for further teaching?
   a. "We should never refer to the medicine as 'candy.'"
   b. "We should never bribe our child to take the medicine."
   c. "He needs to take his medicine or he will lose a privilege."
   d. "We checked that the medicine can be mixed with yogurt or applesauce."

5. A nurse is preparing to administer an intramuscular (IM) injection to an infant as ordered. The nurse prepares which of the following injection sites?
   a. Deltoid
   b. Ventrogluteal
   c. Dorsogluteal
   d. Vastus lateralis

6. The nurse is preparing to remove an IV device from the arm of a six-year-old girl. Which of the following is the best approach to minimize fear and anxiety?
   a. "This won't be painful; you'll just feel a tug and a pinch."
   b. "The first step is for you to give me a hand removing the dressing."
   c. "Be sure to keep your hands clear of the scissors so I don't cut you."
   d. "Please be a big girl and don't cry when I remove this."

7. The nurse is teaching the parents of a five-month-old child how to administer an oral antibiotic. Which of the following responses indicates a need for further teaching?
   a. "We should use the same dropper for all medicines."
   b. "We can follow his medicine with some applesauce or yogurt."
   c. "We can place the medicine along the inside of his cheek."
   d. "We should not forcibly squirt the medication in the back of his throat."

8. What will be the daily maintenance fluid requirement for a child weighing 30 kg?

   a. 1,500 mL

   b. 1,600 mL

   c. 1,700 mL

   d. 1,800 mL

9. The nurse is assessing the aspirate of a gavage feeding tube to confirm placement. Which of the following assessment findings indicates intestinal placement?

   a. Clear aspirate

   b. Tan aspirate

   c. Green aspirate

   d. Yellow aspirate

10. The nurse is preparing to administer medication to a ten-year-old who weighs 70 lbs. The prescribed single dose is 3 to 4 mg/kg per day. Which of the following is the appropriate dose range for this child?

    a. 96 to 128 mg

    b. 105 to 140 mg

    c. 210 to 280 mg

    d. 420 to 560 mg

11. Which of the following is the peripheral IV therapy site?

    a. Thigh

    b. Feet

    c. Buttocks

    d. Upper arms

12. A nurse is required to administer a medicine orally to a three-month-old boy. Which of the following is appropriate for oral administration of medication?

    a. Administer the entire amount at one time

    b. Shake the bottle before administering liquid medication

    c. Try crushing and mixing the tablets with essential foods

    d. Direct the liquid toward the anterior side of the mouth with a dropper

13. Which of the following should a nurse bear in mind while inserting an IV therapy device?

    a. Select a vein in the upper arm

    b. Discourage parental participation during the procedure

    c. Avoid the use of barriers when tying the tourniquet

    d. Ensure adequate pain relief prior to insertion of the device

14. A nurse is caring for a client receiving total parenteral nutrition (TPN). Which of the following measures can the nurse take to reduce the risk of complications? Select all that apply.

    a. Ensure rapid infusion of TPN

    b. Adhere to strict aseptic technique when administering TPN

    c. Administer medication through the TPN lumen only

    d. Ensure that the system remains a closed system at all times

    e. Assess intake and output frequently

15. Which of the following is the preferred site for subcutaneous (SC) administration of medication?

    a. Abdomen

    b. Hands

    c. Forearms

    d. Shoulders

CHAPTER 35

Pain Management in Children

SECTION I: LEARNING OBJECTIVES

1. Identify the major physiologic events associated with the perception of pain.

2. Discuss the factors that influence the pain response.

3. Identify the developmental considerations of the effects and management of pain in the infant, toddler, preschooler, school-age child, and adolescent.

4. Explain the principles of pain assessment as they relate to children.

5. Understand the use of the various pain-rating scales and physiologic monitoring for children.

6. Establish a nursing care plan for children related to management of pain, including pharmacologic and nonpharmacologic techniques and strategies.

SECTION II: ASSESSING YOUR UNDERSTANDING

Activity A *Fill in the blanks.*

1. _____ are specialized receptors at the end of peripheral nerve fibers that become activated when exposed to noxious stimuli.

2. The process of nociceptor activation is called _____.

3. _____ are the substances that change a person's perception of pain.

4. The _____ pain rating scale is similar to the FACES scale, in that it uses facial expressions to indicate increasing degrees of hurt.

5. A nonpharmacologic means of reducing the perception of pain, commonly used in children, is relaxation, which aids in reducing muscle _____ and anxiety.

6. Another nonpharmacologic means of reducing pain in children is _____, which involves having the child focus on a stimulus other than the pain.

7. Cold application results in _____ and alters capillary permeability, leading to a decrease in edema at the site of the injury.

8. Biophysical interventions focus on interfering with the transmission of pain impulses to the _____.

9. _____ analgesia is typically used postoperatively, providing analgesia to the lower body for approximately 12 to 14 hours.

10. Conscious sedation is a medically controlled state of _____ consciousness that allows protective reflexes to be maintained.

Activity B *Consider the following figures.*

OUCHER!

10 —
9 —
8 —
7 —
6 —
5 —
4 —
3 —
2 —
1 —
0 —

1. Identify this pain rating scale.

_____

_____

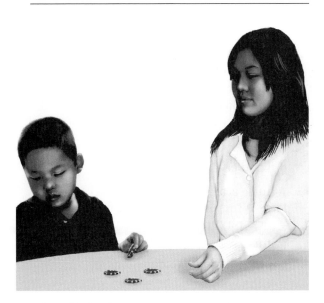

2. Identify the figure.

_____

_____

Activity C *Match the terms in Column A with their definitions in Column B.*

Column A	Column B
____ **1.** Nociceptive pain	**a.** Pain that develops in the tissues
____ **2.** Neuropathic pain	**b.** Pain due to malfunctioning of the peripheral or central nervous system
____ **3.** Somatic pain	
____ **4.** Visceral pain	**c.** Pain that develops within the organs
____ **5.** Chronic pain	**d.** Pain due to the activation of the A-delta fibers and C fibers by noxious stimuli
	e. Pain that continues past the expected point of healing for injured tissue

Activity D *Put the items in correct sequence by writing the letters in the boxes provided below.*

1. Given below are physiologic events that lead to the sensation of pain. Choose the proper sequence of their occurrence.

   a. Modulation

   b. Transmission

   c. Transduction

   d. Perception

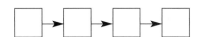

Activity E *Briefly answer the following.*

1. What is the pain threshold?

_____

_____

_____

2. What is the difference between superficial somatic pain and deep somatic pain?

_____

_____

_____

3. What are the medications used for pain management?

_____

_____

_____

4. What is gate control theory?

_____

_____

_____

5. What are the short- and long-term consequences of inadequately treated pain in newborns?

_____

_____

_____

6. How is imagery used in pain management?

_____

_____

_____

SECTION III: APPLYING YOUR KNOWLEDGE

Activity F *Consider this scenario and answer the questions.*

1. Daniel Paul is a five-year-old boy admitted to the pediatric unit for treatment of a respiratory infection. The physician prescribes parenteral antibiotics three times a day. The mother tells the nurse that the child becomes very violent and cries loudly during administration of antibiotics; the child is otherwise playful and not fussy.

   a. What are the principles of pain assessment in the child?

   _____

   _____

   _____

   b. How should the nurse provide pain management for the child when administering the parenteral antibiotic?

   _____

   _____

   _____

SECTION IV: PRACTICING FOR NCLEX

Activity G *Answer the following questions.*

1. The nurse in a postoperative unit is caring for a 15-year-old who underwent a tonsillectomy. The nurse finds that the child is restless and complains of pain in the throat. Which of the following assessment tools should the nurse use to assess pain in the child?

   a. FACES pain rating scale

   b. Word–graphic rating scale

   c. Oucher pain rating scale

   d. Poker chip tool

2. The nurse is conducting the physical examination of an adolescent client. The nurse understands that the client may not exhibit any emotions about having pain. Which of the following changes may indicate pain in the client?

   a. Clenched fists

   b. Physical aggression

   c. Intense emotional upset

   d. Loud cry

3. A nurse is assessing the pain level of an infant. Which of the following findings is a typical physiologic indicator of pain?

   a. Increased oxygen saturation

   b. Decreased heart rate

   c. Palmar sweating

   d. Increased vagal tone

4. A nurse is applying a eutectic mixture of local anesthetics (EMLA) as ordered for a client. In which of the following situations is EMLA contraindicated?

   a. Infants less than 6 weeks of age

   b. Children with dark skin

   c. Infants receiving methemoglobin-inducing agents

   d. Children undergoing venous cannulation

5. The nurse is caring for a child who has received postoperative epidural analgesia. What is the priority nursing assessment?

   a. Constipation

   b. Easy bruising

   c. Occult blood in stool

   d. Respiratory depression

6. The nurse is caring for a child postoperatively. The nurse administers tab morphine to the child as per the physician's order to alleviate pain. For which of the following should the nurse assess after administering tab morphine?

   a. Bowel sounds

   b. Bleeding

   c. Tachycardia

   d. Hypertension

7. A nurse is using a pain-rating scale to assess pain in a toddler. Which of the following should the nurse consider when using a pain-rating scale?

   a. Use any scale available

   b. Use different scales at different times

   c. Use a developmentally appropriate scale

   d. Use within 15 minutes of administering a pain-relief measure

8. The nurse documents the following findings of the Neonatal Infant Pain Scale administered to an infant. Facial expression: relaxed; Cry: whimper; Breathing patterns: change in breathing; Arms: flexed; Legs: flexed; State of arousal: awake. What is the score on the basis of this scale?

   a. 3

   b. 4

   c. 5

   d. 6

9. The nurse is caring for an infant postoperatively. Which of the following tools should the nurse use to assess pain in the infant, because the infant lacks verbal abilities?

   a. Riley Infant Pain Scale

   b. Neonatal Infant Pain Scale

   c. Pain observation scale

   d. CRIES scale

10. A nurse caring for a terminally ill child uses imagery to help manage his pain. What instructions should the nurse give the child for practicing imagery?

    a. Repeat positive statements in your mind

    b. Inhale and exhale slowly

    c. Count in ascending order

    d. Create a pleasurable image in your mind

11. A venipuncture is to be performed for a child. The physician instructs the nurse to apply a eutectic mixture of local anesthetics (EMLA). Which of the following interventions should the nurse adopt when applying EMLA?

    a. Apply the cream 30 minutes before the procedure

    b. Use two thirds of a five-gram tube for an application

    c. Cover the site with a transparent, occlusive dressing

    d. Place a thin layer of cream on the site of application

12. The nurse is caring for a child who has a cast on the hand and forearm for fracture of the radius. Which of the following are signs and symptoms indicating deep somatic pain due to sympathetic nervous system activation? Select all that apply.

    a. Diaphoresis

    b. Tachycardia

    c. Hypertension

    d. Hyperalgia

    e. Allodynia

13. The nurse is assessing pain in an infant, using the CRIES scale. Which of the following parameters should the nurse consider when using the scale? Select all that apply.
    a. Facial expressions
    b. Increased vital signs
    c. Sleeplessness
    d. Consolability
    e. Vocal ability

14. The nurse caring for a client with a sprained leg plans to use biophysical interventions for pain management. Which of the following interventions can the nurse use? Select all that apply.

    a. Biofeedback
    b. Thought-stopping
    c. Heat application
    d. Pressure application
    e. Massage therapy

15. A nurse caring for a preschooler plans to use distraction for pain relief in the client. Which of the following techniques can the nurse use? Select all that apply.
    a. Blowing pinwheels
    b. Computer games
    c. Blowing bubbles
    d. Listening to music
    e. Listening to stories

Nursing Care of the Child With an Infectious or Communicable Disorder

SECTION I: LEARNING OBJECTIVES

1. Discuss anatomic and physiologic differences in children versus adults in relation to the infectious process.

2. Identify nursing interventions related to common laboratory and diagnostic tests used in the diagnosis and management of infectious conditions.

3. Identify appropriate nursing assessments and interventions related to medications and treatments for childhood infectious and communicable disorders.

4. Distinguish various infectious illnesses occurring in childhood.

5. Devise an individualized nursing care plan for the child with an infectious or communicable disorder.

6. Develop patient/family teaching plans for the child with an infectious or communicable disorder.

SECTION II: ASSESSING YOUR UNDERSTANDING

Activity A *Fill in the blanks.*

1. The white blood cells use phagocytosis to ingest and destroy the _____.

2. _____ are often used to lower fever and increase the comfort of the client.

3. The body actually produces a natural antipyretic, called _____.

4. _____ is a systemic overresponse to infection resulting from bacteria, fungi, viruses, or parasites.

5. _____ is an acute respiratory disorder characterized by paroxysmal cough and copious secretions.

6. _____ is an acute, often fatal neurologic disease caused by the toxins produced by *Clostridium tetani*.

7. Many viral infections of the skin in childhood are called viral _____.

8. _____ is a contagious disease caused by paramyxovirus; it is characterized by fever and parotitis.

9. _____ are organisms larger than yeast or bacteria that can cause infection; they live in or on a host.

10. _____ infections seen in children include pinworms, roundworms, and hookworms.

Activity B *Consider the following figures.*

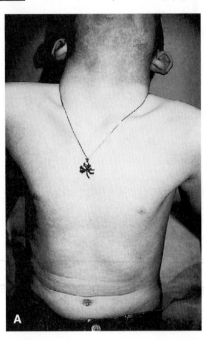

A

1. Identify the image.

_____

_____

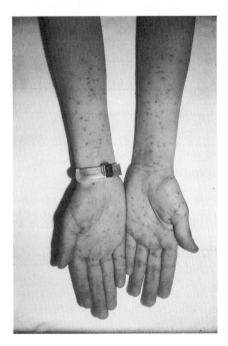

2. Identify the image.

_____

_____

Activity C *Match the chain link in Column A with the proper word or phrase in Column B.*

Column A

____ **1.** Infectious agent

____ **2.** Mode of transmission

____ **3.** Portal of entry

____ **4.** Portal of exit

____ **5.** Reservoir

____ **6.** Susceptible host

Column B

a. Gastrointestinal tract

b. Child

c. Respiratory tract

d. Fomite

e. Rickettsia

f. Animal

Activity D *Put the items in correct sequence by writing the letters in the boxes provided below.*

1. Given below in random order are the stages of infectious diseases. Choose the proper order:

a. Convalescence

b. Illness

c. Incubation

d. Prodrome

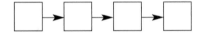

Activity E *Briefly answer the following.*

1. What are the risk factors for sepsis that are related to pregnancy and labor?

_____

_____

_____

2. What are the methods used in the nursing management of mumps?

_____

_____

_____

3. What causes hyperthermia?

_____

_____

_____

4. What is the role of nurses in preventing the spread of infections?

_____

_____

_____

5. What is the function of the white blood cells?

_____

_____

_____

6. What are the factors that could cause sepsis in a hospitalized child?

_____

_____

_____

SECTION III: APPLYING YOUR KNOWLEDGE

Activity F *Consider this scenario and answer the questions.*

1. Seven-year-old Nicholas Croxton is brought to the clinic by his mother. He presents with a history of fever and myalgia. The nurse observes a ring-like rash on the back of his hand.

a. What information should the nurse gather when obtaining the health history of the child?

_____

_____

_____

b. Nicholas is diagnosed with Lyme disease. What would be the typical therapeutic management in this case?

_____

_____

_____

c. List a few preventive measures that a nurse can teach Nicholas and his mother to prevent tick-borne illnesses.

_____

_____

_____

SECTION IV: PRACTICING FOR NCLEX

Activity G *Answer the following questions.*

1. A six-year-old boy is suspected of having late-stage Lyme disease. Which of the following assessments would produce findings supporting this concern?

a. Inspection for erythema migrans

b. Assessment of the child's knees for arthritis

c. Observation of facial palsy

d. Examination for conjunctivitis

2. A ten-year-old girl with long hair is brought to the emergency room because she began acting irritable, complained of a headache, and is very sleepy. What question would be most appropriate to ask the parents?

a. "Has she done this before?"

b. "How long has she been acting like this?"

c. "What were you doing before she began feeling sick?"

d. "What medications is she currently taking?"

3. The nurse is preparing to administer acetaminophen to a four-year-old girl to provide comfort to the child. Which of the following precautions is very specific with antipyretics?

a. Check for medicine allergies

b. Take the entire course of medication

c. Ensure proper dose and interval

d. Warn of possible drowsiness

4. The nurse is caring for a ten-year-old girl admitted to the health care facility with a fever of unknown origin. The nurse needs to obtain a urine sample for culture and sensitivity. Which of the following steps should the nurse take to ensure that the sensitivity result is accurate?

   a. Obtain the entire volume of urine

   b. Obtain three specimens on three different days

   c. Place bags on the perineum

   d. Obtain the specimen before antibiotics are administered

5. The nurse at an outpatient facility is obtaining a blood specimen from a nine-year-old girl. Which of the following techniques should the nurse use?

   a. Puncture a vein on the dorsal side of the hand

   b. Provide oral sucrose before the procedure

   c. Access an indwelling venous access device

   d. Use an automatic lancet device on the heel

6. The pediatric nurse knows that there are a number of anatomic and physiologic differences between children and adults. Which of the following statements about the immune systems of infants and young children is true?

   a. Children have an immature immune response

   b. Cellular immunity is not functional in children

   c. Children have an increased inflammatory response

   d. Passive immunity overlaps immunizations

7. Which of the following children needs to be seen immediately in the pediatrician's office?

   a. A ten-month-old with a fever and petechiae who is grunting

   b. A two-month-old with a slight fever and irritability following immunizations the previous day

   c. A four-month-old with a cough, elevated temperature, and wetting eight diapers every 24 hours

   d. An eight-month-old who is restless, irritable, and afebrile

8. The nurse is caring for a five-year-old girl with scarlet fever. Which of the following interventions will most likely be part of her care?

   a. Exercising both standard and droplet precautions

   b. Palpating for and noting enlarged lymph nodes

   c. Monitoring for changes in respiratory status

   d. Teaching proper administration of penicillin V

9. A nurse is performing a capillary heel puncture for an infant. Which of the following should the nurse do to obtain blood with a capillary specimen collection tube?

   a. Cleanse the site with dry gauze or a cotton ball

   b. Wipe away the first drop of blood with an antiseptic wipe

   c. Avoid squeezing the foot during specimen collection

   d. Hold an antiseptic wipe over the site until bleeding stops

10. A nurse is caring for a five-year-old with pruritus. Which of the following should the nurse perform to provide comfort to the child?

   a. Offer warm fluids such as soup

   b. Apply warm compresses to the area

   c. Provide the child with mitts

   d. Dress the child in warm clothing

11. A nurse is instructing the parents of a three-year-old regarding management of fever. About which of the following should the nurse inform the parents?

   a. Call the physician if temperature is greater than 38°C

   b. Cover the child with blankets

   c. Use cold water to sponge the child

   d. Give an antipyretic prior to sponging

12. The nurse is teaching the parents of a six-year-old about the removal of ticks. Which of the following should the nurse tell the parents? Select all that apply.
    a. Use fine-tipped tweezers to extract the tick
    b. Use a paper towel or latex gloves to protect fingers
    c. Grasp the tick at the end farthest from the skin
    d. Twist and jerk the tick away from the skin
    e. Clean the site with soap and water after removal

13. A nurse is caring for a four-year-old boy at a well-child clinic. About which of the following should the nurse inform the parents of the boy regarding prevention of tetanus?
    a. Booster immunizations are given every five years
    b. Tetanus is manifested as a rash
    c. All wounds should be cleaned thoroughly with antiseptic
    d. Booster immunization should be taken if the wound is contaminated

14. The nurse is caring for a six-year-old with cat scratch disease. About which of the following should the nurse tell the parents of the child? Select all that apply.
    a. Routine infant immunization can prevent the disease
    b. Ensure that cats do not lick open wounds on the child
    c. Wash any bites or scratches with soap and running water
    d. Transmission-based isolation is required
    e. Ensure control of fleas in cats

15. A nurse assessing a seven-year-old girl observes the presence of head lice. Which of the following control measures should the nurse ask the caregiver to perform? Select all that apply.
    a. Avoid sending the child to school
    b. Soak combs in pediculicide, shampoo, or hot water
    c. Wash headgear, towels, and pillowcases in hot water
    d. Wash bedding and clothing worn four days prior to treatment in hot water
    e. Treat bedmates prophylactically

CHAPTER 37

Nursing Care of the Child With a Neurologic Disorder

SECTION I: LEARNING OBJECTIVES

1. Compare how the anatomy and physiology of the neurologic system in children differs from those in adults.

2. Identify various factors associated with neurologic disease in infants and children.

3. Discuss common laboratory and other diagnostic tests useful in the diagnosis of neurologic conditions.

4. Discuss common medications and other treatments used for treatment and palliation of neurologic conditions.

5. Recognize risk factors associated with various neurologic disorders.

6. Distinguish among different neurologic illnesses on the basis of the signs and symptoms associated with them.

7. Discuss nursing interventions commonly used for neurologic illnesses.

8. Devise an individualized nursing care plan for the child with a neurologic disorder.

9. Develop client and family teaching plans for the child with a neurologic disorder.

10. Describe the psychosocial impact of chronic neurologic disorders on children.

SECTION II: ASSESSING YOUR UNDERSTANDING

Activity A *Fill in the blanks.*

1. _____ increases the speed and accuracy of nerve impulses.

2. A smaller-than-normal head circumference may indicate _____.

3. _____ eyes may indicate increased intracranial pressure.

4. A _____ seizure is usually associated with a core temperature that increases rapidly to 39°C or higher.

5. _____ sign is an indication of meningitis.

6. _____ meningitis is the most common type of meningitis affecting children less than five years of age.

7. _____ is the primary problem resulting from near-drowning.

8. _____ are benign, recurring, throbbing headaches often accompanied by nausea, vomiting, and photophobia.

9. Positional _____ refers to asymmetry in head shape without fused sutures.

10. Bruising of cerebral tissue is known as a _____.

Activity B   *Consider the following figures.*

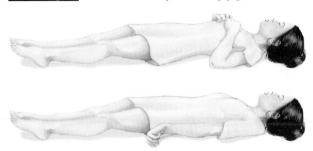

1. Indicate which is decorticate and which is decerebrate posturing.

_____

_____

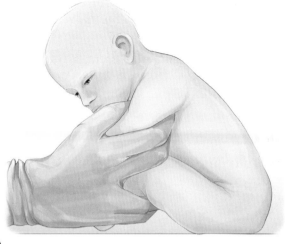

A

3. Explain what is being done in the image.

_____

_____

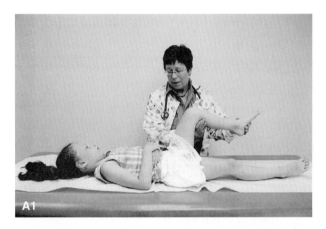

A1

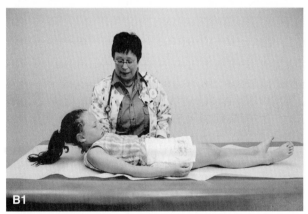

B1

2. Indicate which shows Kernig's sign and which shows Brudzinski's sign.

_____

_____

Activity C   *Match the neurologic disorders in Column A with their proper descriptions in Column B.*

Column A

____ **1.** Meningitis

____ **2.** Craniosynostosis

____ **3.** Epilepsy

____ **4.** Encephalitis

____ **5.** Hydrocephalus

Column B

a. Infection of the lining around the brain and spinal cord

b. Inflammation of the brain, sometimes including the meninges

c. Characterized by two or more unprovoked seizures more than 24 hours apart

d. Not a specific disease but rather the result of other brain disorders

e. Premature closure of the cranial sutures

Activity D *Put the items in correct sequence by writing the letters in the boxes provided below.*

1. Given below, in random order, are the levels of consciousness. Choose the correct order from lowest to highest.

   a. Coma

   b. Confusion

   c. Full consciousness

   d. Obtunded

   e. Stupor

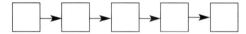

Activity E *Briefly answer the following.*

1. Describe the opisthotonic position and indicate at what age a child would assume this position and what neurologic disorder is implicated.

   _____

   _____

   _____

2. What is the purpose of the Pediatric Glasgow Coma Scale?

   _____

   _____

   _____

3. What kind of precautions should be taken for a child with seizures?

   _____

   _____

   _____

4. What are neonatal seizures?

   _____

   _____

   _____

5. How does breath-holding occur in children?

   _____

   _____

   _____

6. What are cerebral vascular disorders?

   _____

   _____

   _____

SECTION III: APPLYING YOUR KNOWLEDGE

Activity F *Consider this scenario and answer the questions.*

1. Jessica Clark, five years old, is admitted to the neurologic unit at a pediatric hospital after having a seizure at school. From her mother, the nurse learns that Jessica has a history of seizures and is taking phenobarbital to control them. The mother states, "Ever since Jessica started school this year, it has been more difficult to get her to take her medicine."

   a. What additional assessment data should the nurse obtain?

      _____

      _____

      _____

   b. What diagnostic and laboratory tests should the nurse anticipate?

      _____

      _____

      _____

   c. Minutes after leaving the room, the nurse is called back by the mother because Jessica is having another seizure. Identify nursing interventions related to the care of this child during and immediately following a seizure. List them in order of priority.

      _____

      _____

      _____

   d. What teaching should the nurse provide this child's family? Include a discussion on ways to increase compliance with the seizure medication.

      _____

      _____

      _____

SECTION IV: PRACTICING FOR NCLEX

Activity G *Answer the following questions.*

1. A nurse is caring for an infant with positional plagiocephaly on the right side of the head. Which of the following should the nurse do to prevent flattening of the skull?
   a. Place the infant on the abdomen when awake
   b. Place the infant in a supine position most of the time
   c. Place a rolled washcloth along the left side of the head
   d. Place the infant in a left-lateral position most of the time

2. During physical assessment of a two-month-old infant, the nurse notes horizontal nystagmus in the infant's eyes. Which of the following does this indicate?
   a. Increased intracranial pressure
   b. Brain stem dysfunction
   c. Lesions in the brainstem
   d. Intracranial mass

3. A nurse is caring for an infant with suspected botulism. Which of the following should the nurse assess for in the infant? Select all that apply.
   a. Continual vomiting
   b. Poor feeding
   c. Weak cry
   d. Hyperreflexia
   e. Constipation

4. A nurse is caring for an eight-year-old girl who was in a car accident. The CT scan and MRI reports show a contusion in the child's brain. Which of the following symptoms should the nurse assess for in the child?
   a. Trouble focusing when reading
   b. Difficulty concentrating
   c. Vomiting and lethargy
   d. Bleeding from the ear

5. A nurse is assessing the level of consciousness in a six-month-old child. Which of the following states indicates that the child has limited responses to the environment and falls asleep unless stimulated?
   a. Confusion
   b. Obtunded
   c. Stupor
   d. Coma

6. The nurse is caring for a three-year-old boy who is experiencing seizure activity. Which of the following diagnostic tests will determine the seizure area in the brain?
   a. Cerebral angiography
   b. Lumbar puncture
   c. Video electroencephalogram
   d. Computed tomography

7. A nurse assessing an infant with suspected hydrocephalus notes a "cracked pot" sound on percussing the infant's head. Which of the following does this indicate?
   a. Smallness of the skull
   b. Separation of the sutures
   c. Swelling in the brain
   d. Intracranial hemorrhage

8. A nurse notes facial twitching when caring for a newborn and suspects a nonepileptic seizure. Which of the following should the nurse know to recognize these seizures as nonepileptic? Select all that apply.
   a. The EEG may be normal in a nonepileptic seizure
   b. An epileptic seizure is accompanied by tremors and jitteriness
   c. Tachycardia and elevated blood pressure are absent in nonepileptic seizures
   d. Ocular deviation may be seen in a nonepileptic seizure
   e. A nonepileptic movement may be suppressed by gently restraining the limb

9. An eight-year-old child is admitted to the health care facility with high fever and seizures. Which of the following should the nurse expect when assessing the child?

   a. The child's core temperature is likely to decrease

   b. The seizure will stop only after the child receives medication

   c. The seizure will last a few seconds to ten minutes

   d. The seizure is myoclonic in character

10. A nurse is assessing a child with head trauma. Which of the following should the nurse recognize as an early sign of increased intracranial pressure?

    a. Lowered level of consciousness

    b. Projectile vomiting

    c. Bradycardia

    d. Fixed and dilated pupils

11. A nurse is educating the parents of an epileptic child. Which of the following instructions should the nurse provide the parents?

    a. Place the child supine during a seizure

    b. Open the child's jaw with a tongue blade or fingers

    c. Do not restrain the child

    d. Support the child in a sitting position if the seizure occurs while sitting

12. A nurse is caring for an adolescent client with type II Arnold-Chiari malformation. Which of the following signs should the nurse look for in the client?

    a. Choking and gagging

    b. Spasticity and upper extremity weakness

    c. Weight loss

    d. Coarse upper airway sounds

Nursing Care of the Child With a Disorder of the Eyes or Ears

SECTION I: LEARNING OBJECTIVES

1. Differentiate between the anatomic and physiologic difference of the eyes and ears in children as compared with adults.

2. Identify various factors associated with disorders of the eyes and ears in infants and children.

3. Discuss the common laboratory and other diagnostic tests useful in the diagnosis of disorders of the eyes and ears.

4. Discuss the common medications and treatments used for the treatment and palliation of conditions affecting the eyes and ears.

5. Recognize risk factors associated with various disorders of the eyes and ears.

6. Distinguish between different disorders of eyes and ears based on the signs and symptoms associated with them.

7. Discuss nursing interventions commonly used in regard to disorders of the eyes and ears.

8. Devise an individualized nursing care plan for the child with a sensory impairment or other disorder of eyes and ears.

9. Develop patient/family teaching plans for the child with a disorder of the eyes or ears.

10. Describe the psychosocial impact of sensory impairment on children.

SECTION II: ASSESSING YOUR UNDERSTANDING

Activity A *Fill in the blanks.*

1. Inflammation of the bulbar or palpebral conjunctiva is referred to as _____.

2. Often, with upper respiratory infections, there is enlargement of the _____, which contributes to obstruction of the Eustachian tubes, leading to infection.

3. One way to assess for otitis media with effusion is to check the mobility of the _____ membrane. This can be tested with pneumatic otoscopy.

4. _____ refers to chronic scaling and discharge along the eyelid margin.

5. The treatment for both hyperopia and _____ is prescription eyeglasses or contact lenses.

6. In strabismus, the vision in one eye may be "turned off" by the brain to avoid _____.

7. _____ glaucoma is an autosomal recessive disorder that is common in interrelated marriages or relationships.

8. Delayed-onset hearing loss can be _____ hearing loss. It is caused by damage to the hair cells in the cochlea or along the auditory pathway.

9. _____ is used to confirm the diagnosis of otitis media with effusion (OME).

10. Systemic _____ are used to treat periorbital cellulitis.

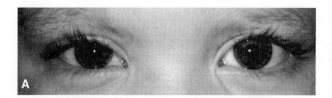

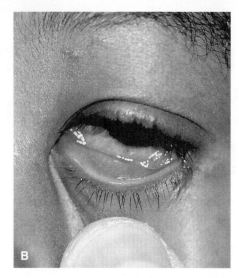

Activity B *Consider the following figures.*

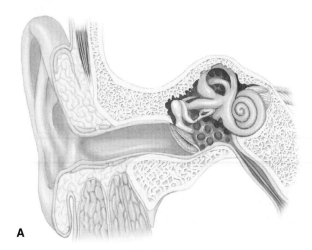

A

2. Identify the types of disorders shown in the figure.

_____

_____

Activity C *Match the type of eye injury in Column A with its characteristics in Column B.*

Column A	Column B
____ **1.** Simple contusion (black eye)	**a.** Vision is usually unaffected
____ **2.** Corneal abrasion	**b.** Appears as erythema in the sclera; can be quite large initially
____ **3.** Eyelid injury	**c.** Photophobia may be present
____ **4.** Foreign body	**d.** Bruising and edema of eyelid
____ **5.** Scleral hemorrhage	**e.** Complaint of "something in the eye"

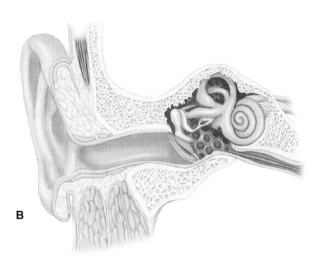

B

1. What does the figure depict?

_____

_____

Activity D *Put the items in correct sequence by writing the letters in the boxes provided below.*

1. Given below, in random order, are vision and hearing milestones in a child. Choose the correct order.

   a. Binocular vision

   b. Eye color

   c. Functional hearing

   d. Visual acuity of 20/20

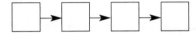

Activity E *Briefly answer the following.*

1. What are the symptoms of astigmatism?

   _____

   _____

   _____

2. What are the common types of strabismus?

   _____

   _____

   _____

3. What is legal blindness?

   _____

   _____

   _____

4. What is conductive hearing loss?

   _____

   _____

   _____

5. What are the risk factors for otitis media with effusion (OME)?

   _____

   _____

   _____

6. What is nystagmus?

   _____

   _____

   _____

SECTION III: APPLYING YOUR KNOWLEDGE

Activity F *Consider this scenario and answer the questions.*

1. Austin Snow, a nine-year-old child, presents in the clinic with severe ear pain. The nurse identifies infection and inflammation of the skin of the external ear canal. Austin is diagnosed with otitis externa.

   a. What interventions should the nurse perform to relieve pain and treat the infection in the child?

   _____

   _____

   _____

   b. What measures should the nurse suggest to the mother to prevent otitis externa?

   _____

   _____

   _____

   _____

SECTION IV: PRACTICING FOR NCLEX

Activity G *Answer the following questions.*

1. A ten-year-old boy has just been treated for otitis externa, and now the nurse is teaching the boy and his parents about prevention. Which of the following recommendations would be included as part of the education?

   a. Using alcohol and vinegar for soreness

   b. Using cotton swabs to keep the inner ear dry

   c. Using antibiotics only for bacterial infection

   d. Washing his hair only when necessary

2. The nurse is educating the parents of a five-year-old girl with infectious conjunctivitis about the disorder. Which of the following is most important to prevent its spread?

   a. Not sharing face cloths with others

   b. Staying home from school during infection

   c. Keeping hands away from eyes

   d. Washing hands frequently after providing care

3. The nurse is teaching the parents of a four-year-old boy with strabismus. Which of the following subjects would be most important?
   a. The importance of complying with patching as prescribed
   b. The possibility that multiple operations may be necessary
   c. The importance of completing the full course of oral antibiotics
   d. The need for ultraviolet-protective glasses postoperatively

4. The nurse is caring for a seven-year-old girl with amblyopia unrelated to any other disorder. Which of the following interventions would be most helpful?
   a. Educating parents on how to use atropine drops
   b. Ensuring follow-up visits with the ophthalmologist
   c. Protecting the operative site with eye patching
   d. Encouraging the child to wear glasses regularly

5. The nurse is caring for a two-year-old boy with regressed retinopathy of prematurity. Which of the following interventions would be the first priority for this child?
   a. Assessing the child for asymmetric corneal light reflex
   b. Observing for signs of visual impairment
   c. Referring the child to the local early intervention program
   d. Teaching the parents to check whether the child's glasses fit

6. A nurse is caring for a three-year-old child who was brought to the health care facility with corneal abrasions. Which of the following should the nurse assess for when performing a physical assessment on the child?
   a. Erythema
   b. Bruising
   c. Edema of the lid
   d. Photophobia

7. The nurse is caring for an eight-year-old boy with otitis media with effusion. Which of the following situations may have caused this disorder?
   a. He has a moist ear canal
   b. He is experiencing recurrent viral URTI
   c. He frequently goes swimming
   d. He recently had bacterial conjunctivitis

8. A child is brought to the emergency department with deep lacerations of the eyelid. The lacerations are sutured. The child should be referred to an ophthalmologist to prevent which of the following conditions?
   a. Scleral hemorrhage
   b. Corneal abrasions
   c. Ptosis
   d. Black eye

9. A nurse is caring for a four-year-old child with acute otitis media. Which of the following conditions should the nurse consider as a complication of acute otitis media?
   a. Chlamydial pneumonia
   b. Orbital cellulitis
   c. Amblyopia
   d. Tympanosclerosis

10. A nurse is caring for a two-year-old child who underwent surgery for congenital cataract. Which of the following signs should the nurse look for as a complication of the cataract surgery?
    a. Glaucoma
    b. Myopia
    c. Blindness
    d. Strabismus

11. The nurse is caring for a two-year-old girl with persistent otitis media with effusion. Which of the following interventions is most important to the developmental health of the child?
    a. Reassessing for language acquisition
    b. Promoting the benefits of breast-feeding
    c. Telling parents not to smoke in the house
    d. Warning against taking nonprescription drugs

12. A three-year-old boy may have strabismus. Which of the following examinations would the nurse expect to assist with first in order to find out if he has strabismus?
    a. Refractive examination
    b. Visual acuity test
    c. Ophthalmologic examination
    d. Corneal light reflex test

13. A nurse is performing a visual acuity test for a three-year-old child. Which of the following should be the visual acuity in the child?
    a. 20/400
    b. 20/100
    c. 20/50
    d. 20/20

14. A nurse is assigned to care for an infant who underwent surgery for infantile glaucoma. Which of the following is the immediate postoperative intervention that the nurse should consider when caring for the infant?
    a. Encourage muscle exercise of the affected eye
    b. Teach the parents how to administer post-operative medications
    c. Apply elbow restraints to prevent the child from rubbing the eyes
    d. Encourage the parents to comply with on-going visual assessment

15. A pediatric nurse is interviewing the parents of a child diagnosed with retinopathy of pre-maturity. Which of the following risk factors should the nurse look for?
    a. Low birth weight
    b. Developmental delay
    c. Astigmatism
    d. Genetic syndrome

CHAPTER 39

Nursing Care of the Child With a Respiratory Disorder

SECTION I: LEARNING OBJECTIVES

1. Compare how the anatomy and physiology of the respiratory system in children differs from those of adults.

2. Identify various factors associated with respiratory illness in infants and children.

3. Discuss common laboratory and other diagnostic tests useful in the diagnosis of respiratory conditions.

4. Discuss common medications and other treatments used for treatment and palliation of respiratory conditions.

5. Recognize risk factors associated with various respiratory disorders.

6. Distinguish different respiratory illnesses based on the signs and symptoms associated with them.

7. Discuss nursing interventions commonly used for respiratory illnesses.

8. Devise an individualized nursing care plan for the child with a respiratory disorder.

9. Develop patient/family teaching plans for the child with a respiratory disorder.

10. Describe the psychosocial impact of chronic respiratory disorders on children.

SECTION II: ASSESSING YOUR UNDERSTANDING

Activity A *Fill in the blanks.*

1. _____ is an enlargement of the terminal phalanx of the finger, resulting in a change in the angle of the nail to the fingertip.

2. _____, a high-pitched, readily audible inspiratory noise, is a sign of upper airway obstruction.

3. When an infant is in respiratory distress you will hear grunting on _____ which is produced by premature glottic closure and is a sign of serious respiratory difficulty.

4. _____ syndrome is an acute encephalopathy that has been associated with aspirin use in the influenza-infected child.

5. Inflammation of the throat mucosa is referred to as _____.

6. Children with pneumonia often have areas of _____ identified on a CXR. These areas are defined as collapsed or airless portions of the lung, causing gas exchange to become impaired.

7. A _____ is the surgical construction of a respiratory opening in the trachea.

8. The first sign of respiratory illness in infants and children is _____.

9. In cystic fibrosis, the _____ enzyme activity is lost and malabsorption of fats, proteins, and carbohydrates occurs.

10. _____ occurs as a result of peripheral vasoconstriction in an effort to conserve oxygen for vital functions.

Activity B *Consider the following figures.*

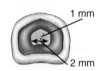
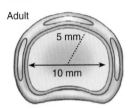
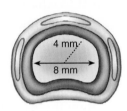

A

B

Infant   2 mm

4 mm

1 mm

2 mm

1 mm circumferential edema causes 50% reduction of diameter and radius, increasing pulmonary resistance by a factor of 16.

Adult

5 mm.

10 mm

4 mm.

8 mm

1 mm circumferential edema causes 20% reduction of diameter and radius, increasing pulmonary resistance by a factor of 2.4.

1. What does the above figure depict?

_____

_____

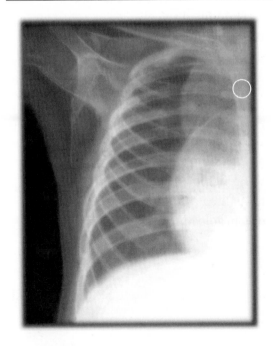

2. Identify the figure.

_____

_____

Activity C *Match the respiratory disorders listed in Column A with the their area of inflammation listed in Column B.*

Column A

___ **1.** Influenza

___ **2.** Pharyngitis

___ **3.** Pneumonia

___ **4.** Allergic rhinitis

___ **5.** Rhinosinusitis

Column B

a. Upper respiratory epithelium

b. Throat mucosa

c. Lung parenchyma

d. Paranasal sinuses

e. Nasal mucosa

Activity D *Put the items in correct sequence by writing the letters in the boxes provided below.*

1. Given below, in random order, are the steps for using a bulb syringe to suction nasal secretions. Choose the correct order:

a. Compress the bulb.

b. Empty the bulb and clean the bulb syringe.

c. Instill saline solution.

d. Place the bulb in the nose.

e. Release pressure on the bulb.

f. Remove the bulb from the nose.

g. Tilt the infant's head back.

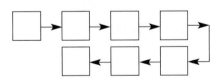

Activity E *Briefly answer the following.*

1. What is nasopharyngitis?

_____

_____

_____

2. What are the genetic reasons for cystic fibrosis?

3. What is pneumothorax?

4. What are the laboratory and diagnostic tests commonly performed in pneumonia?

5. What are the complications involved in respiratory distress syndrome (RDS)?

6. What is the nursing assessment of children with epistaxis?

SECTION III: APPLYING YOUR KNOWLEDGE

Activity F *Consider this scenario and answer the questions.*

1. A three-year-old child was brought to the hospital in an unconscious state following aspiration of a foreign body. The medical team in the emergency unit reacted quickly and removed the foreign body. What precautions should the nurse teach the parents to observe to prevent foreign body aspiration?

SECTION IV: PRACTICING FOR NCLEX

Activity G *Answer the following questions.*

1. A nurse is caring for a newborn with bronchopulmonary dysplasia. Which of the following nursing interventions should the nurse perform?

   a. Provide chest physiotherapy with postural drainage

   b. Keep the newborn well hydrated to prevent dehydration

   c. Provide a light, low-calorie intake

   d. Provide continuous ventilatory and oxygen support

2. A nurse is caring for a three-year-old girl with hypoxemia. Which of the following would be best to relieve these symptoms?

   a. Suctioning

   b. Saline lavage

   c. Saline gargles

   d. Oxygen

3. Upon the examination of a four-year-old child, who is experiencing difficulty in breathing, the nurse finds that the child has wheezing that clears with coughing. Which of the following conditions would this indicate?

   a. Secretions in lower trachea

   b. Obstruction of the bronchioles

   c. Fluid-filled alveoli

   d. Intrathoracic foreign body

4. A nurse is assigned to take care of a child with a high-grade fever. As per the physician's advice, the nurse auscultates the lungs of the child and hears rales. Crackling sounds, or rales, can be heard in which of the following disease conditions?

   a. Pneumonia

   b. Bronchiolitis

   c. Asthma

   d. Chronic lung disease

5. A nurse working in a health care facility receives a five-year-old child with breathing difficulty. Upon examination, the nurse finds that the child has clubbing of the fingers. Which of the following disorders could cause clubbing of the fingers?

   a. Chronic respiratory illness
   b. Epistaxis
   c. Pneumonia
   d. Influenza

6. A nurse is assessing a child with sinusitis. Which of the following is a characteristic of the involvement of the ethmoid sinus?

   a. Irritability
   b. Halitosis
   c. Facial pain
   d. Eyelid edema

7. A nurse is caring for a three-year-old child who is experiencing difficulty in breathing. Upon palpation the nurse notes absence of tactile fremitus. Which of the following conditions would this indicate?

   a. Atelectasis
   b. Pneumonia
   c. Pleural effusion
   d. Cystic fibrosis

8. The nurse is caring for a five-year-old girl showing signs and symptoms of epiglottitis. The nurse recognizes which of the following to be a complication of the disorder?

   a. Respiratory distress
   b. Acute otitis media
   c. Aseptic meningitis
   d. Retraction of chest wall

9. The nurse is caring for a ten-year-old girl with allergic rhinitis. Which of the following interventions help prevent secondary bacterial infection?

   a. Use of oral antihistamines
   b. Use of anti-inflammatory nasal sprays
   c. Avoiding allergens
   d. Performing nasal washes

10. The nurse knows that respiratory disorders in children are due to differences in anatomy and physiology. Which of the following is an accurate statement?

    a. Infants consume twice as much oxygen as adults
    b. Adults have twice as many alveoli as newborns
    c. The tongue is proportionately smaller in infants
    d. Hypoxemia occurs less rapidly in children than in adults

11. The nurse is taking the health history of a three-year-old girl with a fever, chest pain, and cough. Which of the following is a risk factor for pneumonia?

    a. The child is allergic to dust
    b. The child has HIV infection
    c. The child has aspirated a foreign body
    d. The child was born prematurely

12. The nurse is developing a teaching plan for the parents of a 10-year-old boy with cystic fibrosis. Which of the following subjects would be part of the plan?

    a. Using a metered-dose inhaler
    b. Proper use of a nebulizer
    c. Using a flutter valve device
    d. How to work a peak flow meter

13. A nurse is caring for a child who is unable to maintain oxygen saturations after a tracheostomy. Which of the following should the nurse include as a chronic tracheostomy complication?

    a. Pulmonary edema
    b. Anatomic damage
    c. Formation of granulation tissue
    d. Air entry

14. The nurse is caring for a 14-month-old boy with cystic fibrosis. Which of these signs of ineffective family coping requires the most urgent intervention?

    a. Compliance with therapy wanes
    b. Family becomes overly vigilant
    c. Child feels fearful and isolated
    d. Siblings are jealous or worried

CHAPTER 40

Nursing Care of the Child With a Cardiovascular Disorder

SECTION I: LEARNING OBJECTIVES

1. Compare anatomic and physiologic differences of the cardiovascular system in infants and children versus adults.

2. Describe nursing care related to common laboratory and diagnostic tests used in the medical diagnosis of pediatric cardiovascular conditions.

3. Distinguish cardiovascular disorders common in infants, children, and adolescents.

4. Identify appropriate nursing assessments and interventions related to medications and treatments for pediatric cardiovascular disorders.

5. Develop an individualized nursing care plan for the child with a cardiovascular disorder.

6. Describe the psychosocial impact of chronic cardiovascular disorder on children.

7. Devise a nutrition plan for a child with cardiovascular disease.

8. Develop a patient/family teaching plan for the child with a cardiovascular disorder.

SECTION II: ASSESSING YOUR UNDERSTANDING

Activity A *Fill in the blanks.*

1. Cardiac catheterization may be categorized as diagnostic, interventional, or _____.

2. _____ of the aorta is narrowing of the aorta.

3. _____ is a condition in which the myocardium cannot contract properly.

4. _____ disease is an acute systemic vasculitis occurring mostly in infants and young children.

5. _____ and cardiopulmonary bypass required during cardiac surgery for CHD may have a long-term impact on the child's cognitive ability and academic function.

6. _____ is manifested as increased cyanosis, hypoxemia, dyspnea, and agitation.

7. _____ heart disease is defined as structural anomalies that are present at birth.

8. _____ stenosis is a condition causing obstruction of the blood flow between the left ventricle and the aorta.

9. _____ refers to BP that is persistently between the 90th and 95th percentiles.

10. Aortic clicks are best heard at the _____ and can be mitral or aortic in nature.

<hr>

Activity B *Consider the following figures.*

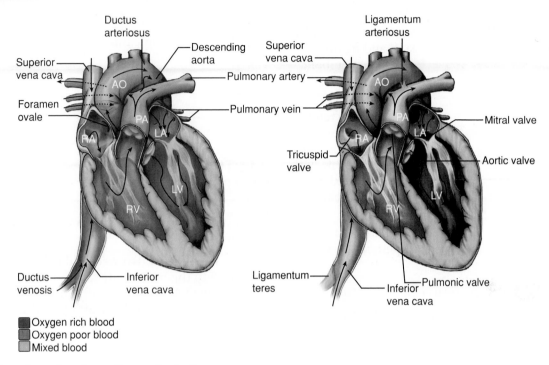

Oxygen rich blood
Oxygen poor blood
Mixed blood

1. What does the above figure depict?

_____

_____

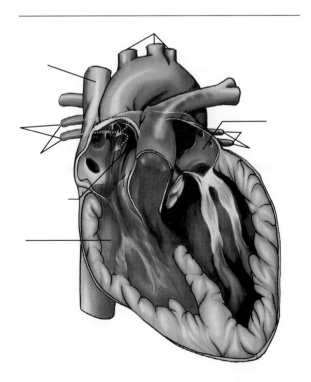

2. Label the figure to the left and identify the congenital heart defect.

_____

_____

Activity C *Match the medications in Column A with their appropriate indication in Column B.*

Column A

___ 1. Alprostadil

___ 2. Furosemide

___ 3. Heparin

___ 4. ACE inhibitors

Column B

a. Used to manage edema associated with heart failure

b. Indicated for prophylaxis and treatment of thromboembolic disorders, especially after cardiac surgery

c. Indicated for temporary maintenance of ductus arteriosus patency in infants with ductal-dependent congenital heart defects

d. For management of hypertension

Activity D *Briefly answer the following.*

1. What are the three types of atrial septal defects?

_____

_____

_____

2. What circulatory changes occur from gestation to birth?

_____

_____

_____

3. What is tetralogy of Fallot?

_____

_____

_____

4. What is total anomalous pulmonary venous connection (TAPVC)?

_____

_____

_____

5. What are the common manifestations of heart failure in a child with congenital heart disease (CHD)?

_____

_____

_____

6. What is orthotopic transplantation?

_____

_____

_____

SECTION III: APPLYING YOUR KNOWLEDGE

Activity E *Consider this scenario and answer the questions.*

1. Amy Gardener, a two-week-old baby, was admitted to the health care facility secondary to suspected tetralogy of Fallot. The physician orders a cardiac catheterization for the baby as a diagnostic procedure.

   a. What preprocedural assessment should be carried out?

   _____

   _____

   _____

   b. How should the nurse care for the baby after the procedure?

   _____

   _____

   _____

SECTION IV: PRACTICING FOR NCLEX

Activity F *Answer the following questions.*

1. The nurse is assessing the heart rate of a healthy four-month-old infant. Which of the following heart rate ranges would the nurse expect?
   a. 120 to 130 bpm
   b. 80 to 105 bpm
   c. 70 to 80 bpm
   d. 60 to 68 bpm

2. A nurse in an outpatient department is assessing a two-year-old child with cardiovascular disease. Which of the following assessment findings suggests presence of congenital heart disease?
   a. Narrow or thready pulse
   b. Prominent precordial chest wall
   c. Edema in lower extremities
   d. Clubbing of toes and fingers

3. A nurse is instructed to administer Aldactone to a child with edema due to heart failure. Which of the following parameters should the nurse monitor in the client?
   a. Serum potassium
   b. Platelet count
   c. Serum glucose
   d. Liver enzymes

4. The nurse is assessing the blood pressure of a healthy 13-year-old boy. Which of the following readings should the nurse expect?
   a. 94–112/56–60 mm Hg
   b. 100–120/50–70 mm Hg
   c. 80–100/64 mm Hg
   d. 80/40 mm Hg

5. The nurse performs a physical examination of a child who is admitted to the health care facility with a diagnosis of coarctation of the aorta. Which of the following findings should the nurse expect during auscultation?
   a. Moderately loud systolic murmur at the base of the heart
   b. Systolic murmur at left sternal border
   c. Systolic ejection murmur at upper left sternal border
   d. Fixed splitting of the second heart sound

6. A nurse is caring for a child with a ventricular septal defect who was admitted for a planned surgical repair of the defect. Which of the following complications of a ventricular septal defect can be avoided by early surgery?
   a. Ventricular dysrhythmia
   b. AV block
   c. Infective endocarditis
   d. Pulmonary hypertension

7. A nurse in an intensive care unit is caring for a postoperative infant who underwent pulmonary artery banding surgery. Which of the following should the nurse monitor in the child?
   a. Monitor for left ventricular dysfunction
   b. Monitor for complete heart block
   c. Monitor for ventricular dysrhythmias
   d. Monitor for atrial dysrhythmias

8. A nurse in the pediatric unit is caring for an infant with heart failure. The nurse is instructed to administer digoxin orally once a day. In which of the following conditions should the nurse withhold the administration of digoxin?
   a. If BP falls more than 15 mm Hg
   b. If serum digoxin level is 0.8 ng/ml
   c. If child shows signs of hypotension
   d. If apical pulse is <90

9. A nurse is reviewing the medication order of a six-year-old child with Kawasaki disease. Which of the following medication orders aims to prevent coronary dilatation in Kawasaki disease?
   a. Aspirin followed by second dose of intravenous immunoglobulin
   b. High dose of aspirin in four divided doses
   c. Single intravenous immunoglobulin dose
   d. Pulsed-dose corticosteroids

10. A nurse is reviewing the CBC of a child in acute phase of Kawasaki disease. Which of the following findings would be expected?
    a. Elevated hematocrit
    b. Elevated RBC count
    c. Elevated platelets counts
    d. Elevated white blood cell count

11. The nurse is assessing the past medical history of an 11-month-old infant with a suspected cardiovascular disorder. Which of the following responses by the mother warrants further investigation?

   a. "I was on a low dose of lithium during pregnancy."

   b. "I had the flu during my last trimester."

   c. "I underwent many x-rays for a broken arm last month."

   d. "I have been using a strong cleaning product since last month."

12. The nurse is palpating the pulse of a child with suspected patent ductus arteriosus. Which of the following assessment findings would the nurse expect to note?

   a. Weak pulses in lower extremity

   b. Presence of bounding pulse

   c. Presence of chest pain similar to angina

   d. Dyspnea and cyanosis

13. The nurse is assessing the skin of a 12-year-old with suspected right ventricular heart failure. Which of the following findings would the nurse expect to note?

   a. Edema of the face

   b. Edema in the presacral region

   c. Edema of the lower extremities

   d. Edema of the hands

14. The nurse is auscultating heart sounds of a child with a mitral valve prolapse. Which assessment finding would the nurse expect?

   a. Abnormal splitting of S2 sounds

   b. Clicks on the upper left sternal border

   c. A mild to late ejection click at the apex

   d. Intensifying of S2 sounds

15. A nurse inspects the skin of a hypertensive client in the cardiology unit. Which of the following findings might the nurse note in the client?

   a. Malar rash

   b. Polymorphus rash

   c. Desquamation

   d. Erythema

Nursing Care of the Child With a Gastrointestinal Disorder

SECTION I: LEARNING OBJECTIVES

1. Compare the differences in the anatomy and physiology of the gastrointestinal system between children and adults.

2. Discuss common medical treatments for infants and children with gastrointestinal disorders.

3. Discuss common laboratory and diagnostic tests used to identify disorders of the gastrointestinal tract.

4. Discuss medication therapy used in infants and children with gastrointestinal disorders.

5. Recognize risk factors associated with various gastrointestinal illnesses.

6. Differentiate between acute and chronic gastrointestinal disorders.

7. Distinguish common gastrointestinal illnesses of childhood.

8. Discuss nursing interventions commonly used for gastrointestinal illnesses.

9. Devise an individualized nursing care plan for infants/children with a gastrointestinal disorder.

10. Develop teaching plans for family/patient education for children with gastrointestinal illnesses.

11. Describe the psychosocial impact that chronic gastrointestinal illnesses have on children.

SECTION II: ASSESSING YOUR UNDERSTANDING

Activity A *Fill in the blanks.*

1. The lower esophageal sphincter prevents _____ of stomach contents up into the esophagus and/or oral cavity.

2. _____ may occur in a child with undeveloped esophageal muscle tone, if edema or narrowing of the esophagus occurs.

3. Vomiting is a reflex with three different phases. The first phase is the prodromal period, the second phase is _____, and the third phase is vomiting.

4. Oral candidiasis is a _____ infection of the oral mucosa that appears as white patches in the mouth.

5. _____ is the presence of stones in the gallbladder.

6. _____ disorders that result in failure of the liver to function result in the need for liver transplantation.

7. Meckel's diverticulum is the result of an incomplete fusion of the _____ duct during embryonic development.

8. Early recognition and treatment of dehydration are critical to prevent progression to _____ shock.

9. _____ is either an increase in the frequency or a decrease in the consistency of stool.

10. In pyloric stenosis, the circular muscle of the _____ becomes hypertrophied.

Activity B *Consider the following figures.*

1. Label the locations of the ileostomy and colostomy shown in the image.

_____

_____

Activity C *Match the observations in Column A with their possible indications in Column B.*

Column A	Column B
____ 1. Distended veins on abdomen	a. Malfunction of liver
____ 2. Areas of ecchymosis	b. High abdominal obstruction or dehydration
____ 3. Icteric eyes	c. Abuse
____ 4. Depressed or concave abdomen	d. Abdominal or vascular obstruction or distention

Activity D *Briefly answer the following.*

1. Explain why infants are at particular risk for dehydration or overhydration.

_____

_____

_____

2. State a few ways to check hydration status.

_____

_____

_____

3. What is appendicitis? How can it be treated?

_____

_____

_____

4. What are the nursing interventions to help maintain appropriate nutrition in children with GI disorders?

_____

_____

_____

5. What is intussusception? How can it be treated?

_____

_____

_____

6. What is GERD?

_____

_____

_____

SECTION III: APPLYING YOUR KNOWLEDGE

Activity E *Consider this scenario and answer the questions.*

1. A nurse is caring for a mother who had delivered a baby with a cleft lip and palate. The anomaly in the infant was unexpected for both parents. The craniofacial team repaired the cleft after some days with facial suture lines.

   a. The nurse observes that the parents find the appearance of the repaired cleft with suture lines appalling. How can the nurse encourage infant-parent bonding?

   _____

   _____

   _____

   b. The nurse sees the need to educate the parents regarding how to prevent injury to the facial suture line and to the palatal operative sites. What measures can the nurse ask the parents to follow?

   _____

   _____

   _____

SECTION IV: PRACTICING FOR NCLEX

Activity F *Answer the following questions.*

1. A nurse is conducting a physical examination for a one-year-old child. Being able to palpate which of the following would need a follow-up?
   a. Liver
   b. Kidneys
   c. Sigmoid colon
   d. Cecum

2. A nurse is interacting with the parents of a two-year-old child using an ostomy pouch following surgery for a gastrointestinal disorder. Which of the following statements indicates a need for further teaching?
   a. "We tie the ostomy pouch loosely around the stoma to prevent irritation."
   b. "We avoid tight or constricting clothing around his stoma site."
   c. "We use powder to protect his skin around the ostomy site."
   d. "We empty the ostomy pouch several times a day."

3. A nurse is caring for a toddler with diarrhea. Which of the following interventions should the nurse perform?
   a. Maintain a clear liquid diet for 24 hours
   b. Encourage milk products
   c. Avoid complex carbohydrate foods
   d. Avoid fatty foods

4. A nurse is interacting with the parents of a child who is to be provided oral rehydration therapy due to moderate dehydration resulting from vomiting. Which of the following statements indicates need for intervention?
   a. "We will withhold oral feeding for one to two hours after his vomiting."
   b. "We can give him candied ginger in case he feels nauseous."
   c. "We can give him things like milk and soup for oral rehydration."
   d. "We want him to resume a regular diet once he is rehydrated."

5. Which of the following is a feature of Crohn's disease?

   a. Continuous distribution of the affected area, distal to proximal

   b. X-ray reveals superficial colitis

   c. Total colon affected

   d. Anorexia

6. A nurse is talking to a mother of a one-month-old boy diagnosed with gastroesophageal reflux disease. Which of the following statements made by the mother would necessitate intervention?

   a. "I should give him smaller, more frequent feedings."

   b. "I should frequently burp him during feedings."

   c. "I can thicken the formula with oatmeal cereal."

   d. "I should keep the crib flat."

7. The parents of a child diagnosed with celiac disease want to know about its treatment. Which of the following would be the best response regarding the treatment?

   a. "Medication and regular exercise can increase his immunity against celiac disease."

   b. "Immunization injections at periodic intervals should help him."

   c. "The only current treatment for celiac disease is a strict gluten-free diet."

   d. "You should restrict intake of gluten until he is an adolescent."

8. A mother of a child with oral candidiasis (thrush) is curious about the factors that could have led to it. Which of the following should the nurse mention as the risk factors that can contribute to thrush? Select all that apply.

   a. Immune disorders

   b. Excessive intake of formula

   c. Use of corticosteroid inhalers

   d. Use of antibiotics

   e. Excessive vomiting

9. A father presents to the clinic with a very ill child. Which of the following assessment findings can strongly suggest the occurrence of intussusception to the nurse? Select all that apply.

   a. Sudden onset of intermittent, crampy abdominal pain

   b. Abdominal distention

   c. Vomiting

   d. Tachycardia

   e. Severe pain

10. A nurse is referring to the health history documented for a client. The mention of which of the following can indicate gastroesophageal reflux disease (GERD)? Select all that apply.

    a. Chest pains

    b. Explosive stools

    c. Halitosis

    d. Poor dentition

    e. Rectal bleeding

11. Which of the following are causes of short bowel syndrome? Select all that apply.

    a. Stretched rectal vault

    b. Lack of ganglion cells in the bowel

    c. Necrotizing enterocolitis

    d. Small intestinal atresia

    e. Gastroschisis

12. Which of the following can a nurse expect during the clinical presentation of a child with autoimmune hepatitis? Select all that apply.

    a. Jaundice

    b. Abdominal distention

    c. Hepatosplenomegaly

    d. Right upper quadrant pain

    e. Steatorrhea

13. Which of the following tests helps determine bleeding in the GI tract?

    a. Endoscopic retrograde cholangiopancreatography (ERCP)

    b. Esophageal manometry

    c. Hemoccult

    d. Small bowel series with upper GI series

14. A nurse is caring for a six-year-old boy with fluid deficit due to excessive losses through vomiting. Which of the following measures should the nurse take to maintain his fluid balance?

   a. Offering large amounts of oral rehydration solution every three hours

   b. Reintroducing regular diet when symptoms have lessened or resolved

   c. Encouraging high-carbohydrate fluids

   d. Encouraging fluids and milk products that contain high levels of sugar

15. Parents of a two-year-old boy with a small umbilical hernia ask a nurse for the best approach to treatment. Which of the following is the ideal response by the nurse?

   a. "An immediate surgical correction is required."

   b. "I will need to assess if the hernia can be reduced."

   c. "A few home remedies can easily reduce the hernia."

   d. "Belly bands should be used to reduce the hernia."

Nursing Care of the Child With a Genitourinary Disorder

SECTION I: LEARNING OBJECTIVES

1. Compare the anatomic and physiologic differences of the genitourinary system in infants and children versus adults.

2. Describe nursing care related to common laboratory and diagnostic testing used in the medical diagnosis of pediatric genitourinary conditions.

3. Distinguish the genitourinary disorders common in infants, children, and adolescents.

4. Identify appropriate nursing assessments and interventions related to medications and treatments for the pediatric genitourinary disorders.

5. Develop an individualized nursing care plan for the children with genitourinary disorder.

6. Describe the psychosocial impact of chronic genitourinary disorders on children.

7. Devise a nutrition plan for the child with renal insufficiency.

8. Develop patient/family teaching plans for the child with a genitourinary disorder.

SECTION II: ASSESSING YOUR UNDERSTANDING

Activity A *Fill in the blanks.*

1. Cytotoxic drugs cause bone marrow _____.

2. _____ refers to the stoma in the abdominal wall to the bladder.

3. *Escherichia coli* is usually found in the perineal and anal region, close to the _____ opening.

4. A voiding _____ is performed to determine the presence of a structural defect that may be causing hydronephrosis.

5. _____ disorders are the most frequent cause of hypertension in children.

6. The decrease in protein and albumin in the bloodstream is called _____.

7. Acute _____ is a condition in which immune processes injure the glomeruli.

8. _____ is a method by which the amount of protein in the urine can be monitored.

9. _____ dialysis uses the child's abdominal cavity as a semipermeable membrane to help remove excess fluid and waste products.

10. _____ is the removal of the excess foreskin of the penis.

Activity B *Consider the following figures.*

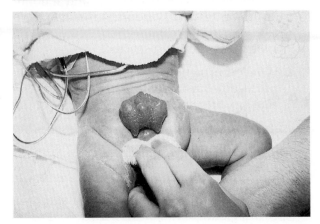

1. What does the figure depict?

_____

_____

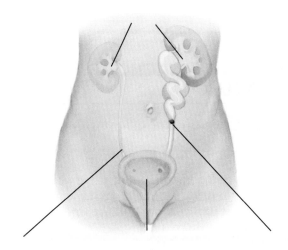

2. Label the figure and identify the type of genitourinary disorder.

_____

_____

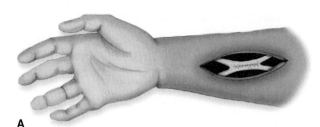

A

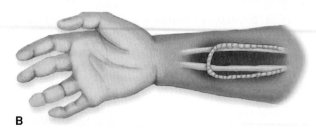

B

3. Identify the figure.

_____

_____

Activity C *Match the terms in Column A with their definitions in Column B.*

Column A

____ **1.** Proteinuria

____ **2.** Anasarca

____ **3.** Cystitis

____ **4.** Pyelonephritis

____ **5.** Hyperlipidemia

Column B

a. Severe generalized edema

b. Lower urinary tract infection

c. Elevated lipid levels in bloodstream

d. Upper urinary tract infection

e. Excess loss of protein in urine

Activity D *Put the items in correct sequence by writing the letters in the boxes provided below.*

1. The procedure of double diapering is given below in random steps. Choose the correct sequence.

a. Unfold both diapers and place the smaller diaper inside the larger one.

b. Cut a hole or a cross-slit in the front of the smaller diaper

c. Carefully bring the penis and catheter/stent together through the hole in the smaller diaper and close the diaper.

d. Place both diapers under the child.

e. Close the larger diaper, making sure the tip of the catheter is inside the larger diaper.

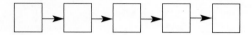

Activity E *Briefly answer the following.*

1. What are the key nursing implications following cystoscopy?

_____

_____

_____

2. What is vesicoureteral reflux?

_____

_____

_____

3. What is hydronephrosis?

_____

_____

_____

4. What are various types of enuresis?

_____

_____

_____

5. What medications/supplements are commonly used to treat the complications of end-stage renal disease?

_____

_____

_____

6. What are hydrocele and varicocele?

_____

_____

_____

SECTION III: APPLYING YOUR KNOWLEDGE

Activity F *Consider this scenario and answer the questions.*

1. Kevin, a four-year-old, is brought to the clinic by his mother. He has had fatigue and abdominal pain for the past 12 hours. A throat culture confirms streptococcal infection. Acute glomerulonephritis is suspected.

a. What other signs and symptoms should a nurse look out for that may help confirm acute glomerulonephritis?

_____

_____

_____

b. Kevin is diagnosed with acute post-streptococcal glomerulonephritis (APSGN). What interventions can the nurse perform when caring for Kevin?

_____

_____

_____

SECTION IV: PRACTICING FOR NCLEX

Activity G *Answer the following questions.*

1. The nurse is caring for a ten-year-old girl presenting with fever, dysuria, flank pain, urgency, and hematuria. The nurse would expect to help obtain which of the following tests first to reveal preliminary information about the urinary tract?

a. Total protein, globulin, and albumin

b. Creatinine clearance

c. Urinalysis

d. Urine culture and sensitivity

2. The nurse is administering cyclophos-phamide as ordered for a ten-year-old boy with nephrotic syndrome. Which of the following instructions is most accurate regarding administration of this cytotoxic drug?

   a. Check for allergy before administering the drug

   b. Monitor for signs of precocious puberty in the client

   c. Encourage fluids and voiding during and after administration

   d. Preferably administer the drug at bedtime

3. A two-year-old boy is brought to the health care facility with complaints of bedwetting. On interviewing the mother, the nurse learns that the child had previously demonstrated bladder control over a period of six consecutive months but has again become incontinent. Which of the following categories of enuresis should the nurse note?

   a. Primary enuresis

   b. Secondary enuresis

   c. Diurnal enuresis

   d. Nocturnal enuresis

4. The nurse is assessing an infant with suspected hemolytic-uremic syndrome. Which of the following characteristics of this condition would the nurse expect to assess, including information from the chart review?

   a. Hemolytic anemia, acute renal failure, and hypotension

   b. Dirty green-colored urine, elevated erythrocyte sedimentation rate, and depressed serum complement level

   c. Hemolytic anemia, thrombocytopenia, and acute renal failure

   d. Thrombocytopenia, hemolytic anemia, and nocturia several times each night

5. The nurse is caring for a child who receives hemodialysis treatment via an AV fistula. Which of the following findings indicates an immediate need to notify the physician?

   a. Absence of a bruit

   b. Presence of a thrill

   c. Dialysate without fibrin or cloudiness

   d. Alterations in blood pressure

6. A nurse is caring for a thirteen-year-old boy with end-stage renal disease who is preparing to have his hemodialysis treatment in the dialysis unit. Which of the following is the appropriate nursing action?

   a. Allow liberal diet and intake of fluid

   b. Take his blood pressure measurement in the extremity with the AV fistula

   c. Withhold his routine medication until after dialysis is completed

   d. Assess the Tenckhoff catheter site

7. A nurse is caring for a child with acute glomerulonephritis. The nephrologist instructs the nurse to administer Lasix to the client. Which of the following measures should the nurse consider when administering Lasix?

   a. Monitor renal function and electrolytes

   b. Monitor for hyperkalemia

   c. Monitor for the development of pulmonary edema

   d. Monitor for the signs of infection

8. A nurse caring for a client with end-stage renal disease is required to send the client's blood sample for testing serum calcium levels. Which of the following should the nurse be aware of when drawing blood for serum calcium?

   a. Ensure that the child is NPO from midnight till morning

   b. Avoid prolonged use of a tourniquet

   c. Obtain a culture specimen before the test

   d. Ensure that the child has a full bladder

9. Upon examination of a newborn, the nurse notes that the baby's urethral opening is on the dorsal surface of the penis. Which of the following terms describes the condition?

   a. Hydronephrosis

   b. Bladder exstrophy

   c. Hypospadias

   d. Epispadias

10. A nurse is caring for a three-year-old child with nephrotic syndrome. The nurse collects the current and past medical history to elicit the risk factors for nephrotic syndrome. Which of the following should the nurse include as a risk factor for nephrotic syndrome?

   a. Prune belly syndrome

   b. Chromosome abnormalities

   c. Neurogenic bladder

   d. History of intrauterine growth retardation

11. A nurse is preparing discharge teaching for a 14-year-old girl admitted to the health care facility with a urinary tract infection. Which of the following measures should the nurse include to help prevent recurrence of urinary tract infection?

   a. Use bubble bath to soothe perineum

   b. Wear cotton underwear to prevent perineal irritation

   c. Wipe from back to front after voiding

   d. Hold the urine from time to time

12. A nurse is newly posted to the surgical unit. Which of the following genitourinary conditions should the nurse consider a surgical emergency?

   a. Testicular torsion

   b. Hydrocele

   c. Phimosis

   d. Varicocele

13. The nurse is caring for a child with renal failure predisposed to developing hypocalcemia. Which of the following signs of hypocalcemia should the nurse monitor for?

   a. Muscle weakness

   b. Abdominal cramps

   c. Muscle twitching

   d. Irregular pulse

14. A nurse is caring for a 12-year-old girl with vulvovaginitis. Which of the following signs indicate that the child has *Trichomonas vaginalis* infection?

   a. White cottage-cheese-like discharge

   b. Thin gray discharge

   c. Yellowish-gray discharge

   d. Brownish-green discharge

15. The nurse is preparing a child for a voiding cystourethrogram. Which of the following conditions is an indication for this procedure?

   a. Vesicoureteral reflux

   b. Urinary outlet obstruction

   c. Kidney tumor

   d. Hydronephrosis

CHAPTER 43

Nursing Care of the Child With a Neuromuscular Disorder

SECTION I: LEARNING OBJECTIVES

1. Compare differences between the anatomy and physiology of the neuromuscular system in children versus adults.

2. Identify nursing interventions related to common laboratory and diagnostic tests used in the diagnosis and management of neuromuscular conditions.

3. Identify appropriate nursing assessments and interventions related to medications and treatments used for childhood neuromuscular conditions.

4. Distinguish various neuromuscular illnesses occurring in childhood.

5. Devise an individualized nursing care plan for the child with a neuromuscular disorder.

6. Develop patient/family teaching plans for the child with a neuromuscular disorder.

7. Describe the psychosocial impact of chronic neuromuscular disorders on the growth and development of children.

SECTION II: ASSESSING YOUR UNDERSTANDING

Activity A *Fill in the blanks.*

1. Dermatomyositis is an _____ disease that results in inflammation of the muscles or associated tissues.

2. Lack of use of extremities leads to muscular _____.

3. Muscular _____ refers to a group of inherited conditions that result in progressive muscle weakness and wasting.

4. As the muscles deteriorate from muscular dystrophy, joints may become fixated, resulting in _____.

5. Children with myelomeningocele often have a _____ bladder, which causes incontinence.

6. Spina bifida occulta is a defect of the spinal cord that is usually present in the _____ area.

7. _____, the less serious form of spina bifida cystica, occurs when the meninges herniate through a defect in the vertebrae.

8. The use of _____ may slow the progression of Duchenne muscular dystrophy.

9. Braces may be used in young children with cerebral palsy to combat _____.

10. _____ is a type of brain damage that may result from neonatal hyperbilirubinemia.

Activity B *Consider the following figures.*

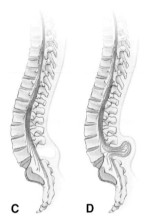

C   D

1. Identify the types of neural defects shown in the images.

_____

_____

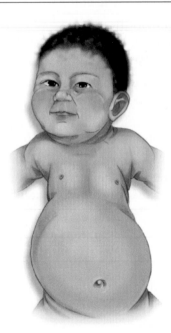

2. Identify the neuromuscular disorder shown in the figure.

_____

_____

Activity C *Match the diagnostic test in Column A with its proper definition in Column B.*

Column A

_____ 1. Muscle biopsy

_____ 2. Dystrophin

_____ 3. Myelography

_____ 4. Creatine kinase

_____ 5. Fluoroscopy

Column B

a. A normal intracellular plasma membrane protein in the muscle

b. Removal of a piece of tissue with a needle

c. X-ray study of the spinal cord

d. Radiographic examination that uses continuous x-rays to show live, real-time images

e. Reflects muscle damage

Activity D *Put the items in correct sequence by writing the letters in the boxes provided below.*

1. Given below, in random order, are the actions exhibited in Gowers' sign by children with Duchenne muscular dystrophy. Choose the correct order of actions.

   a. The child uses his hands to walk up the legs to assume an upright position

   b. The child uses hands to support some of his weight, while raising the posterior

   c. The child rolls onto his hands and knees

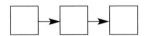

Activity E *Briefly answer the following.*

1. What are the four classifications of cerebral palsy? Which is the most common form? Which is the rarest form?

_____

_____

_____

2. What are the appropriate nursing management focuses for a child with myelomeningocele?

_____

_____

_____

3. What are three common symptoms of Guillain-Barre Syndrome (GBS)? How can the nurse assess for respiratory deterioration?

_____

_____

_____

4. What are the tests used in the diagnosis of muscular dystrophy?

_____

_____

_____

5. What are the risk factors for myelomeningocele?

_____

_____

_____

6. What are the perinatal causes of cerebral palsy?

_____

_____

_____

SECTION III: APPLYING YOUR KNOWLEDGE

Activity F *Consider this scenario and answer the questions.*

1. Elijah Jefferson, a two-year-old boy, was recently diagnosed with cerebral palsy. He was born at 28 weeks' gestation after a complicated and prolonged delivery. Elijah's parents have many questions and concerns about their son's diagnosis. They ask, "Can Elijah outgrow this disorder with proper physical and occupational therapy?"

a. How can you help Elijah's parents to have an accurate perception of cerebral palsy?

_____

_____

_____

b. What are some assessment findings on examination that are characteristic of cerebral palsy (CP)?

_____

_____

_____

c. Discuss the focus of nursing management when caring for a child with cerebral palsy.

_____

_____

_____

SECTION IV: PRACTICING FOR NCLEX

Activity G *Answer the following questions.*

1. The nurse is conducting a physical examination of a nine-month-old baby with a suspected neuromuscular disorder. Which of the following findings would warrant further evaluation?

a. Presence of symmetrical spontaneous movement

b. Slightly flexed resting posture

c. Absence of tonic neck reflex

d. Presence of Moro reflex

2. The nurse is conducting a wellness examination of a six-month-old child. The mother points out some dimpling and skin discoloration in the child's lumbosacral area. How should the nurse respond?

a. "This could be an indicator of spina bifida; we need to evaluate this further."

b. "This can be considered a normal variant with no adverse effects; however, the physician will want to take a closer look."

c. "Dimpling, skin discoloration, and abnormal patches of hair are often indicators of spina bifida occulta."

d. "This is often an indicator of spina bifida occulta as opposed to spina bifida cystica."

3. A nurse is caring for an infant with a meningocele. Which of the following would alert the nurse that the lesion is increasing in size?

a. Leaking cerebrospinal fluid

b. Increasing intracranial pressure

c. Constipation and bladder dysfunction

d. Increasing head circumference

4. A nurse is teaching the parents of a boy with a neurogenic bladder about clean intermittent catheterization. Which of the following responses indicates a need for further teaching?

a. "We must be careful to use latex-free catheters."

b. "The very first step is to apply water-based lubricant to the catheter."

c. "My son may someday learn how to do this for himself."

d. "We need to soak the catheter in a vinegar and water solution each week."

5. At a well-child checkup of a three-year-old the mother mentions that her son was late in learning to walk and now "has difficulty climbing stairs." The nurse would know that these are common findings in a child with Duchenne muscular dystrophy, and she would assess the child for what hallmark finding of DMD?

a. Inability to rise from floor in standard fashion

b. Smaller-than-normal calf muscles

c. Signs of hydrocephalus

d. Lordosis

6. The nurse is caring for a five-year-old child with Guillain-Barre Syndrome (GBS). Which of the following would be the best way to assess the level of paralysis?

a. Gentle tickling

b. Observe for symmetrical flaccid weakness

c. Monitor for ataxia

d. Inquire about sensory disturbances

7. The nurse is providing presurgical care for a newborn with myelomeningocele. Which of the following is the central nursing priority?

a. Maintain the infant's body temperature

b. Prevent rupture or leaking of cerebrospinal fluid

c. Maintain the infant in the prone position

d. Keep the lesion free from fecal matter or urine

8. A nurse is caring for a 13-year-old boy with Duchenne muscular dystrophy affecting the lower extremities. Which of the following should the nurse suggest to maximize the child's quality of life? Select all that apply.

a. Ensure long periods of bed rest

b. Avoid any kind of sport

c. Use a wheelchair for mobility

d. Participate in computer activities

e. Avoid overexertion

9. A nurse is assessing a child with athetoid cerebral palsy. Which of the following characteristics should the nurse assess for in the child?

a. Hypertonicity of affected extremities

b. Continuation of primitive reflexes

c. Uncontrolled writhing movements

d. Exaggeration of deep tendon reflexes

10. A nurse is caring for a child with cerebral palsy. Which of the following may be used to maintain muscle strength in the child?

a. Braces

b. Splinting

c. Serial casting

d. Walkers

11. A nurse is performing a physical assessment of an infant with cerebral palsy. Which of the following should the nurse note during assessment?

a. Relaxed anal sphincter

b. Lack of response to touch and pain stimuli

c. Absence of deep tendon reflexes

d. Scissor-crossing of legs with plantarflexion

12. A nurse is caring for a child with a high cervical injury sustained in a car accident. Which of the following should the nurse know is a result of high cervical injury?

a. Neurogenic bladder

b. Inability to breathe without assistance

c. Muscle weakness and wasting

d. Paradoxical breathing

13. The pediatric nurse is taking report on a client with type 1 SMA (spinal muscular atrophy). The nurse knows that the priority nursing action for this child is which of the following?

    a. Proper positioning to promote support of spine

    b. Maintaining adequate nutrition

    c. Promoting pulmonary function

    d. Promoting mobility

14. The pediatric nurse is planning discharge teaching for a 14-year-old girl diagnosed with dermatomyositis and her family. The nurse knows to include which of the following in the discharge teaching?

    a. Importance of participating in physical activities, especially while the disease is active

    b. Importance of maintaining medication regimen in order to prevent calcinosis and joint deformity

    c. Importance of knowing side effects of anticholinergics and IV IgG

    d. Importance of appropriate stress management and avoidance of extreme temperatures

15. A nurse is educating the parents of a child with cerebral palsy who has had a baclofen pump implanted to manage spasticity. Which of the following postoperative instructions should the nurse provide the parents?

    a. Have the pump refilled with medication every month

    b. Get the pump replaced in a year

    c. Limit activity in your child and encourage bed rest

    d. Complications include infection, rupture, dislodgement, or blockage of catheter

CHAPTER 44

Nursing Care of the Child With a Musculoskeletal Disorder

SECTION I: LEARNING OBJECTIVES

1. Compare the anatomy and physiology of the musculoskeletal system in children versus adults.

2. Identify nursing interventions related to common laboratory and diagnostic tests used in the diagnosis and management of musculoskeletal disorders.

3. Identify appropriate nursing assessments and interventions related to medications and treatments for common childhood musculoskeletal disorders.

4. Distinguish various musculoskeletal disorders occurring in childhood.

5. Devise an individualized nursing care plan for the child with a musculoskeletal disorder.

6. Develop patient/family teaching plans for the child with a musculoskeletal disorder.

7. Describe the impact of chronic musculoskeletal disorders on the growth and development of children.

SECTION II: ASSESSING YOUR UNDERSTANDING

Activity A *Fill in the blanks.*

1. _____ and conversion of cartilage to bone continue throughout childhood and are complete at adolescence.

2. _____ are used to immobilize a bone that has been injured or a diseased joint.

3. _____ analgesics act on receptors in the brain to alter perception of pain.

4. _____ is the x-ray of a joint after direct injection with a radiopaque substance.

5. _____ is the presence of extra digits on the hand and foot.

6. _____ refers to an acetabulum that is shallow or sloping instead of cup-shaped.

7. _____ results from tightness of the sternocleidomastoid muscle, resulting in the infant's head being tilted to one side.

8. _____ disorders in which fat absorption is altered may lead to rickets, because vitamin D is a fat-soluble vitamin.

9. _____ is a lateral curvature of the spine that exceeds 10 degrees.

10. _____ result from a twisting or turning motion of the affected body part and often take as long as a fracture to heal.

Activity B *Consider the following figure.*

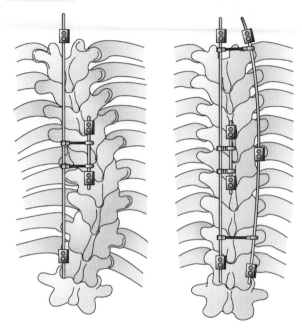

1. What does the figure demonstrate?

_____

_____

Activity C *Match the common medical treatments used in musculoskeletal disorders listed in Column A with their proper descriptions in Column B.*

Column A

_____ **1.** Fixation

_____ **2.** Splinting

_____ **3.** Casting

_____ **4.** Traction

Column B

a. Application of plaster or fiberglass material to form a rigid apparatus to immobilize a body part

b. Temporary stiff support of injured area

c. Surgical reduction of a fracture or skeletal deformity with an internal or external pin or fixation device

d. Application of a pulling force on an extremity or body part

Activity D *Put the items in correct sequence by writing the letters in the boxes provided below.*

1. Given below, in random order, are steps involved in petaling a cast. Choose the correct sequence.

a. Round one end of each strip

b. Apply the first strip by tucking the straight end inside the cast and by bringing the rounded end over the cast edge to the outside

c. Cut several strips of adhesive tape three to four inches in length

d. Repeat the procedure, overlapping each additional strip, until all rough edges are completely covered

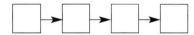

Activity E *Briefly answer the following.*

1. What are pectus excavatum and pectus carinatum?

_____

_____

_____

2. How is clubfoot classified?

_____

_____

_____

3. What treatment is given for the child with rickets?

_____

_____

_____

4. How is osteomyelitis acquired?

_____

_____

_____

5. Children in which age group are mostly affected with transient synovitis?

_____

_____

_____

6. What are the usual laboratory findings in case of septic arthritis?

_____

_____

_____

SECTION III: APPLYING YOUR KNOWLEDGE

Activity F _Consider this scenario and answer the questions._

1. One-year-old Oliver Harn is brought to the clinic by his mother. Oliver fell down while attempting to stand up on his own; this resulted in a fracture. He is diagnosed with osteogenesis imperfecta, following a skin biopsy.

a. What assessments should the nurse perform for Oliver, who is diagnosed with osteogenesis imperfecta?

_____

_____

_____

b. What measures can the nurse teach Oliver's parents to prevent injuries?

_____

_____

_____

SECTION IV: PRACTICING FOR NCLEX

Activity G _Answer the following questions._

1. A nurse is conducting a physical examination of an infant with suspected metatarsus adductus. Which of the following findings would indicate type II metatarsus adductus?

a. Forefoot is inverted and turned slightly upward

b. Forefoot is flexible past neutral actively and passively

c. Forefoot is flexible passively past neutral, but only to midline actively

d. Forefoot is rigid and does not correct to midline even with passive stretching

2. A nurse is reviewing the laboratory investigation report of a 12-year-old diagnosed with rickets. Which of the following should the nurse expect?

a. Elevated alkaline phosphatase levels

b. Elevated white blood cell count

c. Elevated erythrocyte sedimentation rate

d. Elevated C-reactive protein level

3. The nurse is conducting a routine physical examination of a newborn. Which of the following findings would point to a possible abnormal developmental variation?

a. Asymmetry of thigh or gluteal folds

b. Internal tibial torsion

c. In-toeing of feet

d. Genu varum

4. A nurse is providing instructions for home cast care. Which of the following responses from the mother indicates a need for further teaching?

a. "We must avoid causing depressions in the cast."

b. "Pale, cool, or blue skin coloration is to be expected."

c. "The casted arm must be kept still."

d. "We need to be aware of odor or drainage from the cast."

5. The nurse is providing postoperative care for a boy who has undergone surgical correction for pectus excavatum. The nurse should emphasize which of the following to the child and his parents?

a. "Please watch for signs of infection."

b. "Be sure to monitor his vital capacity."

c. "Do not allow him to lie on either side."

d. "You may log-roll the child if necessary."

6. The nurse is caring for a five-month-old girl diagnosed with developmental dysplasia of the hip (DDH). The mother is anxious about the treatment of the condition. Which of the following would best address the mother's concerns?

   a. "Your baby would require skeletal traction."
   b. "Your baby will likely wear a Pavlik harness."
   c. "Your baby might be required to wear a spica cast."
   d. "Your baby might require an open surgical reduction."

7. The nurse is conducting a physical examination of a newborn with suspected osteogenesis imperfecta (OI). Which of the following is a common finding?

   a. Inversion of the heel
   b. Medial deviation of the forefoot
   c. Extra digits on the hand
   d. Blue sclera

8. A nurse is instructed to administer a Ketorolac tablet twice a day to a client who has undergone open reduction internal fixation of the left tibia. Which of the following side effects of the drug should the nurse look for?

   a. Heart burn
   b. Constipation
   c. Abdominal discomfort
   d. Regurgitation

9. A nurse is preparing a client for cast removal. Which of the following signs should the nurse consider as normal after the removal of a cast?

   a. Brown, flaky skin
   b. Skin coolness
   c. Prolonged capillary refill
   d. Pale or blue skin

10. A nurse is caring for a client who has a cervical skin traction applied with a skin strap. Which of the following is an important nursing intervention in this case?

    a. Ensure the ankle and heel are free from pressure
    b. Remove the traction every eight hours to assess skin

    c. Ensure the head halter does not place pressure on the ear
    d. Maintain elbow flexed at 90 degrees

11. A child is put on balanced suspension traction for a femur fracture. What should the nurse's monitoring of the child include?

    a. Avoiding pressure to popliteal area
    b. Ensuring that the leg is slightly abducted
    c. Assessing the fingers and hands for coolness
    d. Ensuring proper replacement of sling

12. A nurse is reviewing the laboratory reports of a five-year-old client with septic arthritis. Which of the following laboratory findings should the nurse expect in the client?

    a. Elevated C-reactive protein
    b. Decreased erythrocyte sedimentation rate
    c. Decreased white blood cell count
    d. Elevated neutrophil count

13. A nurse is collecting history from a seven-year-old boy suspected of having Osgood-Schlatter disease. Which of the following symptoms should the nurse expect to find?

    a. Tenderness in the proximal humerus
    b. Pain over the posterior aspect of calcaneus
    c. Painful swelling in the anterior portion of the tibial tubercle
    d. Pain in the anterior aspect of the middle part of the lower leg

14. A nurse is caring for a child with a Pavlik harness. Which of the following is an important nursing intervention for the child?

    a. Change the diaper with the baby in the harness
    b. Do not wash the harness
    c. Place clothes under the harness
    d. Do not place the child to sleep on the back

15. A nurse is assessing a six-year-old child admitted with rickets. Which of the following is a risk factor for rickets?

    a. Chronic renal disease
    b. Renal osteodystrophy
    c. Orthogenesis imperfecta
    d. Infected varicella lesions

CHAPTER 45

Nursing Care of the Child With an Integumentary Disorder

SECTION I: LEARNING OBJECTIVES

1. Compare anatomic and physiologic differences of the integumentary system in infants and children versus adults.

2. Describe nursing care related to common laboratory and diagnostic tests used in the medical diagnosis of integumentary disorders in infants, children, and adolescents.

3. Distinguish integumentary disorders common in infants, children, and adolescents.

4. Identify appropriate nursing assessments and interventions related to pediatric integumentary disorders.

5. Develop an individualized nursing care plan for the child with an integumentary disorder.

6. Describe the psychosocial impact of a chronic integumentary disorder on children or adolescents.

7. Develop patient/family teaching plans for the child with an integumentary disorder.

SECTION II: ASSESSING YOUR UNDERSTANDING

Activity A *Fill in the blanks.*

1. Diaper-wearing _____ the skin's pH, activating fecal enzymes; this further contributes to skin maceration.

2. Levels of serum _____ may be elevated in the child with atopic dermatitis.

3. _____ is a chronic inflammatory dermatitis that may occur on the skin or scalp. In infants it occurs most often on the scalp and is commonly referred to as cradle cap.

4. Acne neonatorum occurs as a response to the presence of maternal _____.

5. _____ is a localized infection and inflammation of the skin and subcutaneous tissue and is usually preceded by skin trauma.

6. Tinea _____ is a fungal disease of the skin more noticeable in the summer with tanning of unaffected areas; it is known by its oval scaly lesions, especially on the upper back, chest, and proximal arms.

7. _____ is a chronic skin disease with periods of remission and exacerbation, characterized by hyperproliferation of the epidermis, with a rash developing at sites of mechanical, thermal, or physical trauma.

8. Common sites of pressure ulcers in hospitalized children include the occiput and
_____.

9. _____ burns involve only epidermal injury and usually heal without scarring within four to five days.

10. _____ occurs as a result of overexposure to the ultraviolet rays of the sun.

Activity B *Consider the following figures.*

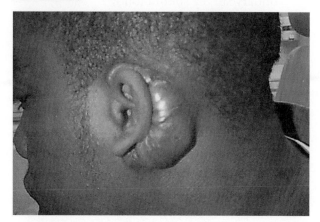

1. What is the integumentary disorder shown in the figure?

_____

_____

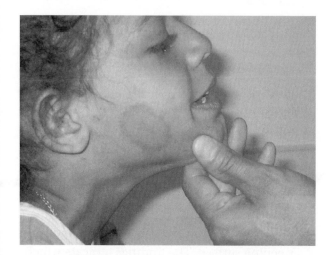

2. Identify the integumentary disorder shown in the figure.

_____

_____

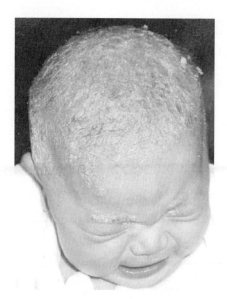

3. What does the figure show?

_____

_____

Activity C *Match the medications in Column A with their integumentary indications in Column B.*

Column A	Column B
____ **1.** Silver sulfadiazine	**a.** Psoriasis, atopic dermatitis
____ **2.** Isotretinoin	**b.** Cystic acne
____ **3.** Coal tar preparations	**c.** 1% Burns
____ **4.** Benzoyl peroxide	**d.** Mild acne vulgaris

Activity D *Put the items in correct sequence by writing the letters in the boxes provided below.*

1. Following are the steps for emergency assessment of a burned child. Arrange the steps in correct sequence.

a. Assess the child's airway

b. Determine the pulse strength, perfusion status, and heart rate

c. Determine the extent and depth of the wound

d. Evaluate the child's skin color, respiratory effort, symmetry of breathing, and breath sounds

☐ → ☐ → ☐ → ☐

Activity E *Briefly answer the following.*

1. What are the cutaneous reactions commonly found in dark-skinned children compared to children with lighter skin?

_____

_____

_____

2. What are the differences between bullous impetigo and nonbullous impetigo?

_____

_____

3. What is the therapeutic management of atopic dermatitis?

_____

_____

_____

4. What are the risk factors for development of pressure ulcers in children?

_____

_____

_____

5. How are burns classified?

_____

_____

_____

6. What precautions should be observed to prevent frostbite?

_____

_____

_____

SECTION III: APPLYING YOUR KNOWLEDGE

Activity F *Consider this scenario and answer the questions.*

1. Billy Cabot, a five-year-old, is brought to the clinic by his mother for an emergency exami-

nation. He was burned by a fire accident in their garage.

a. What are the steps a nurse conducting a primary survey should follow?

_____

_____

_____

b. What are the steps a nurse conducting a secondary survey should follow?

_____

_____

_____

c. Billy is at risk for deficient fluid volume due to the burns. What are the interventions a nurse can take to promote fluid balance?

_____

_____

_____

SECTION IV: PRACTICING FOR NCLEX

Activity G *Answer the following questions.*

1. The nurse is conducting a primary survey of a child with burns. Which of the following assessment findings points to airway injury from burn or smoke inhalation?

a. Cervical spine injury

b. Internal traumatic injuries

c. Presence of stridor

d. Red, dry lesions on the abdomen

2. The nurse is caring for a ten-month-old infant with a rash. The child's mother reports that the onset was abrupt. The nurse assesses diffuse erythema and skin tenderness with ruptured bullae in the axillary area with a red weeping surface. The findings indicate which of the following bacterial infections?

a. Cellulitis

b. Folliculitis

c. Scalded skin syndrome

d. Bullous impetigo

3. A nurse is teaching methods to promote skin hydration to the parents of an infant with atopic dermatitis. Which of the following responses indicates a need for further teaching?

   a. "We need to avoid skin products containing perfumes or fragrances."

   b. "We should use a mild soap like unscented Dove for sensitive skin."

   c. "We should use soap to clean only dirty areas of the body."

   d. "We should bathe our child in hot water, twice a day, to prevent itching."

4. A nurse is caring for a child with tinea pedis. Which of the following assessment findings would the nurse expect to note?

   a. Red scaling rash on soles and between the toes

   b. Patches of scaling on the scalp with central hair loss

   c. Inflamed boggy mass on scalp, filled with pustules

   d. Erythema, scaling, and maceration in the inguinal creases

5. The nurse is conducting the physical examination of a nine-month-old boy diagnosed with erythema multiforme. Which of the following assessment findings would the nurse expect to note?

   a. Hypopigmented, oval, scaly lesions on upper back and chest and proximal arms

   b. Silvery or yellow-white scale plaques and sharply demarcated borders

   c. Thick or flaky greasy yellow scales on the neck and trunk area

   d. Lesions over the extensor surfaces of the extremities with spread to the trunk

6. A two-year-old girl is brought to the health care facility following a wasp sting. What is the priority nursing intervention?

   a. Remove jewelry or restrictive clothing

   b. Apply ice intermittently on the affected area

   c. Administer diphenhydramine as per protocol

   d. Cleanse the wound with mild soap and water

7. The nurse observes blistering with erythema and edema when assessing a child for frostbite. What degree of frostbite does it indicate?

   a. First degree

   b. Second degree

   c. Third degree

   d. Fourth degree

8. A nurse is caring for a child with tinea capitis. The physician prescribes Griseofulvin for the child. Which of the following interventions should the nurse consider when caring for the child?

   a. Monitor for Cushing syndrome

   b. Give the medicine along with fatty food

   c. Monitor for suicidal risk

   d. Taper the medication doses before stopping

9. A nurse is caring for a two-year-old child who is hospitalized for a long time and is at risk of developing pressure ulcers due to immobility. Which of the following interventions should the nurse adopt to prevent pressure ulcers in the child?

   a. Turn the child frequently

   b. Apply topical antibiotics

   c. Apply a cold compress

   d. Dress the client in layers

10. A nurse is educating the parents of a child with diaper dermatitis. Which of the following guidelines should the nurse include in the teaching?

    a. Wash the diaper area with soap

    b. Use rubber pants for the baby

    c. Let the child go diaperless for a period of time

    d. Use baby wipes with preservatives

11. A nurse is examining an adolescent who presented with acne. The nurse is aware that acne involves which of the following components of the integumentary system?

    a. Hair follicle

    b. Pilosebaceous unit

    c. Skin and subcutaneous tissue

    d. Epidermis

12. A nurse assesses an adolescent with severe acne. Which of the following is an appropriate teaching for the adolescent?

   a. Use oil-based cosmetics and hair products

   b. Use alcohol-based cleaners on the acne

   c. Use headbands, helmet and hats

   d. Use noncomedogenic cosmetic products

13. An adolescent girl is prescribed isotretinoin for acne vulgaris. During history collection, the nurse finds that the client is sexually active. Which of the following is an important nursing implication specific for the female client on isotretinoin treatment?

   a. The client should be on a pregnancy prevention program

   b. Lipid profile and complete blood cell count should be done

   c. The client should be monitored for suicidal risk

   d. Beta-human chorionic gonadotropin should be checked

14. On initial examination of a child with burns, the nurse finds the area to be edematous, leathery, and waxy. The child denies any pain on the burnt area. Which of the following types of burns should the nurse document?

   a. Superficial burns

   b. Partial-thickness burns

   c. Deep partial-thickness burns

   d. Full-thickness burns

15. A nurse is examining a five-year-old child who sustained burns. Which of the following pattern of burn would rule out child abuse–induced burns?

   a. Spatter-type

   b. Porcelain-contact sparing

   c. Flexor-sparing

   d. Stocking glove pattern

CHAPTER 46

Nursing Care of the Child With a Hematologic Disorder

SECTION I: LEARNING OBJECTIVES

1. Identify major hematologic disorders that affect children.

2. Determine priority assessment information for children with hematologic disorders.

3. Identify priority interventions for children with hematologic disorders.

4. Analyze laboratory data in relation to normal findings and report abnormal findings.

5. Provide nursing diagnoses appropriate for the child and family with hematologic disorders.

6. Develop a teaching plan for the family of children with hematologic disorders.

7. Identify resources for children and families with hematologic disorders or nutrition deficits.

SECTION II: ASSESSING YOUR UNDERSTANDING

Activity A *Fill in the blanks.*

1. The complete blood cell count is also called the _____ .

2. The fetus receives iron through the _____ from the mother.

3. Failure of the bone marrow to produce cells is known as _____ anemia.

4. The presence of _____ in the bloodstream interferes with the enzymatic processes of the biosynthesis of heme.

5. Sickle cell disease is a group of inherited _____ in which the RBCs do not carry the normal adult hemoglobin, but rather a less effective type.

6. _____ is a complication that occurs in beta-thalassemia major as a result of rapid hemolysis of RBCs, the decrease in hemoglobin production, and the increased absorption of dietary iron in response to the severely anemic state.

7. Excess iron is removed by _____ therapy.

8. Thalassemia _____ leads to mild microcytic anemia, and often no treatment is required.

9. _____ is a group of X-linked recessive disorders that result in deficiency in one of the coagulation factors in the blood.

10. Heme is iron surrounded by _____ .

Activity B *Consider the following figure.*

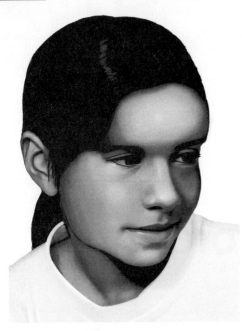

1. a. Identify the disorder to which these characteristics are related.

_____

_____

b. What causes these characteristics?

_____

_____

Activity C *Match the terms in Column A with their definitions in Column B.*

Column A

_____ **1.** Macrocytic

_____ **2.** Poikilocytosis

_____ **3.** Hypochromic

_____ **4.** Platelet

_____ **5.** Purpura

_____ **6.** Splenomegaly

Column B

a. Enlarged red blood cells

b. Less color in the red blood cell

c. Variation in the size and shape of the RBCs, respectively

d. An area of purple discoloration on the skin due to hemorrhage of underlying tissues

e. Enlargement of the spleen

f. A blood component that is a portion of the clotting function of the blood

Activity D *Briefly answer the following.*

1. Explain the difference between folic acid deficiency and pernicious anemia. What is the appropriate management for each?

_____

_____

_____

2. What is the recommended action for a blood lead level of 20 to 44 mcg/dL, according to the American Academy of Pediatrics?

_____

_____

_____

3. What are some of the first signs that indicate the development of problems in the hematologic system?

_____

_____

_____

4. What does the physical examination of a child with iron deficiency anemia include?

_____

_____

_____

5. What are the complications of sickle cell anemia?

_____

_____

_____

6. Why is the preterm infant at an increased risk for anemia?

_____

_____

_____

SECTION III: APPLYING YOUR KNOWLEDGE

Activity E *Consider this scenario and answer the questions.*

1. Jayda Johnson, 15 months old, is brought to the clinic for a routine exam. Her parents state that she has been irritable lately. Assessment findings reveal pallor of the mucous membranes and conjunctivae, heart rate of 120, and a heart murmur heard upon auscultation.

   a. What other assessment information about the home environment is important for the nurse to gather?

   _____

   _____

   _____

   b. Lab results revealed a hemoglobin level of 10 g/100 mL and hematocrit of 29%. The physician decides to start Jayda on a daily dose of ferrous sulfate. What instructions should be given to the child's parents?

   _____

   _____

   _____

   c. What sociocultural influences may be related to the child's condition?

   _____

   _____

   _____

SECTION IV: PRACTICING FOR NCLEX

Activity F *Answer the following questions.*

1. The nurse is caring for a child with disseminated intravascular coagulation (DIC). The nurse notices signs of neurologic deficit. Which of the following is the most appropriate nursing action?

   a. Continue to monitor neurologic signs

   b. Notify the physician

   c. Evaluate respiratory status

   d. Inspect for signs of bleeding

2. The nurse is examining the hands of a child with suspected iron deficiency anemia. Which of the following would the nurse expect to find?

   a. Capillary refill in less than two seconds

   b. Pink palms and nail beds

   c. Absence of bruising

   d. Spooning of nails

3. The nurse is providing dietary instructions for a five-year-old with iron deficiency anemia. Which of the following responses by the mother indicates a need for further teaching?

   a. "Red meat is a good option; he loves the hamburgers from the drive-through."

   b. "He will enjoy tuna casserole and eggs."

   c. "There are many iron-fortified cereals that he likes."

   d. "I must encourage him to eat a variety of iron-rich foods that he likes."

4. A nurse is caring for a seven-year-old boy with hemophilia who requires an infusion of factor VIII. He is fearful about the process and is resisting treatment. How should the nurse respond?

   a. "I would like you to administer this infusion."

   b. "Would you help me dilute this and mix it up?"

   c. "Will you help me apply this Band-Aid?"

   d. "Please be brave; we need to stop the bleeding."

5. The nurse is teaching about iron supplement administration. Which of the following is most important to stress to the parents?

   a. "You must precisely measure the amount of iron."

   b. "Your child may become constipated from the iron."

   c. "Please give him plenty of fluids and encourage fiber."

   d. "Place the liquid behind the teeth; the pigment can cause staining."

6. A nurse in the emergency department is examining a six-month-old with symmetrical swelling of the hands and feet. Which of the following conditions should the nurse suspect?

   a. Cooley's anemia

   b. Idiopathic thrombocytopenia purpura

   c. Sickle cell disease

   d. Hemophilia

7. The nurse is caring for an 18-month-old with suspected iron deficiency anemia. Which of the following lab results confirms the diagnosis?

   a. Decreased hemoglobin and hematocrit

   b. Decreased free erythrocyte protoporphyrin (FEP) level

   c. Increased reticulocyte count

   d. Increased serum iron and ferritin levels

8. A ten-year-old child is admitted to the health care facility with suspected lead poisoning. Which of the following should the nurse assess for in the child? Select all that apply.

   a. Blurred vision

   b. Behavioral problems

   c. Skin pallor

   d. Irritability and hyperactivity

   e. Dehydration

9. The nurse is caring for a child with aplastic anemia. Which of the following should the nurse assess the child for? Select all that apply.

   a. Oxygen-carrying capacity

   b. Increased bleeding with menstruation

   c. Oral ulcerations

   d. Infection

   e. Tachycardia

10. Infants with sickle cell anemia are usually asymptomatic until three to four months of age. The presence of which of the following types of Hgb is the reason for this?

    a. Hgb A

    b. Hgb AA

    c. Hgb AS

    d. Hgb F

11. A nurse is auscultating a child with sickle-cell anemia. Which of the following should the nurse note during auscultation? Select all that apply.

    a. Adventitious breath sounds

    b. Crackles

    c. Heart murmur

    d. Elevated heart rate

    e. Wheezing

12. A nurse is caring for a child with thalassemia major. Which of the following should the nurse assess for in the child? Select all that apply.

    a. Bleeding episodes

    b. Pathologic fractures

    c. Growth retardation

    d. Cardiac complications

    e. Skeletal deformities

13. A nurse is educating the parents of a child with idiopathic thrombocytopenia purpura (ITP). Which of the following instructions should the nurse give the parents? Select all that apply.

    a. Avoid using aspirin

    b. Use acetaminophen for pain control

    c. Use nonsteroidal anti-inflammatory drugs

    d. Discourage participation in swimming

    e. Discourage participation in contact sports

CHAPTER 47

Nursing Care of the Child With an Immunologic Disorder

SECTION I: LEARNING OBJECTIVES

1. Explain anatomic and physiologic differences of the immune system in infants and children versus adults.

2. Describe nursing care related to common laboratory and diagnostic testing used in the medical diagnosis of pediatric immune and autoimmune disorders.

3. Distinguish immune and autoimmune disorders common in infants, children, and adolescents.

4. Identify appropriate nursing assessments and interventions related to the medications and treatments for pediatric immune, autoimmune, and allergic disorders.

5. Develop an individualized nursing care plan for the child with an immune or autoimmune disorder.

6. Describe the psychosocial impact of chronic immune disorders on children.

7. Devise a nutrition plan for the child with immunodeficiency.

8. Develop patient/family teaching plans for the child with an immune or autoimmune disorder.

SECTION II: ASSESSING YOUR UNDERSTANDING

Activity A *Fill in the blanks.*

1. In systemic lupus erythematosus (SLE), _____ react with the child's self-antigens to form immune complexes.

2. Family history may be _____ for primary immune deficiency or auto immune disorder, though only 10% of cases present with a family history of SLE.

3. When an infant is born it exhibits _____ immunity to antigens to which the mother had developed antibodies; this immunity lasts about three months.

4. _____ transmission, or transmission perinatally or via breast milk, accounts for 93% of all cases of pediatric HIV infection.

5. _____ refers to a variety of conditions in which the child does not form antibodies appropriately and results in low or absent levels of one or more of the immunoglobulin classes or subclasses.

6. The malar rash of systemic lupus erythematosus (SLE) resembles the shape of a _____.

7. _____ is an immune-mediated response resulting in an adverse physiologic event or reaction.

8. Severe combined immune deficiency (SCID) is a rare X-linked or autosomal recessive disorder that can occur in either sex, characterized by _____ T-cell and B-cell function.

9. _____ occurring in anaphylaxis results in a rapid decrease in plasma volume, leading to the risk of circulatory collapse.

10. The pathophysiology of latex allergy is similar to that of _____ allergy.

Activity B *Match the tests in Column A with their proper definitions in Column B.*

Column A

____ 1. Antinuclear antibody

____ 2. Erythrocyte sedimentation rate

____ 3. Polymerase chain reaction

____ 4. Delayed hypersensitivity skin test

Column B

a. Measures the presence of activated T cells that recognize certain substances

b. Used to detect HIV DNA and RNA

c. Tests for presence of autoantibodies that react against cellular nuclear material

d. Nonspecific test used to determine presence of infection or inflammation

Activity C *Put the items in correct sequence by writing the letters in the boxes provided below.*

1. Place the following anaphylaxis treatment priorities in the proper sequence.

a. Administration of corticosteroids

b. Injection of intramuscular epinephrine

c. Administration of intravenous diphenhydramine

d. Assessment of airway and support of the airway, breathing, and circulation

☐ → ☐ → ☐ → ☐

Activity D *Briefly answer the following.*

1. What are the different types of hypogammaglobulinemia?

2. Which test is preferable for the detection of HIV infection in infants?

3. What is juvenile idiopathic arthritis?

4. Why are skin test responses (such as PPD for tuberculosis detection) diminished until about one year of age?

5. What is anaphylaxis?

6. What is Wiskott-Aldrich syndrome? What are its complications?

SECTION III: APPLYING YOUR KNOWLEDGE

Activity E *Consider this scenario and answer the questions.*

1. A child diagnosed with severe combined immune deficiency (SCID) is admitted to

the health care facility for bone marrow transplantation.

a. How does the nurse assess presence of infection in the child?

_____

_____

_____

b. What nursing interventions are needed to prevent the child from acquiring infections?

_____

_____

_____

SECTION IV: PRACTICING FOR NCLEX

Activity F *Answer the following questions.*

1. The nurse is preparing to administer IVIG to a child who has not had an IVIG infusion before. Which of the following nursing interventions is important before administering IVIG?
   a. Premedicate with acetaminophen or diphenhydramine
   b. Assess baseline serum blood urea nitrogen and creatinine
   c. Observe for signs of anaphylaxis reaction
   d. Administer epinephrine and corticosteroids

2. A nurse is caring for a newborn whose mother is HIV positive. Which of the following diagnostic test results will be positive even if the child is not infected with the virus?
   a. Rheumatoid factor
   b. Antinuclear antibody
   c. Polymerase chain reaction test
   d. Enzyme-linked immunosorbent assay (ELISA)

3. A nurse is conducting a physical examination of a 12-year-old girl with suspected systemic lupus erythematosus (SLE). How would the nurse best interview the client?
   a. "Have you ever had persistent diarrhea for a long time?"
   b. "Have you ever noticed white patches or sores in your mouth?"
   c. "Have you noticed any new bruising or different color patterns on your skin?"
   d. "Have you noticed any hair loss or redness on your face?"

4. A nurse in the emergency department notes lip edema, urticaria, and stridor in an 18-month-old whose mother informs the nurse that the baby was given shellfish an hour before. Which of the following conditions should the nurse immediately suspect?
   a. Severe polyarticular juvenile idiopathic arthritis
   b. Anaphylaxis
   c. Systemic lupus erythematosus
   d. Severe combined immune deficiency

5. The nurse is teaching the parents of a child who has a latex allergy. The nurse tells them to avoid which of the following foods?
   a. Blueberries
   b. Pumpkin
   c. Banana
   d. Pomegranate

6. The nurse is caring for a child with juvenile idiopathic arthritis. There is a symmetrical involvement of six small joints. What does this finding indicate?
   a. The child has polyarticular JIA
   b. The child has systemic JIA
   c. The child pauciarticular JIA
   d. The child is at risk for anaphylaxis

7. A nurse is reviewing the laboratory investigation reports of a child with systematic lupus erythematosus (SLE). Which of the following would the nurse expect to find?
   a. High WBC count
   b. Elevated IgA concentration
   c. Low IgM concentration
   d. Decreased platelet count

8. The nurse is instructed to administer oral aspirin to a client with juvenile idiopathic arthritis. Which of the following nursing interventions should the nurse follow?
   a. Monitor potassium levels
   b. Monitor liver enzymes
   c. Monitor for serum salicylate level
   d. Monitor the CBC

9. A nurse in the intensive care unit is assessing an eleven-year-old boy with X-linked agam-maglobulinemia. Which of the following should the nurse assess in the client?

   a. Neutropenia

   b. Malabsorption

   c. Autoimmune disorders

   d. Respiratory infections

10. A nurse is performing a physical examination of a four-year-old child with systemic lupus erythematosus (SLE). Which of the following assessment should the nurse perform?

    a. Inspect the skin for nonpruritic macular rashes

    b. Auscultate the lungs for pneumonia

    c. Palpate for the presence of lym-phadenopathy

    d. Observe the skin for butterfly rashes

11. The nurse is providing instructions to the parents of a child with a severe peanut allergy. Which of the following statements by the parents indicates a need for further teaching about the use of the EpiPen® Jr.?

    a. "We must massage the area for 10 seconds after administration."

    b. "We must make sure that the black tip is downward."

    c. "The EpiPen® Jr. should be jabbed into the upper arm."

    d. "The EpiPen® Jr. must be held firmly for 10 seconds."

12. A nurse in the pediatric unit is instructing the parents of a child who is allergic to wheat. Which of the following should the child avoid?

    a. Whey

    b. Casein

    c. Yogurt

    d. Durum

13. A nurse is caring for a ten-year-old client with a latex allergy. Which of the following manifestations should the nurse look for in the client?

    a. Photosensitivity

    b. Skin rashes

    c. Stomatitis

    d. Nasal congestion

14. A nurse is assessing a client with polyarticular juvenile idiopathic arthritis. Which of the following non-joint manifestations should the nurse expect to find in the client?

    a. Lymphadenopathy

    b. Severe anemia

    c. Hepatomegaly

    d. Splenomegaly

15. A nurse is caring for a client with juvenile idiopathic arthritis. Which of the following should the nurse teach the parents to help promote a normal life for the client when he or she is discharged? Select all that apply.

    a. Provide adequate pain relief through medications

    b. Apply warm compresses to affected joints

    c. Encourage the child to attend school

    d. Protect against cold weather with layered clothing

    e. Apply sunscreen daily to the skin to prevent rashes

CHAPTER 48

Nursing Care of the Child With an Endocrine Disorder

SECTION I: LEARNING OBJECTIVES

1. Describe the major components and functions of a child's endocrine system.

2. Differentiate between the anatomic and physiologic differences of the endocrine system in children versus adults.

3. Identify the essential assessment elements, common diagnostic procedures, and laboratory tests associated with the diagnosis of endocrine disorders in children.

4. Identify the common medications and treatment modalities used for palliation of endocrine disorders in children.

5. Distinguish specific disorders of the endocrine system affecting children.

6. Link the clinical manifestations of specific disorders in the endocrine system of a child with the appropriate nursing diagnoses.

7. Establish the nursing outcomes, evaluative criteria, and interventions for a child with specific disorders in the endocrine system.

8. Develop child/family teaching plans for the child with an endocrine disorder.

SECTION II: ASSESSING YOUR UNDERSTANDING

Activity A *Fill in the blanks.*

1. The endocrine system and the nervous system work closely together to maintain an optimal internal environment for the body, known as _____.

2. The _____ releases insulin, glucagon, and somatostatin for regulation of blood glucose levels.

3. The most common initial symptoms of diabetes mellitus reported are _____ and polydipsia.

4. Growth hormone deficiency, also known as _____ or dwarfism, is characterized by poor growth and short stature.

5. _____ is an enlargement of the bones of the head and soft parts of the feet and hands.

6. Congenital hypothyroidism, also known as _____, usually results from failure of the thyroid gland to migrate during fetal development.

7. _____ is used to measure levels of thyroxine (T4), which accurately reflect the child's thyroid status.

8. Cushing's syndrome is characterized by a cluster of signs and symptoms resulting from excess levels of _____ .

9. Exercise has an important influence on the _____ effects of insulin.

10. _____ disorders often cause problems in normal growth and development, as well as behavioral changes.

Activity B *Consider the following figure.*

1 a. Identify the disorder in the newborn.

_____

_____

b. What are the causes of this disorder?

_____

_____

Activity C *Match the location of the endocrine gland in Column A with its major effects in Column B.*

Column A

____ **1.** Hypothalamus

____ **2.** Thymus

____ **3.** Parathyroid

____ **4.** Adrenal

Column B

a. Releases aldosterone, mineralocorticoids, androgens, epinephrine, and norepinephrine

b. Produces humoral factors key to the development of immunity

c. Stimulates the pituitary gland to release or withhold hormones

d. Regulates calcium and phosphorus concentrations

Activity D *Put the items in correct sequence by writing the letters in the boxes provided below.*

1. Given below are insulin types. Choose the proper order of their onset times.

a. Lispro

b. NPH

c. Regular

d. Ultralente

$$\square \rightarrow \square \rightarrow \square \rightarrow \square$$

Activity E *Briefly answer the following.*

1. Explain the process of hormone production and secretion.

_____

_____

_____

2. What are the pituitary disorders in children?

_____

_____

_____

3. What is a bone age radiograph? Why is it performed?

_____

_____

_____

4. What is psychosocial dwarfism?

_____

_____

_____

5. What is an insulin pump?

_____

_____

_____

6. What are the differences observed in clients with hyperglycemia and hypoglycemia?

_____

_____

_____

SECTION III: APPLYING YOUR KNOWLEDGE

Activity F _Consider this scenario and answer the questions._

1. John is a 12-year-old with weakness, fatigue, blurred vision, headaches, and mood and behavior changes. After further assessment, he was diagnosed with diabetes mellitus type 2. John's mother asks, "Isn't type 2 diabetes seen only in adults?"

a. How should the nurse address this question?

_____

_____

_____

b. What should be the focus of nursing management for John and his family?

_____

_____

_____

c. What are the challenges that the nurse might anticipate when educating John?

_____

_____

_____

SECTION IV: PRACTICING FOR NCLEX

Activity G _Answer the following questions._

1. The nurse is providing acute care for an 11-year-old boy with hypoparathyroidism. Which of the following is the priority intervention?

a. Providing administration of calcium and vitamin D

b. Ensuring patency of the IV site to prevent tissue damage

c. Monitoring fluid intake and urinary calcium output

d. Administering intravenous calcium gluconate as ordered

2. The nurse is assessing a four-year-old girl with ambiguous genitalia. Which of the following findings would be consistent with congenital adrenal hyperplasia?

a. Auscultation reveals irregular heartbeat

b. Observing pubic hair and hirsutism

c. Palpation elicits pain from constipation

d. Observing hyperpigmentation of the skin

3. The nurse is caring for a four-year-old boy during a growth hormone stimulation test. Which of the following is a priority task for the care of this child?

a. Providing ice chips to suck on

b. Educating family about side effects

c. Monitoring blood glucose levels

d. Monitoring intake and output

4. The nurse is assessing a seven-year-old girl who complains of headache and is irritable and vomiting. Health history reveals she has had meningitis. Which of the following is the priority intervention?

a. Notifying the physician of the neurologic findings

b. Setting up safety precautions to prevent injury

c. Monitoring urine volume and specific gravity

d. Restoring fluid balance with IV sodium chloride

5. The nurse is assessing a one-month-old girl who, according to the mother, does not feed well. Which of the following would suggest that the child has congenital hypothyroidism?

a. Mother reports frequent diarrhea

b. Observation of an enlarged tongue

c. Auscultation reveals tachycardia

d. Palpation reveals warm, moist skin

6. The nurse is caring for an obese 15-year-old girl who missed two menstrual periods. Which of the following findings would indicate polycystic ovary syndrome?

   a. Palpation reveals hypertrophy and weakness

   b. Complaints of blurred vision and headaches

   c. Auscultation reveals increased respiratory rate

   d. Observation of acanthosis nigricans

7. The nurse is assessing a 16-year-old boy who had had long-term corticosteroid therapy. Which of the following findings would lead to a diagnosis of Cushing's disease after using an adrenal suppression test?

   a. History of rapid weight gain

   b. Observing a round, child-like face

   c. Observing high weight–to-height ratio

   d. Observing delayed dentition

8. The nurse is caring for a ten-year-old girl with hyperparathyroidism. Which of the following would be a priority nursing diagnosis for this child?

   a. Disturbed body image due to hormone dysfunction

   b. Imbalanced nutrition: more than body requirements

   c. Deficient fluid volume due to electrolyte imbalance

   d. Deficient knowledge related to treatment of the disease

9. The nurse is teaching an 11-year-old boy and his family how to manage his diabetes. Which of the following teachings focuses on blood glucose monitoring?

   a. Ensure consistency of food intake

   b. Obtain glucose levels before bedtime snacks

   c. Maintain proper injection schedules

   d. Identify carbohydrate, protein, and fat foods

10. The nurse is caring for a 12-year-old girl with hypothyroidism. Which of the following will be part of the nurse's teaching plan for the child and family?

    a. Teaching them how to recognize vitamin D toxicity

    b. Teaching them how to maintain fluid intake regimens

    c. Teaching them to administer methimazole with meals

    d. Instructing them to report irritability or anxiety

11. A nurse is caring for a child who is to undergo water deprivation study. The child is deprived of fluids for several hours. Which of the following are the nursing implications for this child? Select all that apply.

    a. Monitor for orthostatic hypotension

    b. Weigh the child before, during, and after test

    c. Monitor blood glucose levels during study

    d. Obtain serial blood samples at specific times

    e. Rehydrate the child after test

12. A nurse is observing a child with diabetes for complications related to fluctuations in blood glucose levels. Which of the following are symptoms of hypoglycemia? Select all that apply.

    a. Blurred vision

    b. Palpitations

    c. Fruity breath odor

    d. Diaphoresis

    e. Tremors

13. A nurse is assessing a child with acquired hypothyroidism. Which of the following are common complaints that the family or child would report?

    a. Weight loss

    b. Oily skin

    c. Cold intolerance

    d. Diarrhea

14. Which of the following observations during the nursing assessment in a child indicate Cushing's syndrome? Select all that apply.

a. Cervical fat pad

b. Tendency to bruise

c. Gradual onset of weight loss

d. Dehydration

e. Reddish-purple striae on the abdomen

15. A nurse is educating the parents of an infant diagnosed with congenital hypothyroidism. About which of the following should the nurse inform the parents?

a. Discontinue medication after six months

b. Check the pulse before administering medication

c. Administer medication with soy-based preparations

d. Mix medication with a full bottle of formula

Nursing Care of the Child With a Neoplastic Disorder

SECTION I: LEARNING OBJECTIVES

1. Compare childhood and adult cancers.

2. Describe nursing care related to common laboratory and diagnostic testing used in the medical diagnosis of pediatric cancer.

3. Identify the types of cancer common in infants, children, and adolescents.

4. Identify appropriate nursing assessments and interventions related to medications and treatments for pediatric cancer.

5. Develop an individualized nursing care plan for the child with cancer.

6. Describe the psychosocial impact of the cancer on children and their families.

7. Devise a nutrition plan for the child with cancer.

8. Develop patient/family teaching plans for the child with cancer.

SECTION II: ASSESSING YOUR UNDERSTANDING

Activity A *Fill in the blanks.*

1. _____ is the most common extracranial solid tumor in children, occurring most commonly in the abdomen, mainly in the adrenal gland.

2. _____ is a primary disorder of the bone marrow in which the normal elements are replaced with abnormal white cells.

3. _____ is a soft-tissue tumor that usually arises from the embryonic mesenchymal cells that would ordinarily form striated muscle.

4. Retinoblastoma is a congenital, highly malignant tumor that arises from embryonic _____ cells.

5. _____ infection in the leukemic child may lead to disseminated, overwhelming infection.

6. _____ stage of leukemia treatment is characterized by elimination of all residual leukemic cells.

7. _____ rescue occurs with infusion of the donor or autologous cells.

8. _____ is the time after administration of the drug when bone marrow suppression is expected to be at its greatest and the neutrophil count is expected to be at its lowest.

9. Chemotherapy dosing in children is based on body surface area (BSA); a _____ is a commonly used device for determining body surface area.

10. One of the risks of stem cell therapy is relapse of the original disease process and is highest in _____ hematopoietic stem cell therapy.

Activity B   *Consider the following figures.*

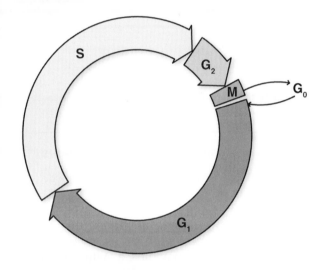

1. Identify the figure.

   _____

   _____

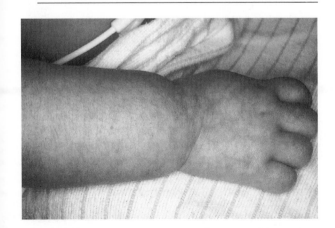

2. What does this figure depict?

   _____

   _____

Activity C   *Match the medical treatment in Column A with the proper description in Column B.*

Column A

____ 1. Biopsy

____ 2. Central venous catheter

____ 3. Implanted port

____ 4. Leukapheresis

____ 5. Radiation therapy

____ 6. Stem cell transplant

Column B

a. IV catheters are inserted into the central circulation

b. A needle-accessible port is implanted under the skin

c. Whole blood is removed from the body, the WBCs are extracted, and the blood is transfused into the child

d. Bone marrow transplant

e. A small piece of the tumor is removed with a needle

f. Ionizing radiation is delivered to the cancerous area

Activity D   *Put the items in correct sequence by writing the letters in the boxes provided below.*

1. Given below, in random order, are phases of the cell cycle. Choose the correct order.

   a. S Chromosomes are copied for new cells

   b. G1 Cell makes more protein in preparation to start to divide

   c. G2 Cell prepares to split into two cells

   d. M Mitosis, cell splits

   e. G0 Resting phase

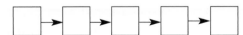

Activity E   *Briefly answer the following.*

1. Describe the signs and symptoms of rhabdomyosarcoma based on the location of the tumor.

   _____

   _____

   _____

2. Name the eight drugs discussed in this chapter that help prevent or palliate the effects of chemotherapy and other tests and therapies.

_____

_____

_____

3. What nursing interventions are needed to avoid the risk of impaired skin integrity related to radiation therapy?

_____

_____

_____

4. What are the general guidelines related to the preparation and administration of chemotherapy?

_____

_____

_____

5. How is the absolute neutrophil count (ANC) calculated? Give an example.

_____

_____

_____

6. How is massive hepatomegaly managed?

_____

_____

_____

SECTION III: APPLYING YOUR KNOWLEDGE

Activity F *Consider this scenario and answer the questions.*

1. Nikita, a toddler, was brought to the clinic by her parents after they noticed a glow in the pupil of the right eye.

a. What should be the priority nursing assessments?

_____

_____

_____

b. Diagnostic evaluation for the child includes an ophthalmologic examination under anesthesia and CT, magnetic resonance imaging (MRI), or ultrasound of the head and eyes to visualize the tumor. What are the nursing implications during magnetic resonance imaging?

_____

_____

_____

c. What care should the nurse take in the post-operative phase?

_____

_____

_____

SECTION IV: PRACTICING FOR NCLEX

Activity G *Answer the following questions.*

1. The nurse is assessing a four-year-old girl whose mother complains that she is not eating well, is losing weight, and has started vomiting after eating. Which of the following risk factors from the health history would suggest the child may have a Wilms' tumor?

a. The child has Down syndrome

b. The child has Beckwith-Wiedemann syndrome

c. The child has Schwachman syndrome

d. The child has a family history of neurofibromatosis

2. The nurse is assessing a three-year-old boy whose mother complains that he is listless and has been having trouble swallowing. Which of the following findings would suggest the child has a brain tumor?

a. Observation reveals nystagmus and head tilt

b. Vital signs show blood pressure measures 120/80

c. Examination shows temperature of 101.3°F and headache

d. Observation reveals a cough and labored breathing

3. The nurse is caring for a six-year-old girl with leukemia. Which of the following signs and symptoms would indicate hyperleukocytosis?

   a. Increased heart rate and distinct S1 and S2 sounds

   b. Wheezing and diminished breath sounds

   c. Respiratory distress and poor perfusion

   d. Increased heart rate and respiratory distress

4. The nurse is teaching a group of 13-year-old boys and girls about screening and prevention of reproductive cancers. Which of the following subjects should the nurse include in her teaching plan?

   a. Self-examination is an effective screening method for testicular cancer

   b. Testicular cancer is one of the most difficult cancers to cure

   c. A Papanicolaou smear requires parental consent in most states

   d. Cervical cancer has a low response rate to therapy

5. The nurse is assessing a 14-year-old girl suspected of having a tumor. Which of the following findings would indicate Ewing's sarcoma?

   a. Child complains of dull bone pain just below her knee

   b. Palpation reveals swelling and erythema on the right ribs

   c. Child complains of persistent pain from a minor ankle injury

   d. Palpation discloses an asymptomatic mass on the upper back

6. The nurse is providing preoperative care to a seven-year-old boy with a brain tumor. Which of the following is the priority intervention?

   a. Assessing for increase in intracranial pressure

   b. Providing a tour of the intensive care unit

   c. Educating the child and parents about shunts

   d. Having him talk to a child who has had this surgery

7. A child has a body weight of 35 kgs and height of 150 cms. Which of the following is the body surface area (BSA) of the child?

   a. 1.02

   b. 1.08

   c. 1.20

   d. 1.80

8. The nurse is teaching the parents of a 15-year-old boy, who is being treated for acute myelogenous leukemia, about the side effects of chemotherapy. For which of the following symptoms should the parents seek medical care immediately?

   a. Earache, stiff neck, or sore throat

   b. Blisters, ulcers, or a rash

   c. A temperature of 101°F or greater

   d. Difficulty or pain when swallowing

9. A nurse is reviewing the laboratory analysis of a client with tumor lysis syndrome. Of which of the following findings should the nurse inform the oncologist?

   a. Decreased bicarbonate levels

   b. Decreased serum calcium levels

   c. Decreased platelet count levels

   d. Decreased pH levels

10. A nurse is assessing a client with superior vena cava syndrome associated with neuroblastoma. Which of the following signs and symptoms should the nurse expect to find in the client?

    a. Dyspnea

    b. Anorexia

    c. Back pain

    d. Hypotension

11. A nurse caring for a three-year-old child with leukemia is instructed to administer cytarabine intravenously during chemotherapy. Which of the following nursing implications should the nurse follow when administering cytarabine?

    a. Use corticosteroid eye drops

    b. Maintain adequate hydration

    c. Monitor urine for change of color

    d. Monitor for Cushing syndrome

12. A client who is on chemotherapy is experiencing nausea and vomiting. The physician instructs the nurse to administer ondansetron intravenously. Which of the following side effects should the nurse be aware of while administering ondansetron intravenously?

 a. Dry mouth

 b. Drowsiness

 c. Mucositis

 d. Wheezing

13. A nurse is caring for a five-year-old child who is scheduled for stem cell transplantation. Which of the following medications is given in the pretransplantation phase?

 a. Gammaglobulin

 b. Mycophenolate

 c. Cyclosporine

 d. Tacrolimus

14. A nurse is assessing a fourteen-year-old boy who is admitted with osteosarcoma. Which of the following assessment findings should the nurse expect on inspection?

 a. Petechiae and purpura

 b. Bluish-gray papular lesions

 c. Salmon-colored lesions

 d. Erythema and swelling

15. A nurse is assessing a child suspected of having a brain tumor. Which of the following risk factors would indicate a brain tumor?

 a. Neurofibromatosis

 b. Down syndrome

 c. Ataxiatelangiectasia

 d. Shwachman syndrome

CHAPTER 50

Nursing Care of the Child With a Genetic Disorder

SECTION I: LEARNING OBJECTIVES

1. Discuss the nurse's role and responsibilities when caring for a child diagnosed with a genetic disorder and his or her family.

2. Identify nursing interventions related to common laboratory and diagnostic tests used in the diagnoses and management of genetic conditions.

3. Distinguish various genetic disorders occurring in childhood.

4. Devise an individualized nursing care plan for the child with a genetic disorder.

5. Develop patient/family teaching plans for the child with a genetic disorder.

SECTION II: ASSESSING YOUR UNDERSTANDING

Activity A *Fill in the blanks.*

1. An enlargement of the spleen and liver is known as _____

2. The risk for autosomal trisomies increases with advanced _____ age.

3. Approximately 3% of all cases of congenital heart disease are caused by a single _____ gene.

4. Trisomy 21 is also known as _____ syndrome.

5. _____ associated with obstructive sleep apnea syndrome has been correlated with lower IQ testing.

6. Females with Turner syndrome may present with some _____ .

7. White spots on the iris of the eye in children with Down syndrome are known as _____ spots.

8. _____ disorders, also referred to as hamartoses, are a group of disorders characterized by abnormalities of both the skin and the central nervous system.

9. Marfan syndrome is a disorder of connective tissue that is caused by a mutation in the gene _____ .

10. Homocystinuria is a deficiency in the enzyme needed to digest a component of food called _____ .

Activity B *Consider the following figures.*

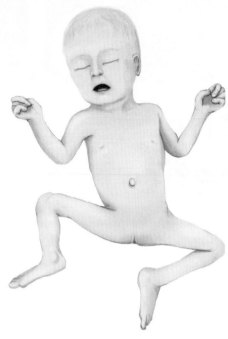

1. Identify the genetic disorder shown in the above image.

   _____

   _____

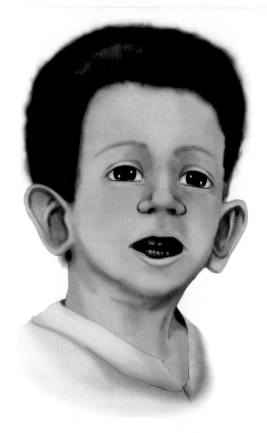

2. a. Identify the genetic disorder shown in the preceding image.

   _____

   _____

   b. What are the behavior problems associated with this disorder?

   _____

   _____

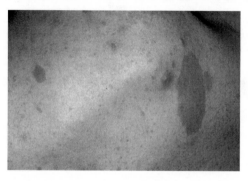

3. Identify the genetic disorder shown in the above figure.

   _____

   _____

Activity C *Match the errors of metabolism in Column A with their associated odors in Column B.*

Column A	Column B
___ 1. Tuberous sclerosis	a. Maple syrup
___ 2. Maple syrup urine disease	b. Benign tumors present in the brain and skin
___ 3. Tyrosinemia	c. Rotting fish
___ 4. Trimethylaminuria	d. Cabbage-like, rancid butter

Activity D *Briefly answer the following.*

1. Describe a few major complications a child with Down syndrome can experience.

   _____

   _____

   _____

2. What should the nurse include when eliciting the health history of a child with a genetic disorder?

_____

_____

_____

3. What is the significance of major and minor anomalies in the assessment of congenital disorders?

_____

_____

_____

4. What is included in the multidisciplinary therapeutic management of children with Down syndrome?

_____

_____

_____

5. How is Turner syndrome diagnosed?

_____

_____

_____

6. What are inborn errors of metabolism?

_____

_____

_____

SECTION III: APPLYING YOUR KNOWLEDGE

Activity E _Consider this scenario and answer the questions._

1. Chloe O'Grady, one week old, is seen in the clinic secondary to abnormal newborn screening results. Her mother states, "Chloe has been doing great. She eats well, every 2 to 3 hours. I don't understand why we're here today. The nurse called and mentioned something about an inborn error of metabolism. I don't understand what that is and how Chloe could have that. She isn't even sick." The newborn screen came back positive for a fatty acid oxidation disorder, medium-chain acyl-CoA dehydroge-

nase deficiency. After further testing, the diagnosis was confirmed.

a. How should the nurse address the mother's concerns?

_____

_____

_____

b. What education and nursing management should the nurse provide?

_____

_____

_____

SECTION IV: PRACTICING FOR NCLEX

Activity F _Answer the following questions._

1. The nurse is assessing a newborn boy. Which of the following findings is the most dependable sign or symptom of neurofibromatosis?

a. History shows a grandparent had neurofibromatosis

b. Measurement shows a slightly larger head size

c. Inspection discloses café-au-lait spots on the trunk

d. Observation reveals freckles in the child's axilla

2. The nurse is assessing a two-week-old boy who was born at home and has not had metabolic screening. Which of the following signs or symptoms would indicate phenylketonuria?

a. Palpation reveals increased reflex action

b. Observation shows signs of jaundice

c. There is a mousy odor to the urine

d. The parents report the child has seizures

3. The nurse is assessing infants in the newborn nursery. Which of the following assessments would be indicative of a major anomaly?

a. A white boy with café-au-lait macules on his trunk

b. An African-American boy with polydactyly

c. A set of identical Indian twin girls with syndactyly

d. An Asian girl with protruding ears

4. The nurse is caring for a newborn girl with galactosemia. Which of the following interventions will be necessary for her health?

   a. Adhering to a low-phenylalanine diet

   b. Eliminating dairy products from her diet

   c. Eating frequent meals and never fasting

   d. Lifetime supplementation with thiamine

5. The nurse is caring for an eight-year-old girl who has just been diagnosed with fragile X syndrome. Which of the following would be the first clue that the nurse should assess in the child?

   a. Low self-esteem

   b. Delay in attaining developmental milestones

   c. Problems with abstract reasoning

   d. Gaze aversion

6. The nurse is assessing a three-year-old boy with Sturge-Weber syndrome. Which of the following findings would be present? Select all that apply.

   a. Port wine stain

   b. Intracranial calcification

   c. Vision and hearing loss

   d. Hemiparesis

   e. Scoliosis

7. A nurse is educating the parents of a three-year-old diagnosed with neurofibromatosis. Which of the following information should the nurse give the parents?

   a. Offspring of persons with neurofibromatosis do not inherit the disorder

   b. Neurofibromatosis can be cured with treatment

   c. Surgical interventions can help remove bone malformations

   d. Neurofibromatosis tends to subside in adulthood

8. The nurse is examining a two-year-old girl with CHARGE syndrome. Which of the following signs or symptoms would be noted?

   a. Tall stature with long limbs

   b. Hypoplastic labia

   c. Minimal subcutaneous fat

   d. Long, narrow face

9. A nurse is assessing a child with VATER association. Which of the following anomalies should the nurse note?

   a. Craniocystosis

   b. Bilateral symmetrical syndactyly

   c. Prominent forehead

   d. Hypoplastic vertebrae

10. The nurse is examining an eight-year-old boy with chromosomal abnormalities. Which of the following signs and symptoms suggest the boy has Angelman syndrome?

    a. Observation reveals short stature

    b. Observation reveals a moonlike round face

    c. History shows surgery for cleft palate repair

    d. Observation shows jerky ataxic movement

11. A nurse is assessing an infant with Down syndrome. Which of the following signs should the nurse look for? Select all that apply.

    a. Wide-spaced nipples

    b. Epicanthal folds

    c. Low posterior hairline

    d. Arched palate

    e. Flattened occiput

12. A nurse is assessing an adolescent male client with Klinefelter syndrome. Which of the following should the nurse look for in the client?

    a. Mental retardation

    b. Short, stubby limbs

    c. Increased breast size

    d. Increased pubic hair

13. A nurse is caring for a child with homocystinuria. Which of the following dietary interventions may be necessary for the child? Select all that apply.

    a. Adhering to methionine-restricted diet

    b. Adhering to special low-protein diet

    c. Ensuring frequent meals

    d. Including cystine supplements in the diet

    e. Including vitamin B6 and B12 supplements

14. A nurse is educating the parents of a six-year-old girl diagnosed with Turner syndrome. Which of the following information should the nurse give? Select all that apply.

a. Your child may have a learning disability

b. Your child's growth may be slow but fertility will not be affected

c. There is a risk of recurrence in future pregnancies

d. There is no cure for Turner syndrome

e. Your child may be prone to skeletal disorders

15. A nurse is caring for a 20-year-old male client who has been diagnosed with Klinefelter syndrome during a routine health checkup. Which of the following is a reason for late diagnosis of the syndrome?

a. Signs are not reported by family members because of social stigma

b. Findings are nonspecific during childhood

c. Prenatal diagnosis is not possible

d. There are no visible signs; all signs are covert

CHAPTER 51

Nursing Care of the Child With a Cognitive or Mental Health Disorder

SECTION I: LEARNING OBJECTIVES

1. Discuss the impact of alterations in mental health upon the growth and development of infants, children, and adolescents.

2. Describe techniques used to evaluate the status of mental health in children.

3. Identify appropriate nursing assessments and interventions related to therapy and medications for the treatment of childhood and adolescent mental health disorders.

4. Distinguish mental health disorders common in infants, children, and adolescents.

5. Develop an individualized nursing care plan for the child with a mental health disorder.

6. Develop patient/family teaching plans for the child with a mental health disorder.

SECTION II: ASSESSING YOUR UNDERSTANDING

Activity A *Fill in the blanks.*

1. Children with _____, a learning disability, have trouble with reading, writing, and spelling.

2. Burns that appear in a stocking or glove pattern are highly suspicious of _____ burns.

3. _____ is defined as failure to provide a child with appropriate food, clothing, shelter, medical care, and schooling.

4. Ritalin is a _____ that increases synaptic levels of dopamine and norepinephrine.

5. _____ is a treatment that uses deep relaxation with suggestibility remarks.

6. _____ causes problems with manual dexterity and coordination.

7. Most children with attention-deficit/ hyperactivity disorder (ADHD) also have _____ such as oppositional defiant disorder, conduct disorder, or anxiety disorder.

8. When caring for a child with Tourette syndrome, therapeutic management involves _____ and behavioral therapies.

9. _____ is an eating disorder that refers to a cycle of normal food intake, followed by binge eating and then purging.

10. _____ therapy uses a specially structured setting for a very ill or very aggressive child to promote his/her adaptive or social skills.

Activity B *Match the term in Column A with its definition in Column B.*

Column A	Column B
____ **1.** Affect	**a.** Feelings of dread, worry, discomfort
____ **2.** Anxiety	**b.** Rapid excessive consumption of food or drink
____ **3.** Binging	
____ **4.** Dysgraphia	**c.** Emotional reaction associated with an experience
____ **5.** Dyscalculia	**d.** Difficulty producing the written word
	e. Problems with math and computation

Activity C *Briefly answer the following.*

1. What are some common behavior management techniques that can be used in the hospital, clinic, classroom, or home setting?

_____

_____

_____

2. What laboratory and diagnostic studies are commonly ordered for the assessment of abuse?

_____

_____

_____

3. Describe generalized anxiety disorder.

_____

_____

_____

4. Write a brief note on mental retardation.

_____

_____

_____

5. What are the warning signs of Münchausen syndrome by proxy?

_____

_____

_____

6. What indications will require a nurse to refer a child for evaluation for a learning disability?

_____

_____

_____

SECTION III: APPLYING YOUR KNOWLEDGE

Activity D *Consider this scenario and answer the questions.*

1. Greg Gauger, a 15-year-old, visits a clinic, accompanied by his father. Greg's father states, "I've noticed some changes in Greg's behavior. He avoids us and his friends, remains shut in his room for long hours, and always appears cheerless." What further assessment information should the nurse gather?

_____

_____

_____

2. A mother brings her two-year-old girl for a wellness checkup. The mother states, "I have seen so much about autism in the news lately. How would I know if Elisa has this disorder?" Address this mother's concerns.

_____

_____

_____

3. A nurse is providing a routine wellness examination for Rob Benson, a 10-year-old boy. The nurse notes that the increase in his stature and weight is less than expected. On further discussion, his mother states, "He never finishes his meals. Lately, he has even started skipping meals." Further evaluation reveals that Rob has an eating disorder. Suggest the steps the nurse or Rob's parents can take to improve his nutritional intake.

_____

_____

_____

SECTION IV: PRACTICING FOR NCLEX

Activity E *Answer the following questions.*

1. The nurse is conducting a well-child assessment of a three-year-old. Which of the following statements by the parents would warrant further investigation?
   a. "He spends a lot of time playing with his little cars."
   b. "He will spend hours repeatedly lining up his cars."
   c. "He is very active and keeps very busy."
   d. "He would rather run around than sit on my lap and read a book."

2. The mother of a ten-year-old boy with attention-deficit/hyperactivity disorder contacts the school nurse. She is upset because her son has been made to feel different by his peers because he has to visit the nurse's office for a lunchtime dose of medication. The boy is threatening to stop taking his medication. How should the nurse respond?
   a. "He should ignore the children; he needs this medication."

   b. "I can have the teacher speak with the other children."
   c. "Remind him that his schoolwork may deteriorate if he stops taking the medication."
   d. "Talk to your physician about an extended-release medication."

3. The nurse is conducting an examination of a boy with Tourette syndrome. Which of the following would the nurse expect to observe?
   a. Toe walking
   b. Sudden, rapid stereotypical sounds
   c. Spinning and hand-flapping
   d. Lack of eye contact

4. A nurse is providing a routine wellness examination and follow-up for a three-year-old recently diagnosed with autism spectrum disorder. Which of the following responses by the parent indicates a need for additional referral or follow-up?
   a. "We try to be flexible and change his routine from day to day."
   b. "We really like the treatment plan that has been created by his school."
   c. "We have recently completed his individualized education plan."
   d. "We have a couple of babysitters who know how to handle his needs."

5. A nurse is caring for a child with mental retardation. The medical chart indicates an IQ of 37. This degree of mental retardation is classified as which of the following?
   a. Mild
   b. Moderate
   c. Severe
   d. Profound

6. A nurse is caring for a ten-year-old mentally retarded girl hospitalized for a scheduled cholecystectomy. The girl expresses fear related to her hospitalization and unfamiliar surroundings. How should the nurse respond?
   a. "Don't worry; you'll be going home soon."
   b. "Tell me about a typical day at home."
   c. "Have you talked to your parents about this?"
   d. "Do you want some art supplies?"

7. The nurse is caring for an adolescent girl with anorexia. Which of the following assessment findings would the nurse expect to note?
   a. Headache
   b. Mouth ulcers
   c. Abdominal pain
   d. High blood pressure

8. A nurse is conducting a physical examination of an adolescent girl with suspected bulimia. Which of the following assessment findings would the nurse expect to note?
   a. Eroded dental enamel
   b. Dry, sallow skin
   c. Soft, sparse body hair
   d. Thinning scalp hair

9. A nurse is caring for a preschooler with injuries in various sites. Which of the following injury sites is suspicious of abuse?
   a. Abdomen
   b. Soles
   c. Palms
   d. Stomach

10. The nurse is providing teaching about medication management of attention-deficit/hyperactivity disorder. Which of the following responses from the parent indicates a need for further teaching?
    a. "We should give it to him with his meals."
    b. "This may cause him to have difficulty sleeping."
    c. "If he takes this medicine he will no longer have ADHD."
    d. "We should see an improvement in his schoolwork."

11. A three-year-old boy has been diagnosed with autism spectrum disorder. His parents ask a nurse for an approach that can completely cure it. Which of the following will be the correct response for the nurse?
    a. "There are no medications or treatments available to cure autism."
    b. "The child should be put on a restrictive diet to guarantee the success of medication."
    c. "Nutritional supplements can cure him but he is too young for them."
    d. "Music therapy by a certified professional can cure him completely."

12. A nurse is caring for a 19-year-old girl diagnosed with bulimia. Which of the following complications can the nurse expect in the client?
    a. Partial paralysis
    b. Hernia
    c. Severe acne
    d. Menstrual problems

13. An eight-year-old boy is diagnosed with post-traumatic stress disorder following a car accident. Which of the following approaches can help him?
    a. Psychostimulants
    b. Antipsychotic medications
    c. Individual psychotherapy
    d. Sensory integration technique

14. A nurse is assessing a 17-year-old girl with behavioral problems. The mention of which of the following in her health history will be indicative of a bipolar disorder?
    a. Social phobia
    b. Poor performance at school
    c. Decreased sleep
    d. Vocal tics

15. A nurse is assessing a 15-year-old girl who admits that she is stressed out with her studies and part-time job. She also has problems relating with people and has no meaningful friendships. Which steps can the nurse take to help her improve her coping skills? Select all that apply.
    a. Encourage suppression of thoughts and feelings
    b. Provide positive feedback for appropriate discussion
    c. Demonstrate unconditional acceptance
    d. Remove all limits on behavior
    e. Teach problem-solving skills

Nursing Care During a Pediatric Emergency

SECTION I: LEARNING OBJECTIVES

1. Identify various factors contributing to emergency situations among infants and children.

2. Discuss common treatments and medications used for a child experiencing an emergency.

3. Conduct a health history of a child experiencing an emergency situation, specific to the emergency.

4. Perform a rapid cardiopulmonary assessment.

5. Discuss common laboratory and other diagnostic tests used during pediatric emergencies.

6. Integrate the principles of the American Heart Association (AHA) and Pediatric Advanced Life Support (PALS) in the comprehensive management of a child with an emergent medical situation.

SECTION II: ASSESSING YOUR UNDERSTANDING

Activity A *Fill in the blanks.*

1. _____ is a process by which a breathing tube is inserted into the airway to assist with breathing.

2. When a child has an abnormal, life-threatening cardiac rhythm, it is necessary to use electrical energy to terminate it. This is called _____

3. If a three-year-old child is breathing at a rate of 40 breaths a minute and is breathing deeply with each breath, this would be charted as _____.

4. _____ occurs when there is no cardiac electrical activity.

5. A decreased amount of carbon dioxide in the blood is called _____.

6. _____ tachycardia is a rare arrhythmia in children that usually is associated with a congenital or acquired cardiac abnormality.

7. _____ is a heart rate significantly slower than the patient's normal heart rate for his or her age.

8. Children in emergency situations commonly have _____ shock that occurs in association with fluid losses.

9. When assisting with ventilating a child, you must be careful not to use too high a rate or volume or you can cause _____, which is defined as the trauma caused by changes in pressure.

10. Paleness around the mouth is known as _____ pallor.

Activity B *Consider the following figures.*

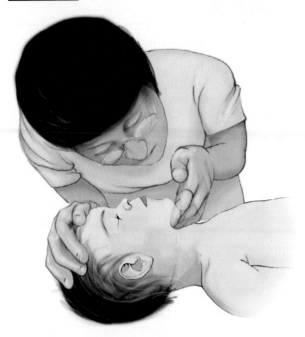

1. What does the figure depict?

_____

_____

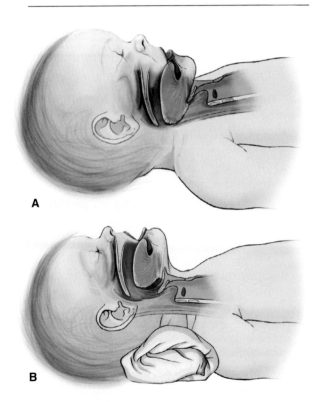

A

B

2. Identify the figure.

_____

_____

Activity C *Match the common medical treatments for pediatric emergencies in Column A with their descriptions in Column B.*

Column A

____ **1.** Bag valve mask

____ **2.** Blood product transfusion

____ **3.** Intubation

____ **4.** IV fluid therapy

____ **5.** Oxygenation

Column B

a. If adverse reaction, stop, infuse saline, reassess the child, and notify physician

b. Ensures adequate chest rise with ventilation

c. Monitor response via color, work of breathing, respiratory rate, pulse oximetry, and level of consciousness

d. Femoral route is optimal during CPR

e. Watch for yellow CO_2 monitor display

Activity D *Put the items in correct sequence by writing the letters in the boxes provided below.*

1. Given below, in random order, are some steps involved in cardiopulmonary resuscitation (CPR). Choose the correct sequence:

a. Administer 100% oxygen

b. Evaluate heart rate and pulses

c. Look, listen, feel for respirations

d. Position airway

e. Suction

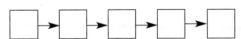

Activity E *Briefly answer the following.*

1. What are the ABCs implied in rapid cardiopulmonary assessment?

_____

_____

_____

2. Define cricoid pressure.

_____

_____

_____

3. List the standard laboratory and diagnostics tests performed in most emergency departments.

_____

_____

_____

4. What is the airway management for a child with no cervical spine injury?

_____

_____

_____

5. What is cardioversion?

_____

_____

_____

6. What are the causes of respiratory emergencies in infants and young children?

_____

_____

_____

SECTION III: APPLYING YOUR KNOWLEDGE

Activity F *Consider this scenario and answer the question.*

1. A seven-year-old boy has a respiratory arrest. The nurses immediately start bag-valve-mask ventilation. How can the nurse assess the child's response to the resuscitative efforts during the course of resuscitation?

_____

_____

_____

SECTION IV: PRACTICING FOR NCLEX

Activity G *Answer the following questions.*

1. According to Pediatric Advanced Life Support (PALS), calculate the minimum acceptable systolic BP for a five-year-old boy.
   a. 80
   b. 90
   c. 70
   d. 60

2. The nurse is examining a ten-month-old girl who has fallen from the back porch. Which assessment will directly follow the evaluation of the ABCs?
   a. Observing skin color and perfusion
   b. Palpating the abdomen for soreness
   c. Auscultating for bowel sounds
   d. Palpating the anterior fontanel

3. The nurse is caring for a ten-month-old boy with signs of respiratory distress. Which is the best way to maintain this child's airway?
   a. Inserting a small towel under his shoulders
   b. Placing a hand under his neck
   c. Using the head-tilt/chin-lift technique
   d. Employing the jaw-thrust maneuver

4. Cardiopulmonary resuscitation (CPR) is in progress on an eight-year-old boy who is in shock. Which is the priority nursing intervention?
   a. Obtaining central venous access via the femoral route
   b. Using a large-bore catheter for peripheral venous access
   c. Inserting an indwelling urinary catheter to measure urine output
   d. Drawing a blood sample for an arterial blood gas analysis

5. The nurse is examining a ten-year-old boy with tachypnea and increased work of breathing. Which finding is a late sign that the child is in shock?

   a. Significantly decreased skin elasticity
   b. Blood pressure slightly less than normal
   c. Equally strong central and distal pulses
   d. Delayed capillary refill with cool extremities

6. Calculate the tracheal tube size for a six-year-old child, in millimeters.

   a. 6.0
   b. 5.0
   c. 4.5
   d. 5.5

7. A three-year-old girl had a near-drowning incident when she fell into a wading pool. Which intervention would be of the highest priority?

   a. Suctioning the upper airway to ensure airway patency
   b. Inserting a nasogastric tube to decompress the stomach
   c. Covering the child with warming blankets
   d. Ensuring the child stays still during an x-ray

8. A three-year-old child is brought to the emergency department with accidental poisoning. Which of the following tests should be performed to assess renal function in the client?

   a. Chemistry panel
   b. Urine toxicology screens
   c. Blood toxicology screens
   d. Serum electrolytes

9. A nurse is assigned to care for a seven-year-old child with collapsed rhythms or pulse-less rhythms. During physical examination, the nurse auscultates breath sounds near the tricuspid area. Which of the following is the appropriate area for auscultating the tricuspid area?

   a. Second right interspace
   b. Second left interspace
   c. Fifth interspace, midclavicular line
   d. Left lower sternal border

10. The nurse is ventilating a nine-year-old girl with a bag valve mask. Which action would most likely reduce the effectiveness of ventilation?

    a. Checking the tail for free flow of oxygen
    b. Pressing down on the mask below the mouth
    c. Referring to Broselow® tape for bag size
    d. Setting the oxygen flow rate at 15 L/minute

11. A five-year-old child is brought to the emergency department following a fall from the terrace. The nurse notes that the child has no pulse. What should be the priority intervention?

    a. Initiate CPR
    b. Administer epinephrine
    c. Administer oxygen
    d. Start IV fluids

12. A two-year-old boy is in respiratory distress. Which nursing assessment finding would suggest the child has aspirated a foreign body?

    a. Hearing dullness when percussing a lung lobe
    b. Auscultating a low-pitched, grating breath sound
    c. Hearing a hyperresonant sound on percussion
    d. Noting absent breath sounds in one lung

13. When resuscitating a child, the nurse inserts a tracheal tube to facilitate ventilation. What should the nurse do to rule out accidental esophageal intubation?

    a. Auscultate over the lung fields for equal breath sounds
    b. Observe for symmetrical rise of the chest
    c. Auscultate over the abdomen while the child is being ventilated
    d. Inspect the tube for presence of water vapor on the inside

14. Which of the following types of shock results in a decrease in cardiac output with an increase in systemic vascular resistance (SVR)?

    a. Warm shock

    b. Cardiogenic shock

    c. Cold shock

    d. Distributive shock

15. A nurse is assigned to care for a client with septic shock. Which of the following tests is conducted to assess for a viral or bacterial infection in septic shock?

    a. Complete blood cell count with differential

    b. Blood culture

    c. C-reactive protein

    d. Toxicology panel

Answers

CHAPTER 1

Activity A

1. doula
2. Intrauterine
3. breast
4. family
5. emancipated
6. specialty
7. discipline
8. competence
9. anticipatory
10. Morbidity

Activity B

1. c   2. b   3. d   4. a   5. e

Activity C

1.

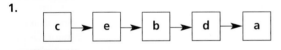

Activity D

1. Nurses need to take care to look beyond the obvious "crushing chest pain" symptom that heralds a heart attack in men, because women present symptoms of CVD in a very different way, and the diagnosis is missed if CVD is not on their list of possibilities. Nurses therefore should monitor the following risk factors in women that could lead to CVD:
   - Cigarette smoking
   - Smoking and use of oral contraceptives or hormone replacement therapy
   - Obesity
   - A diet high in saturated fats
   - Stress
   - Sedentary lifestyle
   - Hypertension
   - Hyperlipidemia
   - Strong family history
   - Diabetes mellitus
   - Postmenopausal status
2. Case management is a collaborative process involving assessment, planning, implementation, coordination, monitoring, and evaluation. It includes advocacy, communication, resource management, client-focused comprehensive care across a continuum, and coordinated care with an interdisciplinary approach.
3. Involvement in social activities, a strong commitment to school and academic performance, and ability to discuss problems with a supportive adult are some of the protective factors that boost resilience in children.
4. Evidence-based nursing practice involves the use of research or evidence in establishing a plan of care and implementing that care. It is a problem-solving approach to nursing clinical decisions. This concept of nursing practice includes the use of the best current evidence in making decisions about the care of women, children, and their families.
5. Maternal mortality rate measures the number of deaths from any cause during the pregnancy cycle per 100,000 live births.
6. Low birth weight and prematurity are major indicators of infant health and significant predictors of infant mortality. The lower the birth weight, the higher the risk of infant mortality.

Activity E

1. Parenting styles vary in the amount of control exerted over the child. The husband seems to fit into the authoritarian parenting style, in which the parent expects obedience from the children without questioning the family rules. He also expects the children to accept the family's beliefs and values. Whatever the style of parenting, it is important that caregiving is sensitive and responsive in order to promote appropriate physical, neurophysiologic, and psychological development. The recent change in family structure may be difficult for the child, especially if there are differing views and practices related to discipline. It may be helpful to discuss this with the child's stepfather. Parenting is more effective if parents adjust their style to meet the needs of their children at different developmental levels and temperaments. The American Academy of Pediatrics (1998) suggests three components: 1) maintain a positive, supportive, nurturing caregiver–child relationship; 2) provide positive reinforcement techniques to increase desirable

behaviors; and 3) remove the positive reinforcement techniques or use punishment to reduce or eliminate undesirable behaviors. Corporal punishment such as spanking may stop the negative behavior but it also increases the chance for physical injury and may lead to altered caregiver–child relationships. Some positive strategies for effective discipline include setting clear, consistent, and developmentally appropriate expected behaviors and providing age-appropriate explanations of the consequences of unacceptable behavior. Always administer the consequence soon after the unacceptable behavior. Make sure the consequence is appropriate to the age of the child and situation. Stay calm but firm without showing anger when administering consequences. Catch the child displaying appropriate behavior and praise the child. Ensure that the environment is set to help the child accomplish the appropriate behavior.

2. With the recent changes in family structure, especially if there are different views and practices related to child care and health practices, family conflict may arise. It is important as a parent to understand this and place the children's interest in the forefront. This can help minimize negative effects.

Activity F

1. **Answer: b**
   RATIONALE: Breastfeeding reduces the rates of infection in infants and helps to improve long-term maternal health. Placing the infant on his or her back to sleep prevents sudden infant death syndrome (SIDS) but does not prevent infections in the infant. Feeding foods high in starch or feeding liquids frequently will not prevent infections either.

2. **Answer: a**
   RATIONALE: The nurses should advocate adequate intake of folic acid supplements during pregnancy to reduce the prevalence of neural defects in infants. Taking vitamin E supplements, engaging in mild exercises during pregnancy, and regularly consuming citrus fruits are healthy habits for the mother and infant, but they do not reduce the infants' risk of developing neural defects.

3. **Answer: d**
   RATIONALE: According to the ANA's code of ethics, the nurse could make arrangements for alternate care providers for a client undergoing an abortion, if the nurse ethically opposes the procedure. Nurses need to make their values and beliefs known to their managers before the situation occurs so alternate staffing arrangements can be made. Under the ANA's code of ethics for nurses, the nurse need not provide emotional support to the client, nor should he or she involve the client's family in convincing the client against an abortion.

4. **Answer: d**
   RATIONALE: The nurse should instruct the client to place her infant on his or her back to sleep to prevent SIDS. Draping the infant in warm clothes, providing very soft bedding, or feeding a mixture of salts, sugar, and water will not prevent SIDS.

5. **Answer: b**
   RATIONALE: Lung cancer has no early symptoms, making its early detection almost impossible. Lung cancer is equally fatal for both men and women; it is not more deadly in men. Women do not have a stronger resistance to lung cancer. It is the most common cancer in women because of the increasing frequency of smoking. Though the early detection of lung cancer is very difficult, its diagnosis is not more challenging in women than in men.

6. **Answer: c**
   RATIONALE: Children living with their grandparents may experience emotional stress if the biological parents are in and out of the child's life. Teaching basic childcare skills is appropriate for an adolescent's family. Identifying the decision-maker may be important for an extended family, and financial aid may be important for single parents.

7. **Answer: c**
   RATIONALE: In the Arab-American culture, women are subordinate to men and children are subordinate to the parents. The nurse would deal directly and exclusively with the father. This family would not place much emphasis on preventive care, either. Inquiring about folk remedies used may be appropriate with African-American families. Coordinating care through the mother might be appropriate with a Hispanic family.

8. **Answer: b**
   RATIONALE: Ignoring the child's temper tantrum is an example of extinction discipline; positive reinforcement is eliminated for inappropriate behavior. Going out for ice cream, praising the child for displaying appropriate behavior, and letting the child go to a friend's house are all types of positive reinforcement.

9. **Answer: d**
   RATIONALE: The nurse should tell the client that it is important for both parents to discuss with the children how things will work after the divorce. The children should not be made to act like adults. The nurse should also ask the client to inform her children about the divorce ahead of time, and tell them the reasons in nonjudgmental terms that they can understand.

10. **Answer: c**
    RATIONALE: In cases of abuse and violence, nurses can serve their clients best by not trying to rescue them but by helping them build on their strengths, providing support, and empowering them to help themselves. Counseling the client's partner against abuse, helping her know the legal impact of her situation, and introducing the client to a women's rights group to garner support are not the best ways of serving the client.

11. **Answer: a & c**
    RATIONALE: To ensure that the client keeps her appointments for good follow-up care, the nurse

should ensure that there is no delay before her examination and that the client should not be examined in a hurry. Scheduling appointments to match the client's comfort and encouraging telephone consultation services may not be the most appropriate interventions to encourage the client to continue her appointments.

12. Answer: a, b, & c
   RATIONALE: The diagnosis of CVD in women is more challenging and therefore difficult because of the prevalence of common myths: CVD is still thought of as a "man's disease" and as being more deadly in males than in females. Symptoms of CVD present differently in females than in males, and this makes the diagnosis even more difficult. CVD has early symptoms and can be detected. In addition, CVD occurring in women younger than 65 years of age is not rare.

13. Answer: a & d
   RATIONALE: To reduce the risk of cardiovascular disease, the nurse should instruct the client to undertake stress management to control her stress levels and to exercise regularly to achieve her ideal weight. Increasing fluid intake will not reduce the risk of CVD. Consumption of simple carbohydrates will not prevent the occurrence of CVD.

14. Answer: a & b
   RATIONALE: The nurse should ask the client if she smokes, because cigarette smoking increases the risk of developing cardiovascular disease. Risk of CVD also increases with weight fluctuations and diabetes; therefore, the nurse also should ask questions related to these. The risk of CVD increases in clients who consume a diet high in saturated fats but not among those who consume a diet high in starch. Having one's first child after the age of 30 increases the risk of developing breast cancer but does not increase the risk of developing CVD.

15 Answer: b, c, & d
   RATIONALE: The nurse should be aware that many pregnant teenage clients develop complications such as anemia, preterm labor, and cephalopelvic disproportion. Dystocia may be associated with pregnancy after 35 years of age. Cardiovascular disease is associated with menopause but not with pregnancy.

CHAPTER 2

Activity A
1. Nonverbal
2. Case
3. Community
4. Outpatient
5. prevention
6. Epidemiology
7. competence
8. encounters
9. Health
10. fragile

Activity B
1. The figure depicts the three levels of prevention in community-based nursing. At the primary level, the nurse provides anticipatory guidance and family teaching. Secondary prevention is the early detection and treatment of adverse health conditions. Tertiary prevention is designed to reduce or limit the progression of a disease or disability after an injury.
2. The figure shows a school nurse in the school setting. The school nurse provides nursing assessment as well as health education to students.

Activity C
1. d   **2.** a   **3.** e   **4.** b   **5.** c

Activity D
1.

$$ e \rightarrow b \rightarrow a \rightarrow c \rightarrow d $$

Activity E
1. Some of the techniques that the nurse can use to enhance learning are slowing down and repeating information often; speaking in conversational style, using plain, nonmedical language; "chunking" information and teaching it in small bites, using logical steps; prioritizing information and teaching "survival skills" first; using visuals, such as pictures, videos, and models; and using an interactive, "hands-on" approach.
2. School nursing is a specialized practice of professional nursing and focuses on improving student health to impact the achievement and success of students. School nurses facilitate positive student responses to normal development; promote health and safety; intervene with actual and potential health problems; provide case management services; and actively collaborate with others to build student and family capacity for adaptation, self-management, self-advocacy, and learning.
3. A triage nurse in a pediatric office must be able to determine from the call whether or not the child needs to be evaluated and if that evaluation should be made emergently. The nurse must carefully question the parent or caregiver about the specifics of the child's condition to determine whether it fits into a low- or high-risk category.
4. Nurses in the school setting develop an Individualized Health Plan (IHP). It is used to formalize the plan of support for a student with complex health care needs. It is a written agreement developed with an interdisciplinary collaboration of school staff along with the student, the student's family, and the student's health care provider. The plan describes the student's needs and how the school plans to meet these needs.
5. During the past several years, the health care delivery system has changed dramatically. With a focus on cost containment, people are spending less time

in the hospital. Patients are being discharged "sicker and quicker" from their hospital beds. The health care system has moved from reactive treatment strategies in hospitals to a proactive approach in the community. This has resulted in an increasing emphasis on health promotion and illness prevention within the community.

6. A birthing center provides a cross between a home birth and a hospital birth. Birthing centers offer a home-like setting with close proximity to a hospital in case of complications. Midwives often are the sole care providers in freestanding birthing centers, with obstetricians as backups in case of emergencies. Birthing centers usually have fewer restrictions and guidelines for families to follow and allow for more freedom in making laboring decisions. Birthing centers aim to provide a relaxing home-like environment and promote a culture of normalcy.

Activity F

1. The nurse should adapt to different cultural beliefs and practices by being flexible and accepting of others' points of view; by listening to clients and learning about their beliefs on health and wellness; and by knowing, understanding, and respecting culturally influenced health behaviors.

2. Some of the cultural characteristics that would be important for a nurse to understand are values, beliefs of the various people to whom they deliver care, time orientation, personal space, language, and family orientation.

3. To ensure culturally competent nursing care to diverse families, the nurse should develop cultural self-awareness; gain cultural knowledge about various world views of different cultures; and participate in cultural encounters.

Activity G

1. **Answer: d**
   RATIONALE: Case management focuses on coordinating health care services while balancing quality and cost outcomes. Helping a family member learn how to perform a procedure is part of the teaching role. Assessing sanitary conditions is done during discharge planning, and establishing eligibility for Medicaid is resource management.

2. **Answer: a**
   RATIONALE: Having a child life specialist play with the child would provide the greatest support for the child and make the greatest contribution to atraumatic care. It is important to explain the procedure to the child and parents, let the child have a favorite toy, and keep the parents calm, but these interventions are not as effective for atraumatic care.

3. **Answer: c**
   RATIONALE: Asking questions or having private conversations with the interpreter may make the family uncomfortable and destroy the patient–nurse relationship. Translation takes longer than a same-language appointment, and this must be considered so that the family is not rushed. A nonprofessional may be unable to adequately translate medical terminology. Using an older sibling can upset the family relationships or cause legal problems.

4. **Answer: a**
   RATIONALE: Recognizing family strengths and individuality is a key element of family-centered home care. Ensuring a safe, nurturing environment is part of the assessment process prior to preparing the nursing plan of care. Information should be shared completely and openly with parents, not "managed." The nurse should respect different methods of coping rather than correcting them.

5. **Answer: b**
   RATIONALE: Promoting the health and safety of a group of children is a common goal of nurses in all community settings. Removing health barriers to learning is the school nurse's goal. Determining the type of care a child needs is the goal of telephone triage. Ensuring the health and well-being of children and families is a goal of family-centered home care.

6. **Answer: b**
   RATIONALE: The nurse should monitor for the incidence of hydrocephalus in the high-risk newborn. Hydrocephalus, along with conditions such as cerebral palsy, retinopathy, and ongoing oxygen dependency, is likely to persist after discharge in a high-risk newborn. Anencephaly and fetal distress syndrome are not conditions that persist after discharge. Spina bifida is most often noted at birth and would not to need to be assessed for by the nurse.

7. **Answer: b**
   RATIONALE: The nurse should instruct the client to take folic acid supplements, because consumption of folic acid supplements reduces the risk of NTDs developing in the growing fetus. Taking vitamin E supplements and consuming legumes or citrus fruits regularly during pregnancy do not reduce the risk of NTDs.

8. **Answer: d**
   RATIONALE: The nurse should inform the women that comprehensive community-centered care should be given to women during their reproductive years. This is because as their reproductive goals change, so do their health care needs. A women's immune system does not weaken immediately after birth. Similarly, women do not have more health problems specifically during their reproductive years. They are not more susceptible to stress during their reproductive years.

9. **Answer: b**
   RATIONALE: The nurse should include the monitoring of the physical and emotional well-being of the client's family members as part of her postpartum care in the home environment. The nurse should provide hands-on experience in infant care instead of providing self-help books to the client.

The nurse should include parental needs along with the infant needs and focus on each of these areas while preparing her discharge plan, because the nurse should identify potential or developing complications not only in the infant but also in the client.

10. **Answer: a**

    RATIONALE: A nurse who thinks stereotypically may assign a client to a staff member who is of the same culture as the client because the nurse assumes that all people of that culture are alike. The nurse also may believe that clients with the same skin color may react in the same manner in similar social situations. Because stereotypes are preconceived ideas unsupported by facts, they may not be real or accurate. In fact, they can be dangerous because they are dehumanizing and interfere with accepting others as unique individuals.

11. **Answer: a, b, & d**

    RATIONALE: When caring for this client, the nurse should convey empathy for what the client is experiencing; she should listen actively by giving verbal and body language clues; and she should show respect by valuing the client and viewing her as special. The nurse should not interact with the client only when required. She should also not respond to the client only in simple answers of "yes" and "no," because it is important for the nurse to establish rapport by initiating social, friendly conversation.

12. **Answer: a, c, & e**

    RATIONALE: To maximize the home care visit, the nurse should plan by prioritizing the client's needs by their potential to threaten the client's health. The nurse should also bear in mind the client's readiness to accept intervention and education, and she should develop goals that reflect primary, secondary, and tertiary prevention levels. Additionally, instead of making an individualized plan of client care, the nurse should review previous interventions made during home visits to eliminate unsuccessful ones. The nurse should check previous home visit narratives to validate interventions

as well as communicate with previous nurses to ask questions and clarify. Instead of training the family, the nurse should obtain the necessary materials or supplies before making the home visit.

13. **Answer: c**

    RATIONALE: Coordinating the services of therapists and other professionals is a primary role for the home care nurse. Although the nurse may prepare the child to see a physician, conduct health screening, or collaborate with teachers, these activities are not unique to home care nursing.

14. **Answer: b**

    RATIONALE: Asking questions is a valid way to evaluate learning. However, it is far more effective to ask open-ended questions because they will better expose missing or incorrect information. As with teaching, evaluation of learning that involves active participation is more effective. This includes the child and family demonstrating skills, teaching skills to each other, and acting out scenarios.

15 **Answer: a**

    RATIONALE: If the client does not comply with treatment regimens, it could indicate that he or she has poor literacy skills. Clients who avoid asking questions for fear of looking "stupid," clients who miss appointments, and clients who are unable to answer queries regarding medications may have poor literacy skills.

CHAPTER 3

Activity A

1. rugae
2. Prolactin
3. epididymis
4. urethra
5. endometrium
6. Skene's
7. episiotomy
8. prostate
9. uterus
10. scrotum

Activity B

1. a. The figure shows the lateral view of the internal female reproductive organs.

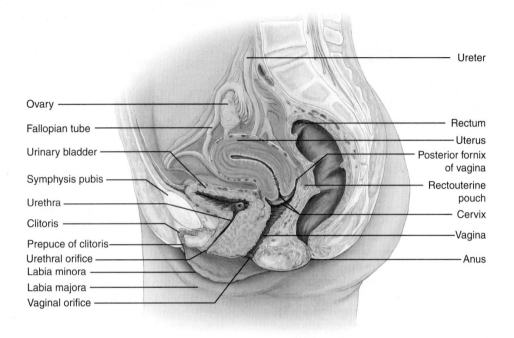

Ureter

Ovary

Fallopian tube

Urinary bladder

Symphysis pubis

Urethra

Clitoris

Prepuce of clitoris

Urethral orifice

Labia minora

Labia majora

Vaginal orifice

Rectum

Uterus

Posterior fornix of vagina

Rectouterine pouch

Cervix

Vagina

Anus

b. The internal female reproductive organs consist of the vagina, uterus, fallopian tubes, and ovaries. The vagina is a canal that connects the external genitals to the uterus. It receives the penis and the sperm ejaculated during sexual intercourse, and it serves as an exit passageway for menstrual blood and for the fetus during childbirth. The uterus is a pear-shaped muscular organ at the top of the vagina. It is the site of menstruation, implantation of a fertilized ovum, development of the fetus during pregnancy, and labor. The fallopian tubes are hollow, cylindrical structures that extend 2 to 3 inches from the upper edges of the uterus toward the ovaries. The fallopian tubes convey the ovum from the ovary to the uterus and sperm from the uterus toward the ovary. The ovaries are a set of paired glands resembling unshelled almonds set in the pelvic cavity below and to either side of the umbilicus. The development and release of the ovum and the secretion of the hormones estrogen and progesterone are the two primary functions of the ovary.

2. a. The figure shows the lateral view of the internal male reproductive organs.

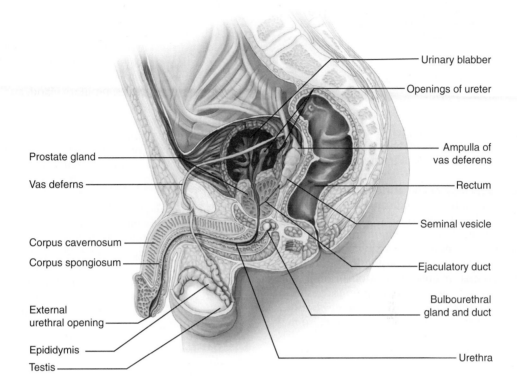

- Urinary blabber
- Openings of ureter
- Ampulla of vas deferens
- Rectum
- Seminal vesicle
- Ejaculatory duct
- Bulbourethral gland and duct
- Urethra
- Prostate gland
- Vas deferns
- Corpus cavernosum
- Corpus spongiosum
- External urethral opening
- Epididymis
- Testis

b. The internal structures include the testes, the ductal system, and accessory glands. The testes are oval bodies the size of large olives that lie in the scrotum. They produce sperm and synthesize testosterone. The vas deferens is a cordlike duct that transports sperm from the epididymis. The seminal vesicles, which produce nutrient seminal fluid, and the prostate gland, which produces alkaline prostatic fluid, are both connected to the ejaculatory duct leading into the urethra.

The bulbourethral glands secrete a mucus-like fluid in response to sexual stimulation and lubricate the head of the penis in preparation for sexual intercourse.

3. The figure shows the internal structures of a testis.

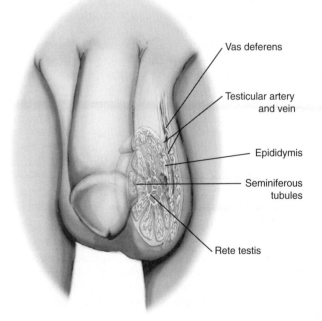

- Vas deferens
- Testicular artery and vein
- Epididymis
- Seminiferous tubules
- Rete testis

Activity C

1. e   **2.** c   **3.** b   **4.** d   **5.** a

Activity D

1.

b → a → d → c

2.

c → b → a → d

Activity E

1. The external female reproductive organs collectively are called the vulva. The vulva serves to protect the urethral and vaginal openings. The structures that make up the vulva include the mons pubis, the labia majora and minora, the clitoris, the structures within the vestibule, and the perineum.

2. Soon after childbirth, colostrum is secreted for approximately a week, with gradual conversion to mature milk. Colostrum is a dark yellow fluid that contains more minerals and protein, but less sugar and fat, than mature breast milk. Colostrum is rich in maternal antibodies, especially immunoglobulin A (IgA), which offers protection for the newborn against enteric pathogens. Colostrum secretion may continue after childbirth.

3. During the perimenopausal years, women may experience physical changes associated with decreasing estrogen levels, which may include vasomotor symptoms of hot flashes, irregular menstrual cycles, sleep disruptions, forgetfulness, irritability, mood disturbances, decreased vaginal lubrication, fatigue, vaginal atrophy, and depression.

4. Nurses can play a major role in assisting menopausal women by educating and counseling them about the multitude of options available for disease prevention, treatment for menopausal symptoms, and health promotion during this time of change in their lives.

5. The testes produce sperm and synthesize testosterone, which is the primary male sex hormone. Sperm is produced in the seminiferous tubules of the testes.

6. The bulbourethral (Cowper's) glands are two small structures about the size of peas, located inferior to the prostate gland. They are composed of several tubes whose epithelial linings secrete a mucus-like fluid. It is released in response to sexual stimulation and lubricates the head of the penis in preparation for sexual intercourse. They gradually diminish in size with advancing age.

Activity F

1. **a.** The nurse should inform Susan about the following: the main function of the reproductive cycle is to stimulate growth of a follicle to release an egg and prepare a site for implantation if fertilization occurs; menstruation, the monthly shedding of the uterine lining, marks the beginning of a new cycle; the menstrual cycle involves a complex interaction of hormones; the ovarian cycle is the series of events associated with a developing oocyte (ovum, or egg) within the ovaries; at ovulation, a mature follicle ruptures in response to a surge of LH, releasing a mature oocyte (ovum); the endometrial cycle is divided into three phases: the follicular or proliferative phase, the luteal or secretory phase, and the menstrual phase; the endometrium, ovaries, pituitary gland, and hypothalamus are all involved in the cyclic changes that help to prepare the body for fertilization; the menstrual cycle results from a functional hypothalamic-pituitary-ovarian axis and a precise sequencing of hormones that lead to ovulation; if conception doesn't occur, menses ensues; and the one thing to remember is that whether a women's cycle is 28 days or 120 days, ovulation takes place 14 days before menstruation.

   b. The nurse should inform Susan that cycles vary in frequency from 21 to 36 days; bleeding lasts 3 to 8 days; blood loss averages 20 to 80 mL; the average cycle is 28 days long, but this varies; and irregular menses can be associated with irregular ovulation, stress, disease, and hormonal imbalances.

Activity G

1. **Answer: b**

   RATIONALE: To increase the chances of conceiving, the best time for intercourse is one or two days before ovulation. This ensures that the sperm meets the ovum at the right time. The average life of a sperm cell is two to three days, and the sperm cells will not be able to survive until ovulation if intercourse occurs a week before ovulation. The chances of conception are minimal for intercourse after ovulation.

2. **Answer: d**

   RATIONALE: Bartholin's glands, when stimulated, secrete mucus that supplies lubrication for intercourse. Endocrine glands secrete hormones for various bodily functions. The pituitary gland releases follicle-stimulating hormone (FSH) to stimulate the ovary to produce follicles. Skene's glands secrete a small amount of mucus to keep the opening to the urethra moist and lubricated for the passage of urine.

3. **Answer: a**

   RATIONALE: The endometrium is the mucosal layer that lines the uterine cavity in nonpregnant women. The fundus is the convex portion above the uterine tubes. The mons pubis is the elevated, rounded, fleshy prominence over the symphysis pubis. The clitoris is a small, cylindrical mass of erectile tissue and nerves located at the anterior junction of the labia minora.

4. **Answer: b**

   RATIONALE: The nurse should inform the client that the yellow fluid is called colostrum, and it contains more minerals and protein, but less sugar and fat, than mature breast milk and is also rich in maternal antibodies. The nurse should inform the client that, gradually, the production of colostrum stops and the production of regular breast milk begins, but there is no need to avoid breastfeeding when colostrum is being produced, if the client's culture allows for it. There is no need to modify diet or to feed formula to the infant.

5. **Answer: c**
RATIONALE: During ovulation, some women can feel a pain around the time the egg is released on one side of the abdomen. The pain is not a sign of pregnancy, as the client experiences this pain regularly during ovulation. The pain is also not related to an irregular menstruation cycle or the client's exercise regimen.

6. **Answer: b**
RATIONALE: The nurse should inform the client that there will be a significant increase in temperature, usually 0.5 to 1° F, within a day or two after ovulation has occurred. The temperature remains elevated for 12 to 16 days, until menstruation begins. During ovulation, some women can feel a pain on one side of the abdomen around the time the egg is released. There is no significant correlation between ovulation and lack of sleep or feeling uneasiness or sickness.

7. **Answer: b**
RATIONALE: After menopause, the uterus shrinks and gradually atrophies. A full bladder, not menopause, causes the uterus to tilt backward. Cervical muscle content does not increase during menopause. Menopause has no significant effect on the outer layer of the cervix.

8. **Answer: d**
RATIONALE: Progesterone is called the hormone of pregnancy because it reduces uterine contractions, thus producing a calming effect on the uterus, allowing pregnancy to be maintained. Follicle-stimulating hormone (FSH) is primarily responsible for the maturation of the ovarian follicle. Luteinizing hormone (LH) is required for both the final maturation of preovulatory follicles and luteinization of the ruptured follicle. Estrogen is crucial for the development and maturation of the follicle.

9. **Answer: c**
RATIONALE: During cold conditions, the scrotum is pulled closer to the body for warmth or protection. The cremaster muscles in the scrotal wall contract to allow the testes to be pulled closer to the body. Frequency of urination has no significant impact in maintaining the scrotal temperature. Increase in blood flow to the genital area occurs primarily during erection and is not due to climatic conditions.

10. **Answer: a**
RATIONALE: With age, the prostate gland gradually enlarges, leading to difficulty during urination. Production of semen never stops, even though the quantity of semen produced may decrease. The

prostate gland is not associated with painful erection. During the normal aging process, the prostate gland does not stop functioning, even though its capacity may be somewhat diminished.

11. **Answer: b**
RATIONALE: The epididymis provides the space and environment for sperm to mature. The testes produce sperm, but they have to mature in the epididymis to become capable of impregnating the ovum. The vas deferens is the organ that transports sperm from the epididymis. The Cowper's glands secrete mucus-like fluid for lubrication during sexual intercourse.

12. **Answer: c**
RATIONALE: The nurse should inform the client that the duration of the flow is about 3 to 7 days. An average cycle length is about 21 to 36 days, not 15 to 20 days. In the ovary, 2 million oocytes are present at birth, and about 400,000 follicles are still present at puberty. Blood loss averages 20 to 80 mL, not 120 to 150 mL.

13. **Answer: c**
RATIONALE: At ovulation, a mature follicle ruptures, releasing a mature oocyte (ovum). Ovulation always takes place 14 days, not 10 days, before menstruation. The lifespan of the ovum is only about 24 hours, not 48 hours; unless it meets a sperm on its journey within that time, it will die. When ovulation occurs, there is a drop, not a rise, in estrogen levels.

14. **Answer: b**
RATIONALE: Gonadotropin-releasing hormone is secreted from the hypothalamus in a pulsatile manner throughout the reproductive cycle. It induces the release of follicle-stimulating hormone and luteinizing hormone to assist with ovulation, both of which are secreted by the anterior pituitary gland. Estrogen is secreted by the ovaries and is crucial for the development and maturation of the follicle.

CHAPTER 4

Activity A

1. Adenomyosis
2. prostaglandin
3. Laparoscopy
4. perimenopause
5. vasectomy
6. medical
7. Osteoporosis
8. spinnbarkeit
9. basal
10. minipills

Activity B

1. This is a diaphragm. A diaphragm is used in conjunction with a spermicidal jelly or cream and inserted into the vagina to prevent the sperm from reaching the ovum.

2. a. The vas deferens is being cut with surgical scissors during a vasectomy.

b. After a vasectomy, the semen no longer contains sperm, because the vas deferens (which carries sperm from the testes to the penis) is surgically cut.

Activity C

1. c   **2.** d   **3.** a   **4.** e   **5.** b

Activity D

1.

b → c → a → e → d

2.

a → e → d → b → c

Activity E

1. Common laboratory tests ordered to determine the cause of amenorrhea are karyotype, ultrasound to detect ovarian cysts, pregnancy test, thyroid function studies, prolactin level, follicle-stimulating hormone level, luteinizing hormone level, 17-ketosteroids tests, laparoscopy, and CT scan of head.

2. Menopause refers to the cessation of regular menstrual cycles. It is the end of menstruation and childbearing capacity. Natural menopause is defined as one year without a menstrual period. The average age at which it occurs is 51 years.

3. The risk factors associated with endometriosis are increasing age, family history of endometriosis, short menstrual cycle, long menstrual flow, young age at menarche, and few or no pregnancies.

4. Infertility is defined as the inability to conceive a child after one year of regular sexual intercourse unprotected by contraception, or the inability to carry a pregnancy to term.

5. In the Two-Day Method, women observe the presence or absence of cervical secretions by examining toilet paper or underwear or by monitoring their physical sensations. Every day, the woman asks two simple questions: "Did I note any secretions yesterday?" and "Did I note any secretions today?" If the answer to either question is yes, she considers herself fertile and avoids unprotected intercourse. If the answers are no, she is unlikely to become pregnant from unprotected intercourse on that day.

6. Intrauterine systems (IUSs) are small, plastic, T-shaped objects that are placed inside the uterus to provide contraception. They prevent pregnancy by making the endometrium of the uterus hostile to implantation of a fertilized ovum, by causing a nonspecific inflammatory reaction.

Activity F

1. Amenorrhea is a normal feature in prepubertal, pregnant, and postmenopausal women. The two categories of amenorrhea are primary and secondary amenorrhea. Primary amenorrhea is defined as either (1) absence of menses by age 14, with absence of growth and development of secondary sexual characteristics, or (2) absence of menses by age 16, with normal development of secondary sexual characteristics. Ninety-eight percent of American girls menstruate by age 16.

2. Causes of primary amenorrhea related to Alexa may include extreme weight gain or loss, stress from a major life event, excessive exercise, or eating disorders such as anorexia nervosa or bulimia. Primary amenorrhea is also caused by congenital abnormalities of the reproductive system, Cushing's disease, polycystic ovarian syndrome, hypothyroidism, and Turner syndrome; other causes are imperforate hymen, chronic illness, pregnancy, cystic fibrosis, congenital heart disease, and ovarian or adrenal tumors.

3. The treatment of primary amenorrhea involves correcting any underlying disorders as well as providing estrogen replacement therapy to stimulate the development of secondary sexual characteristics. If a pituitary tumor is the cause, it might be treated with drug therapy, surgical resection, or radiation therapy. Surgery might be needed to correct any structural abnormalities of the genital tract.

4. The nurse should address the diverse causes of amenorrhea, the relationship to sexual identity, and the possibility of infertility and more serious problems. In addition, the nurse should inform Alexa about the purpose of each diagnostic test, how it is performed, and when the results will be available. Sensitive listening, interviewing, and presenting treatment options are paramount to gaining the client's cooperation and understanding. Nutritional counseling is also vital in managing this disorder, especially when the client has findings suggestive of an eating disorder. Although not all causes can be addressed by making lifestyle changes, the nurse can still emphasize maintaining a healthy lifestyle.

Activity G

1. **Answer: d**
   RATIONALE: When assessing a client for amenorrhea, the nurse should document facial hair and acne as possible evidence of androgen excess secondary to a tumor. The nurse may observe and should document hypothermia, bradycardia, hypotension, and reduced subcutaneous fat in women with anorexia nervosa; however, these are not symptoms of excess androgen.

2. **Answer: b**
   RATIONALE: The nurse should explain to the client that the fertility awareness method relies on the assumption that the "unsafe period" is approximately 6 days; 3 days before and 3 days after ovulation. The method also assumes that sperm can live up to 5 days, not just 24 hours after intercourse. An ovum lives up to 24 hours after being released from the ovary. The exact time of ovulation cannot be determined, so two to three days are added to the beginning and end to avoid pregnancy.

3. Answer: b, d, & e
RATIONALE: When instructing a client with dysmenorrhea on how to manage her symptoms, the nurse should ask her to increase water consumption, use heating pads or take warm baths, and increase exercise and physical activity. Water consumption serves as a natural diuretic; heating pads or warm baths help increase comfort; and exercise increases endorphins and suppresses prostaglandin release. The nurse should also tell the client to limit salty foods to prevent fluid retention during menstruation and to keep legs elevated while lying down, because this helps increase comfort.

4. Answer: d
RATIONALE: The nurse should prepare the client for a laparoscopy to obtain a definitive diagnosis; laparoscopy allows for direct visualization of the internal organs and helps confirm the diagnosis. A hysterosalpingogram (HSG) assesses tubal patency, and a clomiphene citrate challenge test determines ovarian function; these tests are not used to determine the extent of endometriosis.

5. Answer: d
RATIONALE: The nurse should instruct the client to deliver the semen sample to the laboratory for analysis within 1 to 2 hours after ejaculation. The client should also be instructed to collect the sample in a specimen container, not a condom or plastic bag. The client needs to abstain from sexual activity for at least 24 hours before giving the sample, but he need not avoid strenuous activity.

6. Answer: c
RATIONALE: The nurse should explain that during ovulation the cervix is high or deep in the vagina. The os is slightly open during ovulation. Under the influence of estrogen during ovulation, the cervical mucus is copious and slippery and can be stretched between two fingers without breaking. It becomes thick and dry after ovulation, under the influence of progesterone.

7. Answer: c
RATIONALE: If the FSH level is greater than 15, the test is considered abnormal and the likelihood of conception with the client's own eggs is very low. Therefore, the nurse could suggest the use of donor eggs or gamete intrafallopian transfer as an option. Artificial insemination will not help solve the couple's problem. Also, it would be incorrect for the nurse to imply that the couple has no choice other than adoption.

8. Answer: c
RATIONALE: Recent studies have shown that the extended use of active OC pills carries the same safety profile as the conventional 28-day regimen. This option helps reduce the number of periods and is as effective as the conventional regimen. There is no evidence to suggest that discontinuation of active oral contraceptives will not ensure restoration of fertility. Depo-Provera, not active oral contraceptive pills, prevents pregnancy for three months at a time.

9. Answer: d
RATIONALE: The client should be instructed to take her temperature before rising and record it on a chart. If using this method by itself, the client should avoid unprotected intercourse until the BBT has been elevated for three days. The client should be informed that other fertility awareness methods should be used along with BBT for better results. The oral method is better suited than the axillary method for taking the temperature in this case.

10. Answer: d
RATIONALE: The best option for a client who is not well-educated would be the Standard Days Method with CycleBeads, since the 32 color-coded Cycle-Beads are easy to use and understand. An injection of Depo-Provera would also suit this client, since it works by suppressing ovulation and the production of FSH and LH by the pituitary gland and prevents pregnancy for 3 months at a time. Basal body temperature requires the client to take and chart her body temperature; this may be difficult for the client to follow. Coitus interruptus is a method in which the man controls his ejaculation and ejaculates outside the vagina; this suggests that the client rely solely on the cooperation and judgment of her spouse. The lactational amenorrhea method (LAM) works as a temporary method of contraception only for breastfeeding mothers.

11. Answer: a, c, & e
RATIONALE: The nurse should tell the client to inspect the cervical cap prior to insertion for cracks, holes, or tears and to wait approximately 30 minutes after insertion before engaging in sexual intercourse to be sure that a seal has formed between the rim and the cervix. In addition, the cap should not be used during menses because of the potential for toxic shock syndrome; an alternative method such as condoms should be used during this time. The client should be told not to apply spermicide to the rim since it may interfere with the seal. It should be left in place for a minimum of 6 hours after sexual intercourse.

12. Answer: b
RATIONALE: Because of the client's smoking habit, combination oral contraceptives may be contraindicated. Oral contraceptives are highly effective when taken properly but can aggravate many medical conditions, especially in women who smoke. The Lunelle injection, Depo-Provera, or copper intrauterine devices are not contraindicated in this client and can be used with certain precautions. Implantable contraceptives are subdermal time-release implants that deliver synthetic progestin; these are highly effective and are not contraindicated in this client.

13. Answer: b
RATIONALE: The client is seeking a medical abortion. The nurse should inform the client that such medications are effectively used to terminate a pregnancy only during the first trimester, not the

- Does the client have any nipple discharge? If yes, describe its color and consistency.
- Does the client have a feeling of fullness in the breast?
- Is the pain dull, burning, or itchy?
- Is there any skin dimpling or nipple retraction?

b. Mrs. Taylor needs the following education regarding breast health:
- Monthly breast self-examination
- Yearly clinical breast examination
- Yearly mammography

c. The treatment modalities available to Mrs. Taylor in case of a malignancy are:
- Local treatments such as surgery, and radiation
- Systemic treatments such as chemotherapy, hormonal therapy, and immunotherapy

d. Mrs. Taylor will need the following community referrals:
- Telephone counseling by the nurse
- ACS's Reach for Recovery
- Organizations or charities that support cancer research
- Participation in breast cancer walks to raise awareness
- Emotional support groups

Activity F

1. Answer: c
   RATIONALE: During menstrual cycles, hormonal stimulation of the breast tissue causes the glands and ducts to enlarge and swell. The breasts feel swollen, tender, and lumpy during this time, but after menses the swelling and lumpiness decline. This is why it is best to examine the breasts a week after the menses, when they are not swollen. For determining fibrocystic breast changes, it is not best to schedule the breast examination in the second phase of menstrual cycle or immediately after the client has completed her menses.

2. Answer: b
   RATIONALE: Since the physician suspects fibroadenomas, it is important for the nurse to know if the client is pregnant or lactating since the incidence of fibroadenomas is more frequent among pregnant and lactating women. Taking oral contraceptives assists a client with fibrocystic breast changes but is not necessary for a client with fibroadenomas. Fibroadenomas usually occur in women between 20 and 30 years of age. Smoking and a high-fat diet will make the client more susceptible to cancer, not fibroadenomas.

3. Answer: a
   RATIONALE: The nurse should instruct the client with mastitis to increase her fluid intake. A client with mastitis is instructed to continue breastfeeding as tolerated and to frequently change positions while nursing. The nurse should also instruct the client to apply warm, not cold, compresses to the affected breast area or to take a warm shower before breastfeeding.

4. Answer: b
   RATIONALE: When preparing a client for mammography, the nurse should ensure the client has not applied deodorant or powder on the day of testing because they can appear on the x-ray film as calcium spots. It is not necessary for the client to avoid fluid intake an hour prior to testing. Mammography has to be scheduled just after the client's menses to reduce chances of breast tenderness, not when the client is going to start her menses. The client can take aspirin or Tylenol after the completion of the procedure to ease any discomfort, but these medications are not taken before mammography.

5. Answer: d
   RATIONALE: The side effects of chemotherapy are constipation, hair loss, weight loss, vomiting, diarrhea, immunosuppression, and, in extreme cases, bone marrow suppression. The nurse should monitor for these side effects when caring for the client undergoing chemotherapy. Vaginal discharge, headache, and chills are not side effects of chemotherapy. Vaginal discharge is one of the side effects of SERMs (selective estrogen receptor modulators) as a part of hormonal therapy, which is used to prevent cancer from spreading further into the body. Headache is a side effect of aromatase inhibitors under hormonal therapy to counter cancer. Chills are a side effect of immunotherapy.

6. Answer: d
   RATIONALE: The nurse should inform the client that intraductal papillomas and fibrocystic breasts, although considered benign, carry a cancer risk with prolific masses and hyperplastic changes within the breasts. Other benign breast disorders such as mastitis, mammary duct ectasia, and fibroadenomas carry little risk.

7. Answer: a
   RATIONALE: The nurse should inform the client that removing only the sentinel lymph node prevents side effects such as lymphedema, which is otherwise associated with a traditional axillary lymph node dissection. It does not help reveal the hormonal status of the cancer. Hormone-receptor status can be revealed through normal breast epithelium, which has hormone receptors and responds specifically to the stimulatory effects of estrogen and progesterone. A sentinel lymph node biopsy will determine how powerful a chemotherapy regimen the client will have to undergo, but undergoing a sentinel lymph node biopsy will not lessen the aggressiveness of the chemotherapy. Degree of HER-2/neu oncoprotein will be revealed through the HER-2/neu genetic marker, not through a sentinel lymph node biopsy.

8. Answer: b
   RATIONALE: When providing care to the client, the nurse should instruct the client to elevate the affected arm on a pillow. As part of the respiratory care, the nurse should instruct the client to turn,

cough, and breathe deeply every 2 hours; rapid breathing is not encouraged. Active range-of-motion and arm exercises are necessary. To counter any pain experienced by the client, analgesics are administered as needed; intake of medication is not restricted.

9. **Answer: c**

   RATIONALE: Skin edema, redness, and warmth of the breast are symptoms of inflammatory breast cancer. Induced discharge is an indication of benign breast conditions, which are noncancerous. Cancer involves spontaneous nipple discharge. Papillomas and palpable mobile cysts are characteristics of fibroadenomas, intraductal papilloma, and mammary duct ectasia, which are benign breast conditions and are noncancerous.

10. **Answer: d**

    RATIONALE: The symptom of mammary duct ectasia that the nurse should assess for is the presence of green, brown, straw-colored, reddish, gray, or cream-colored nipple discharge with a consistency of toothpaste. Increased warmth of the breasts along with redness is a manifestation of mastitis but not mammary duct ectasia. Skin retractions on pulling are a sign of cancer, not mammary duct ectasia. The nurse has to observe nipple retraction. Tortuous tubular swellings are found only beneath the areola, not in the upper half of the breast, in mammary duct ectasia.

11. **Answer: c**

    RATIONALE: When caring for a client who is being administered selective estrogen receptor modulator, the nurse should monitor for side effects such as hot flashes, vaginal discharge, bleeding, and cataract formation. Weight loss is one of the side effects of chemotherapy, and fever and chills are the side effects of immunotherapy, not of SERM.

12. **Answer: a, c, & d**

    RATIONALE: The modifiable risk factors for breast cancer are postmenopausal use of estrogen and progestins, not having children until after the age of 30, and failing to breastfeed for up to a year after pregnancy. Early menarche or late menopause and previous abnormal breast biopsy are the nonmodifiable risk factors for breast cancer.

13. **Answer: d**

    RATIONALE: When performing the breast self-examination, the nurse should instruct the client to apply hard pressure down to the ribs. Light, not medium, pressure should be applied when moving the skin without moving the tissue underneath. Medium, not light, pressure should be applied midway into the tissue. Client need not specifically palpate the areolar area during breast self-examination.

14. **Answer: b**

    RATIONALE: Adverse effects of trastuzumab include cardiac toxicity, vascular thrombosis, hepatic failure, fever, chills, nausea, vomiting, and pain with first infusion. The nurse should monitor for these adverse effects with the first infusion of trastuzumab. Dyspnea, stroke, and myelosuppression are not side effects caused with the first infusion of trastuzumab. Dyspnea is a side effect of aromatase inhibitors as part of hormonal therapy. Stroke is an adverse effect of selective estrogen receptive modulator (SERM), again as part of hormonal therapy. Myelosuppression is an extreme side effect of chemotherapy.

15. **Answer: a**

    RATIONALE: A nurse should closely monitor for signs of anorexia since it is a likely side effect of radiation therapy, along with swelling and heaviness of the breast, local edema, inflammation, and sunburn-like skin changes. Infection, fever, and nausea are not the side effects of radiation therapy. Infection and fever are the side effects of brachytherapy. Nausea is one of the side effects of chemotherapy.

16. **Answer: b**

    RATIONALE: When caring for a client who has just undergone surgery for intraductal papilloma, the nurse should instruct the client to continue monthly breast self-examinations along with yearly clinical breast examinations. Applying warm compresses to the affected breast and wearing a supportive bra 24 hours a day are instructions given in cases of mastitis but not for intraductal papilloma. The nurse should instruct clients to refrain from consuming salt in the diet in cases of fibrocystic breast changes but not in cases of intraductal papilloma.

17. **Answer: b, d, & e**

    RATIONALE: Lumpectomy is contraindicated for women who have previously undergone radiation to their affected breast, those whose connective tissue is reported to be sensitive to radiation, and those whose surgery will not result in a clean margin of tissue. Clients who have had an early menarche or late onset of menopause and clients who have failed to breastfeed for up to a year after pregnancy are at risk for developing breast cancer. Lumpectomy is a treatment option for clients with breast cancer.

18. **Answer: a, b, & d**

    RATIONALE: The client is more susceptible to lymphedema if the affected arm is used for drawing blood or measuring blood pressure, if she engages in activities like gardening without using gloves, or if she's not wearing a well-fitted compression sleeve to promote drainage return. Consuming foods rich in phytochemicals is essential to prevent the incidence of cancer, not lymphedema. Not consuming a diet high in fiber and protein will not make the client susceptible to lymphedema.

19. **Answer: b, d, & e**

    RATIONALE: The nurse should instruct the client with fibrocystic breast changes to avoid caffeine. Caffeine acts as a stimulant that can lead to discomfort. It is important to maintain a low-fat diet rich in fruits, vegetables, and grains to maintain a healthy body weight. Taking diuretics is important to counteract fluid retention and swelling of the breasts. Practicing good hand-washing techniques and increasing fluid intake are important for clients with mastitis but may not help clients with fibrocystic breast changes.

20. **Answer: a, b, & c**
    RATIONALE: The nurse should instruct the client to restrict intake of salted foods, limit intake of processed foods, and consume seven or more daily portions of complex carbohydrates, not proteins. Increasing liquid intake to 3 liters daily will not reduce her risk of developing breast cancer.

CHAPTER 7

Activity A

1. Cystocele
2. prolapse
3. pessary
4. Polyps
5. leiomyomas
6. Kegel
7. rectum
8. urethra
9. Metrorrhagia
10. Transvaginal

Activity B

1. The figure shows uterine prolapse, which occurs when the uterus descends through the pelvic floor and into the vaginal canal.
2. The figure shows submucosal, intramural, and subserosal fibroids.

Activity C

1. a   **2.** e   **3.** b   **4.** c   **5.** d

Activity D

1. Pelvic organ prolapse could be caused by the following:
   - Constant downward gravity because of erect human posture
   - Atrophy of supporting tissues with aging and decline of estrogen levels
   - Weakening of pelvic support related to childbirth trauma
   - Reproductive surgery
   - Family history of pelvic organ prolapse
   - Young age at first birth
   - Connective tissue disorders
   - Infant birth weight of greater than 4500 grams
   - Pelvic radiation
   - Increased abdominal pressure secondary to lifting of children or heavy objects, straining due to chronic constipation, respiratory problems or chronic coughing, or obesity
2. Kegel exercises strengthen the pelvic-floor muscles to support the inner organs and prevent further

prolapse. They help increase the muscle volume, which will result in a stronger muscular contraction. These exercises might limit the progression of mild prolapse and alleviate mild prolapse symptoms, including low back pain and pelvic pressure. Clients with severe uterine prolapse may not benefit from Kegel exercises.

3. Several factors contribute to urinary incontinence:
   - Intake of fluids, especially alcohol, carbonated drinks, and caffeinated beverages
   - Constipation, which alters the position of pelvic organs and puts pressure on the bladder
   - Habitual preventive emptying, which may result in training the bladder to hold small amounts of urine
   - Anatomic changes due to advanced age, which decrease pelvic support
   - Pregnancy and childbirth, which cause damage to the pelvis structure during birthing process
   - Obesity, which increases abdominal pressure

4. The Colpexin Sphere is a polycarbonate sphere with a locator string that is fitted above the hymenal ring to support the pelvis floor muscle. The sphere is used in conjunction with pelvic floor muscle exercises, which should be performed daily. The sphere supports the pelvic floor muscle and facilitates rehabilitation of the pelvic floor muscles.

5. Uterine fibroids may be medically managed by uterine artery embolization (UAE). UAE is an option in which polyvinyl alcohol pellets are injected into selected blood vessels via a catheter to block circulation to the fibroid, causing shrinkage of the fibroid and resolution of the symptoms. After treatment, most fibroids are reduced by 50% within 3 months, but they might recur. The failure rate is approximately 10% to 15%, and this therapy should not be performed on women desiring to retain their fertility.

6. Bartholin's glands are two mucus-secreting glandular structures with duct openings bilaterally at the base of the labia minora, near the opening of the vagina, that provide lubrication during sexual arousal. A Bartholin's cyst is a fluid-filled, swollen, saclike structure that results from a blockage of one of the ducts of the Bartholin gland. The cyst may become infected and an abscess may develop in the gland. Bartholin's cysts are the most common cystic growths in the vulva, affecting approximately 2% of women at some time in their lives.

Activity E

1. **a.** Pelvic support disorders increase with age and are a result of weakness of the connective tissue and muscular support of the pelvic organs. Vaginal childbirth, obesity, lifting, chronic cough, straining at defecation secondary to constipation, and estrogen deficiency all contribute to pelvic support disorders.
   b. Symptoms of uterine prolapse include low back pain, pelvic pressure, urinary frequency, reten-

tion, and/or incontinence. These symptoms are likely to affect Mrs. Scott's daily activities.

c. Nonsurgical interventions include regular Kegel exercises, estrogen replacement therapy, dietary and lifestyle modifications, and pessaries. Kegel exercises might limit the progression of mild prolapse and alleviate mild prolapse symptoms, including low back pain and pelvic pressure. Estrogen replacement therapy may help to improve the tone and vascularity of the supporting tissue in perimenopausal and menopausal women by increasing blood perfusion and elasticity to the vaginal wall. Dietary and lifestyle modifications may help prevent pelvic relaxation and chronic problems later in life. Pessaries may be indicated for uterine prolapse or cystocele, especially among elderly clients for whom surgery is contraindicated. Surgical interventions include anterior and posterior colporrhaphy and vaginal hysterectomy. Anterior and posterior colporrhaphy may be effective for a first-degree prolapse. A vaginal hysterectomy is the treatment of choice for uterine prolapse because it removes the prolapsed organ that is bringing down the bladder and rectum with it.

Activity F

1. **Answer: c**
   RATIONALE: Weakening of the pelvic-floor muscles causes a feeling of dragging and a "lump" in the vagina; these are symptoms of pelvic organ prolapse. These symptoms do not indicate urinary incontinence, endocervical polyps, or uterine fibroids. Urinary incontinence is the involuntary loss of urine. The symptoms of endocervical polyps are abnormal vaginal bleeding or discharge. In cases of uterine fibroids, the uterus is enlarged and irregularly shaped.

2. **Answer: b**
   RATIONALE: Before starting estrogen replacement therapy, each woman must be evaluated on the basis of a thorough medical history to validate her risk for complications such as endometrial cancer, myocardial infarction, stroke, breast cancer, pulmonary emboli, or deep vein thrombosis. The effective dose of estrogen required, the dietary modifications, and the cost of estrogen replacement therapy can be discussed at a later stage when the client understands the risks associated with estrogen replacement therapy and decides to use hormone therapy.

3. **Answer: a**
   RATIONALE: The nurse should instruct the client to increase dietary fiber and fluids to prevent constipation. A high-fiber diet with an increase in fluid intake alleviates constipation by increasing stool bulk and stimulating peristalsis. Straining to pass a hard stool increases intra-abdominal pressure, which, over time, causes the pelvic organs to prolapse. Avoiding caffeine products would not help

substantially; instead, the client should give up smoking to minimize the risk for a chronic "smoker's cough." In addition to recommending increasing the amount of fiber in her diet, the nurse should also encourage the woman to drink eight 8-oz glasses of fluid daily. The nurse should instruct the client to avoid high-impact aerobics to minimize the risk of increasing intra-abdominal pressure.

4. **Answer: d**
   RATIONALE: The disadvantage of myomectomy is that the fibroids may grow back in the future. Fertility is not jeopardized, because this procedure leaves the uterine wall intact. Weakening of the uterine walls, scarring, and adhesions are caused by laser treatment, not myomectomy.

5. **Answer: b**
   RATIONALE: Kegel exercises might limit the progression of mild prolapse and alleviate mild prolapse symptoms, including low back pain and pelvic pressure. Intake of food is not required before performing Kegel exercises. Surgical interventions do not interfere with Kegel exercises. Kegel exercises do not cause an increase in blood pressure.

6. **Answer: a, b, & d**
   RATIONALE: The predisposing factors for uterine fibroids are age (late reproductive years), nulliparity, obesity, genetic predisposition, and African-American ethnicity. Smoking and hyperinsulinemia are not predisposing factors for uterine fibroids.

7. **Answer: b**
   RATIONALE: Vaginal dryness is one of the side effects of GnRH medications. The other side effects of GnRH medications are hot flashes, headaches, mood changes, musculoskeletal malaise, bone loss, and depression. Increased vaginal discharge, urinary tract infections, and vaginitis are side effects of a pessary, not GnRH medications.

8. **Answer: c**
   RATIONALE: The nurse should instruct the client using a pessary to report any discomfort or difficulty with urination or defecation. Avoiding high-impact aerobics, jogging, jumping, and lifting heavy objects, as well as wearing a girdle or abdominal support, are recommended for a client with prolapse as part of lifestyle modifications and may not be necessary for a client using a pessary.

9. **Answer: b**
   RATIONALE: The most common recommendation for pessary care is removing the pessary twice weekly and cleaning it with soap and water. In addition, douching with diluted vinegar or hydrogen peroxide helps to reduce urinary tract infections and odor, which are side effects of using a pessary. Estrogen cream is applied to make the vaginal mucosa more resistant to erosion and strengthen the vaginal walls. Removing the pessary before sleeping or intercourse is not part of the instructions for pessary care.

10. **Answer: d**
    RATIONALE: The nurse should monitor the client with ultrasound scans every 3 to 6 months. Monitoring gonadotropin level and blood sugar level and scheduling periodic Pap smears are not important assessments for the client with small ovarian cysts.

11. **Answer: a**
    RATIONALE: The nurse should teach the client turning, deep breathing, and coughing prior to the surgery to prevent atelectasis and respiratory complications such as pneumonia. Reducing activity level and the need for pelvic rest are instructions related to discharge planning after the client has undergone a hysterectomy. A high-fat diet need not be avoided before undergoing hysterectomy; avoiding a high-fat diet is required for clients with pelvic organ prolapse to reduce constipation.

12. **Answer: b, c, & e**
    RATIONALE: If the client is at high risk of recurrent prolapse after a surgical repair, is morbidly obese, or has chronic obstructive pulmonary disease, then the client is not a good candidate for surgical repair. Low back pain and pelvic pressure are common to almost all pelvic organ prolapses and do not help to decide whether the client should opt for surgical repair. A client with severe pelvic organ prolapse may be a candidate for surgical repair.

13. **Answer: a, b, & d**
    RATIONALE: The teaching guidelines include continuing pelvic floor (Kegel) exercises, increasing fiber in the diet to reduce constipation, and controlling blood glucose levels to prevent polyuria. The nurse should instruct the client to reduce the intake of fluids and foods that are bladder irritants, such as orange juice, soda, and caffeine, and the client should wipe from front to back to prevent urinary tract infections.

14. **Answer: a, d, & e**
    RATIONALE: The postoperative care plan for a client who has undergone a hysterectomy includes administering analgesics promptly and using a PCA pump, changing linens and gown frequently to promote hygiene, and administering antiemetics to control nausea and vomiting. The nurse should change the position of the client frequently and use pillows for support to promote comfort and pain management. An excess of carbonated beverages in the diet does not affect the postoperative healing process.

15. **Answer: a**
    RATIONALE: The nurse should stress follow-up care to the client with polycystic ovarian syndrome so that the client does not overlook this benign disorder. Increasing intake of fiber-rich foods, increasing fluid intake, and performing Kegel exercises help to control pelvic organ prolapse, not PCOS.

CHAPTER 8

Activity A
1. dysplasia
2. Colposcopy
3. Cryotherapy
4. Endometrial
5. Bethesda
6. Hysterectomy
7. CA-125
8. simplex
9. epithelium
10. Squamous

Activity B
1. a. The image shows ovarian cancer.
   b. The treatment options available for ovarian cancer are as follows:
      - Surgery includes a total abdominal hysterectomy, bilateral salpingo-oophorectomy, peritoneal biopsies, omentectomy, and pelvic para-aortic lymph node sampling to evaluate cancer extension.
      - Aggressive management involving debulking or cytoreductive surgery is commonly performed for advanced-stage ovarian cancer.
      - Additional therapy with radiation may be warranted.
      - Chemotherapy is recommended for all stages of ovarian cancer.
2. a. The image shows vulvar cancer.
   b. Treatment for vulvar cancer varies, depending on the extent of the disease. Laser surgery, cryosurgery, or electrosurgical incision may be used. Larger lesions may need more extensive surgery and skin grafting. The traditional treatment for vulvar cancer has been radical vulvectomy, but more conservative techniques are being used to improve psychosexual outcomes.

Activity C
1. b   2. a   3. d   4. c

Activity D
1.

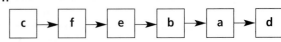

Activity E
1. Risk factors for developing cervical cancer are as follows:
   - Early age of first intercourse (within 1 year of menarche)
   - Lower socioeconomic status
   - Promiscuous male partners
   - Unprotected sexual intercourse
   - Family history of cervical cancer (mother or sisters)
   - Sexual intercourse with uncircumcised men
   - Female offspring of mothers who took diethylstilbestrol (DES)

- Infections with genital herpes or chronic chlamydia
- History of multiple sex partners
- Cigarette smoking
- Immunocompromised state
- HIV infection
- Oral contraceptive use
- Moderate dysplasia on Pap smear within past 5 years
- HPV infection

2. Treatment options for endometrial cancer are as follows:
- Treatment of endometrial cancer depends on the stage of the disease and usually involves surgery, with adjunct therapy based on pathologic findings.
- Surgery most often involves removal of the uterus (hysterectomy) and the fallopian tubes and ovaries (salpingo-oophorectomy).
- In more advanced cancers, radiation and chemotherapy are used as adjunct therapies to surgery.
- Routine surveillance intervals for follow-up care are typically every 3 to 4 months for the first 2 years, since 85% of recurrences occur in the first two years after diagnosis.

3. The following are possible risk factors for ovarian cancer:
- Nulliparity
- Early menarche (<12 years old)
- Late menopause (>55 years old)
- Increasing age (>50 years of age)
- High-fat diet
- Obesity
- Persistent ovulation over time
- First-degree relative with ovarian cancer
- Use of perineal talcum powder or hygiene sprays
- Older than 30 years at first pregnancy
- Positive BRCA-1 and BRCA-2 mutations
- Personal history of breast, bladder, or colon cancer
- Hormone replacement therapy for more than 10 years
- Infertility

4. Transvaginal ultrasound can be used to evaluate the endometrial cavity and measure the thickness of the endometrial lining. It can be used to detect endometrial hyperplasia.

5. The following are the nursing interventions in caring for clients with cancers of the female reproductive tract:
- Validate the client's feelings and provide realistic hope.
- Use basic communication skills in a sincere way during all interactions.
- Provide useful, nonjudgmental information to all women.
- Individualize care to address the client's cultural traditions.
- Carry out postoperative care and instructions as prescribed.

- Discuss postoperative issues, including incision care, pain, and activity level.
- Instruct the client on health maintenance activities after treatment.
- Inform the client and family about available support resources.

6. The following are the diagnostic options for endometrial cancer:
- Endometrial biopsy: An endometrial biopsy is the procedure of choice to make the diagnosis. It can be done in the health care provider's office without anesthesia. A slender suction catheter is used to obtain a small sample of tissue for pathology. It can detect up to 90% of cases of endometrial cancer in the woman with postmenopausal bleeding, depending on the technique and experience of the health care provider. The woman may experience mild cramping and bleeding after the procedure for about 24 hours, but typically mild pain medication will reduce this discomfort.
- Transvaginal ultrasound: A transvaginal ultrasound can be used to evaluate the endometrial cavity and measure the thickness of the endometrial lining. It can be used to detect endometrial hyperplasia. If the endometrium measures less than 4 mm, then the client is at low risk for malignancy.

Activity F

1. a.
- Back pain
- Abdominal bloating
- Fatigue
- Urinary frequency
- Constipation
- Abdominal pressure

b. The most common early symptoms include abdominal bloating, early satiety, fatigue, vague abdominal pain, urinary frequency, diarrhea or constipation, and unexplained weight loss or gain. The later symptoms include anorexia, dyspepsia, ascites, palpable abdominal mass, pelvic pain, and back pain. Early detection of ovarian cancer is possible if the clients are informed about yearly bimanual pelvic examination and transvaginal ultrasound to identify ovarian masses.

c. Disturbed body image related to:
- Loss of body part
- Loss of good health
- Altered sexuality patterns
Anxiety related to:
- Threat of malignancy
- Potential diagnosis
- Anticipated pain/discomfort
- Effect of condition treatment on future
Deficient knowledge related to:
- Disease process and prognosis
- Specific treatment options
- Diagnostic procedures needed

d. In Stage I, the ovarian cancer is limited to the ovaries. In Stage II, the growth involves one or both ovaries, with pelvic extension. In Stage III, the cancer spreads to the lymph nodes and other organs or structures inside the abdominal cavity. In Stage IV, the cancer has metastasized to distant sites. Treatment options for ovarian cancer vary, depending on the stage and severity of the disease. Usually a laparoscopy (abdominal exploration with an endoscope) is performed for diagnosis and staging, as well as evaluation for further therapy.

Activity G

1. Answer: a
RATIONALE: The client should have Papanicolaou tests regularly to detect cervical cancer during the early stages. Blood tests for mutations in the BRCA genes indicate the lifetime risk of the client of developing breast or ovarian cancer. CA-125 is a biologic tumor marker associated with ovarian cancer, but it is not currently sensitive enough to serve as a screening tool.

2. Answer: a
RATIONALE: Early onset of sexual activity, within the first year of menarche, increases the risk of acquiring cervical cancer later on. Obesity, infertility, and hypertension are risk factors that are associated with endometrial cancer.

3. Answer: c
RATIONALE: The nurse should inform the client that surgery most often involves removal of the uterus (hysterectomy) and the fallopian tubes and ovaries (salpingo-oophorectomy). Removal of the tubes and ovaries, not just the uterus, is recommended because tumor cells spread early to the ovaries, and any dormant cancer cells could be stimulated to grow by ovarian estrogen. In advanced cancers, radiation and chemotherapy are used as adjuvant therapies to surgery. Routine surveillance intervals for follow-up care are typically every 3 to 4 months for the first 2 years.

4. Answer: b
RATIONALE: The client's present age increases her risk of developing ovarian cancer, as women who are older than 50 are at a greater risk. The client's age at menarche (older than 12) and menopause (younger than 55) are both normal. The client is underweight and not obese, so her weight is not a risk factor for ovarian cancer.

5. Answer: c
RATIONALE: To identify ovarian masses in their early stages, the client needs to have yearly bimanual pelvic examinations and a transvaginal ultrasound. Pap smears are not effective enough to detect ovarian masses. The U.S. Preventive Services Task Force (USPSTF) recommends against routine screening for ovarian cancer with serum CA-125, because the potential harm could outweigh the potential benefits. X-rays of the pelvic area do not detect ovarian masses.

6. Answer: a
RATIONALE: Only 5% of ovarian cancers are genetic in origin. However, the nurse needs to tell the client to seek genetic counseling and thorough assessment to reduce her risk of ovarian cancer. Oral contraceptives reduce the risk of ovarian cancer and should be encouraged. Breastfeeding should be encouraged as a risk-reducing strategy. The nurse should instruct the client to avoid using perineal talc or hygiene sprays.

7. Answer: c
RATIONALE: The nurse should instruct the client to avoid wearing tight, restrictive undergarments. The nurse should teach the client genital self-examination to assess for any unusual growths in the vulvar area. The nurse should instruct the client to seek care for any suspicious lesions and to avoid self-medication. The client should use barrier methods of birth control (such as condoms) to reduce the risk of contracting sexually transmitted infections that may increase the risk of vulvar cancer.

8. Answer: b, c, & e
RATIONALE: To reduce the risk of cervical cancer, the nurse should encourage clients to avoid smoking and drinking. In addition, because STIs such as HPV increase the risk of cervical cancers, care should be taken to prevent STIs. Teenagers also should be counseled to avoid early sexual activity, because it increases the risk of cervical cancer. The use of barrier methods of contraception, not IUDs, should be encouraged. Avoiding stress and high blood pressure will not have a significant impact on the risk of cervical cancer.

9. Answer: a, c, & d
RATIONALE: The responsibilities of a nurse while caring for a client with endometrial cancer include ensuring that the client understands all the treatment options available, suggesting the advantages of a support group and providing referrals, and offering the family explanations and emotional support throughout the treatment. The nurse should also discuss changes in sexuality with the client as well as stress the importance of regular follow-up care after the treatment and not just in cases where something unusual occurs.

10. Answer: b, d, & e
RATIONALE: Irregular vaginal bleeding, persistent low backache not related to standing, and elevated or discolored vulvar lesions are some of the symptoms that should be immediately brought to the notice of the primary health care provider. Increase in urinary frequency and irregular bowel movements are not symptoms related to cancers of the reproductive tract.

11. Answer: b
RATIONALE: The nurse should explain to the client that the colposcopy is done because the physician has observed abnormalities in Pap smears. The nurse should also explain to the client that the procedure is painless and there are no adverse ef-

fects, such as pain during urination. There is no need to avoid intercourse for a week after the colposcopy.

12. Answer: b
RATIONALE: According to the 2001 Bethesda system for classifying Pap smear results, a result of ASC-H means that the client is to be referred for colposcopy without HPV testing. ASC-US means that the test has to be repeated in 4 to 6 months or the client has to be referred for colposcopy. AGC or AIS results indicate immediate colposcopy, with the follow-up based on the results of findings.

13. Answer: a
RATIONALE: Abnormal and painless vaginal bleeding is a major initial symptom of endometrial cancer. Diabetes mellitus and liver disease are the risk factors, not symptoms, for endometrial cancer. Back pain is associated with ovarian cancer.

14. Answer: a, b, & d
RATIONALE: Although direct risk factors for the initial development of vaginal cancer have not been identified, associated risk factors include advancing age (>60 years old), HIV infection, smoking, previous pelvic radiation, exposure to diethylstilbestrol (DES) in utero, vaginal trauma, history of genital warts (HPV infection), cervical cancer, chronic vaginal discharge, and low socioeconomic level. Persistent ovulation over time and hormone replacement therapy for more than 10 years are risk factors associated with ovarian cancer.

15 Answer: a
RATIONALE: The skin condition Lichen sclerosus has been linked with risk of vulvar cancer. Previous pelvic radiation and exposure to diethylstilbestrol (DES) in utero are risk factors associated with vaginal rather than vulvar cancer, and tamoxifen use is a risk factor for endometrial cancer.

CHAPTER 9

Activity A

1. battered
2. Incest
3. Statutory
4. Rohypnol
5. circumcision
6. Acquaintance
7. sexual
8. hyperarousal
9. avoidance
10. dermoid

Activity B

1. d   2. b   3. a   4. c

Activity C

1.

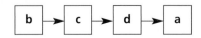

Activity D

1. The cycle of violence occurs in an abusive relationship. It includes three distinct phases: the tension-building phase, the acute battering phase, and the honeymoon phase. The cyclic behavior begins with a time of tension-building arguments, progresses to violence, and settles into a making-up or calm period. With time, this cycle of violence increases in frequency and severity as it is repeated over and over again. The cycle can cover a long or short period of time. The honeymoon phase gradually shortens and eventually disappears altogether.

2. An abuser may financially abuse the partner in the following ways:
   • Preventing the woman from getting a job
   • Sabotaging the current job
   • Controlling how all money is spent
   • Refusing to contribute financially

3. The potential nursing diagnoses related to violence against women include the following:
   • Deficient knowledge related to understanding of the cycle of violence and availability of resources
   • Fear related to possibility of severe injury to self or children during cycle of violence
   • Low self-esteem related to feelings of worthlessness
   • Hopelessness related to prolonged exposure to violence
   • Compromised individual and family coping related to persistence of victim–abuser relationship

4. Posttraumatic stress disorder (PTSD) develops when an event outside the range of normal human experience occurs that produces marked distress in the person. Symptoms of PTSD are divided into 3 groups:
   • Intrusion (re-experiencing the trauma, including nightmares, flashbacks, recurrent thoughts)
   • Avoidance (avoiding trauma-related stimuli, social withdrawal, emotional numbing)
   • Hyperarousal (increased emotional arousal, exaggerated startle response, irritability)

5. The nurse should screen the client for the following signs to determine if she is a victim of abuse:
   • Injuries: bruises, scars from blunt trauma, or weapon wounds on the face, head, and neck
   • Injury sequelae: headaches, hearing loss, joint pain, sinus infections, teeth marks, clumps of hair missing, dental trauma, pelvic pain, breast or genital injuries
   • The reported history of the injury doesn't seem to add up to the actual presenting problem
   • Mental health problems: depression, anxiety, substance abuse, eating disorders, suicidal ideation, or suicide attempts
   • Frequent health care visits for chronic, stress-related disorders such as chest pain, headaches, back or pelvic pain, insomnia, and gastrointestinal disturbances
   • Partner's behavior at the health care visit: appears overly solicitous or overprotective, unwilling to

leave client alone with the health care provider, answers questions for her, and attempts to control the situation in the health care setting

6. Abuse during pregnancy threatens the well-being of the mother and fetus. Physical violence to the pregnant woman brings injuries to the head, face, neck, thorax, breasts, and abdomen. Mental health consequences are also significant. Women assaulted during pregnancy are at a risk for depression, chronic anxiety, insomnia, poor nutrition, excessive weight gain or loss, late entry into prenatal care, preterm labor, miscarriage, stillbirth, premature and low-birth-weight infants, placental abruption, uterine rupture, chorioamnionitis, vaginitis, sexually transmitted infections, urinary tract infections, or smoking and substance abuse.

Activity E

1. **a.** Some of the common symptoms of physical abuse include depression, sexual dysfunction, backaches, sexually transmitted infections, fear or guilt, or phobias.
   b. Suzanne may not seek help in the abusive relationship for the following reasons:
   - She may feel responsible for the abuse.
   - She may feel she deserved the abuse.
   - She may have been abused as a child and has low self-esteem.
   c. The following strategies may help Suzanne to manage the situation:
   - Teaching coping strategies to manage stress
   - Encouraging the establishment of realistic goals
   - Teaching problem-solving skills
   - Encouraging social activities to connect with other people
   - Explaining that abuse is never OK

Activity F

1. **Answer: c**
   RATIONALE: The nurse should inform the client that alcohol, drugs, money problems, depression, or jealousy do not cause violence and are excuses given by the abuser for losing control. Even though violence against women was common in the past, the police, justice system, and society are beginning to make domestic violence socially unacceptable. The nurse also needs to emphasize that physical abuse is not the result of provocation from the female but an expression of inadequacy of the perpetrator. Violence against women is widespread, and whatever the cause of the assault, there is no justification for physical or sexual assault.

2. **Answer: a**
   RATIONALE: The nurse should clearly explain to the client that whatever the cause of the incident, no one deserves to be a victim of physical abuse. Even though the partner appears to be genuinely contrite, most people who attack their spouses are serial abusers and there is no certainty that they will not

repeat their actions. The client should realize that even if she tries her best not to upset her partner, her partner may abuse her again. The client should never accept battering as a normal part of any relationship.

3. **Answer: c**
   RATIONALE: Attacking pets and destroying valued possessions are examples of emotional abuse. Observing the client's movements closely may be a sign of suspicion. Throwing objects at the client is physical abuse. Forcing the client to have intercourse against her will is an act of sexual abuse.

4. **Answer: b**
   RATIONALE: Abusers are most likely to exhibit antisocial behavior or childlike aggression. They use aggression to control their victims. Abusers come from all walks of life; they are not just restricted to low-income groups, nor are they necessarily products of divorced parents. The physical characteristics of the abusers vary, and they are not necessarily physically imposing.

5. **Answer: d**
   RATIONALE: For every rape victim who turns up, the nurse should ensure that the appropriate law enforcement agencies are apprised of the incident. Victims should not be made to wait long hours in the waiting room, as they may leave if no one attends to them. Victims of rape should be treated with more sensitivity than other clients. While the primary job of a nurse is to medically care for the rape victim, a nurse should also pay due attention to collecting evidence to substantiate the victim's claim in a court of law.

6. **Answer: c**
   RATIONALE: The nurse should tell the client that she is a victim of sexual abuse because her partner forces her to have intercourse against her will. The nurse should also explain to the client that she is in no way responsible for such incidents and that she has a right to refuse sexual intimacy. There is no justification for sexual abuse and the client should not regard it as "normal" behavior.

7. **Answer: c**
   RATIONALE: The nurse should use pictures and diagrams to ensure that the client understands what is being explained. Instead of using medical terms, the nurse should use simple, accurate terms as much as possible. The nurse should look directly at the client while speaking to her and not at the interpreter. The nurse should not place any judgment on the cultural practice.

8. **Answer: b**
   RATIONALE: If the nurse suspects physical abuse, the nurse should attempt to interview the woman in private. Many abusers will not leave their partners for fear of being discovered. The nurse should use subtle ways of doing this, such as telling the woman a urine specimen is required and showing her the way to the restroom, providing the nurse and client some private time. Asking the partner directly if he was responsible will not help because the partner

may not admit his culpability. Telling the partner to leave the room immediately may rouse the suspicions of the partner. Questioning the client about the injury in front of the partner may trigger another abusive episode and should be avoided. Precaution should be taken to prevent the abuser from punishing the woman when she returns home.

9. **Answer: a**
RATIONALE: The nurse should use direct quotes and specific language as much as possible when documenting. The nurse should not obtain photos of the client without informed consent. The nurse should, however, document the refusal of the client to be photographed. Documentation must include details as to the frequency and severity of abuse and the location, extent, and outcome of injuries, not just a description of the interventions taken. The nurse is required by law to inform the police of any injuries that involve knives, firearms, or other deadly weapons or that present life-threatening emergencies. Hence, the nurse should explain to the client why the case has to be reported to the police.

10. **Answer: a**
RATIONALE: The nurse should offer referrals to the client, such as support groups or specialists, so that the client gets professional help in recovering from the incident. The nurse should help the client cope with the incident rather than telling the client to forget about it. The nurse should also educate the client about the connection between the violence and some of the symptoms that she has developed recently, like palpitations. Confirming with the partner whether the client's story is true will create further problems for the client, and the nurse may lose the client's trust.

11. **Answer: a**
RATIONALE: To minimize risk of pregnancy, the nurse should ensure that the client takes a double dose of emergency contraceptive pills: the first dose within 72 hours of the rape and the second dose 12 hours after the first dose, if not sooner. It is better to use contraceptive measures immediately than to wait for signs of pregnancy. Using spermicidal creams or gels or regular oral contraceptive pills will not prove effective in preventing unwanted pregnancies.

12. **Answer: b, c, & d**
RATIONALE: Some of the factors that may lead to abuse during pregnancy are resentment toward the interference of the growing fetus and change in the woman's shape, perception of the baby as a competitor once he or she is born, and insecurity and jealousy of the pregnancy and the responsibilities it brings. Concern for the child will never result in physical abuse, as the unborn child is also at risk through assault during pregnancy. Serial abusers may exhibit violent tendencies during pregnancy, and such behavior is unacceptable.

13. **Answer: a, b, & e**
RATIONALE: Victims of human trafficking have restrictions on their daily movements, so the nurse should ask questions to learn whether the client can move around freely. The nurse should also find out if the client could leave her present job or situation if she wants to. Asking clients what their parents do or what their educational background is does not help determine whether they are victims of human trafficking.

14. **Answer: b, c, & e**
RATIONALE: To screen for abuse, the nurse should assess for mental health problems or injuries. The nurse should also be alert for inconsistencies regarding the reporting of the injury and the actual problem. Having sexually transmitted infections frequently is not a sign of physical or sexual abuse. Usually, partners of suspected victims seem overprotective and they do not leave the client alone.

15 **Answer: a, b, & c**
RATIONALE: To learn whether the client is having physical symptoms of PTSD, the nurse should ask the client if she is having trouble sleeping and whether she is emotionally stable or given to bursts of irritability. The nurse should also find out if the client experiences heart palpitations or sweating. Asking the client if she is feeling numb emotionally assesses the presence of avoidance reactions, not physical manifestation of PTSD. The nurse should ask the client whether she has upsetting thoughts and nightmares to assess for the presence of intrusive thoughts.

CHAPTER 10

Activity A

1. Allele
2. mutation
3. autosomes
4. amnion
5. Chromosomes
6. morula
7. karyotype
8. Polyploidy
9. genome
10. phenotype

Activity B

1. The figure shows spermatogenesis. One spermatogonium gives rise to four spermatozoa.
2. The figure shows oogenesis. One mature ovum and three abortive cells are produced from each oogonium.
3. a. The figure shows fetal circulation. The arrows indicate the path of blood.
   b. The umbilical vein carries oxygen-rich blood from the placenta to the liver and through the ductus venosus. From there it is carried to the inferior vena cava to the right atrium of the heart. Some of the blood is shunted through the foramen ovale to the left side of the heart, where it is routed to the brain and upper extremities. The

rest of the blood travels down to the right ventricle and through the pulmonary artery. A small portion of the blood travels to the nonfunctioning lungs, while the remaining blood is shunted through the ductus arteriosus into the aorta to supply the rest of the body.

Activity C

1. c   **2.** b   **3.** a   **4.** e   **5.** d

Activity D

1. For conception or fertilization to occur, a healthy ovum from the woman has to be released from the ovary. It passes into an open fallopian tube and starts its journey downward. Sperm from the male must be deposited into the vagina and be able to swim approximately seven inches to meet the ovum, where one spermatozoa penetrates the ovum's thick outer membrane. Fertilization takes place in the outer third of the ampulla of the fallopian tube.

2. The three different stages of fetal development during pregnancy are as follows:
   - Preembryonic stage: Begins with fertilization and continues through the second week
   - Embryonic stage: Begins 15 days after conception and continues through the eighth week
   - Fetal stage: Begins from the end of the eighth week and lasts until birth

3. The sex of the zygote is determined at fertilization. It depends on whether the ovum is fertilized by a Y-bearing sperm or an X-bearing sperm. An XX zygote will become a female and an XY zygote will become a male.

4. Concurrent with the development of the trophoblast and implantation, further differentiation of the inner cell mass of the zygote occurs. Some of the cells become the embryo itself, and others give rise to the membranes that surround and protect it. The three embryonic layers of cells formed are:
   - Ectoderm—forms the central nervous system, special senses, skin, and glands
   - Mesoderm—forms skeletal, urinary, circulatory, and reproductive organs
   - Endoderm—forms respiratory system, liver, pancreas, and digestive system

5. Amniotic fluid is derived from fluid transported from the maternal blood across the amnion and fetal urine. Its volume changes constantly as the fetus swallows and voids. Amniotic fluid is composed of 98% water and 2% organic matter. It is slightly alkaline and contains albumin, urea, uric acid, creatinine, bilirubin, lecithin, sphingomyelin, epithelial cells, vernix, and fine hair called lanugo.

6. The placenta produces hormones that control the basic physiology of the mother in such a way that the fetus is supplied with the necessary nutrients and oxygen needed for successful growth. The placenta produces the following hormones necessary for normal pregnancy:

- Human chorionic gonadotropin (or hCG)
- Human placental lactogen (hPL)
- Estrogen (estriol)
- Progesterone (progestin)
- Relaxin

Activity E

1. The nurse should explain the following functions of the amniotic fluid:
   - Helps maintain a constant body temperature for the fetus
   - Permits symmetric growth and development of fetus
   - Cushions the fetus from trauma
   - Allows umbilical cord to be free of compression
   - Promotes fetal movement to enhance musculoskeletal development
   - Amniotic fluid volume can be important in determining fetal well-being.

The nurse should explain the following functions of the placenta:
   - Makes hormones to ensure implantation of the embryo and to control mother's physiology to provide adequate nutrients and water to the growing fetus
   - Transports oxygen and nutrients from the mother's bloodstream to the developing fetus
   - Protects the fetus from immune attack by the mother
   - Removes fetal waste products
   - Near term, it produces hormones to mature fetal organs in preparation of extrauterine life.

The nurse should also explain these facts about the umbilical cord:
   - It is a lifeline from the mother to the fetus
   - It is formed from the amnion and contains one large vein and two small arteries
   - Wharton's jelly surrounds the vessels to prevent compression
   - At term, the average length is 22 inches long and an inch in width

Shana should be reassured that she will continue to feel fetal movement throughout her pregnancy and that it is not common for a fetus to get "tangled in its umbilical cord."

Activity F

1. Answer: b

   RATIONALE: This disorder is not X-linked. Either the father or the mother can pass the gene along, regardless of whether their mate has the gene or not. The only way that an autosomal dominant gene is not expressed is if it does not exist. If only one of the parents has the gene, then there is a 50% chance it will be passed on to the child.

2. Answer: c

   RATIONALE: The nurse should instruct the client to stop using drugs, alcohol, and tobacco, as these harmful substances may be passed on to the fetus from the mother. There is no need to avoid exercise during pregnancy as long as the client follows the prescribed regimen. Wearing comfortable clothes is not as important as the client's health. The client need not stay indoors during pregnancy.

3. **Answer: c**

   RATIONALE: The nurse should find out the cause and age of death for deceased family members, as it will help establish a genetic pattern. Instances of premature birth or depression during pregnancy are not related to any genetically inherited disorders. A family history of drinking or drug abuse does not increase the risk of genetic disorders.

4. **Answer: a**

   RATIONALE: The risk of trisomies such as Klinefelter syndrome increase with the age of the mother at the time of pregnancy. Klinefelter syndrome occurs only in males. Having twins does not increase the risk of Klinefelter syndrome for the babies, nor does the client's previous smoking habit have any bearing on the risk for Klinefelter syndrome.

5. **Answer: b**

   RATIONALE: Down syndrome is due to an extra chromosome present in the body. Down syndrome is not genetically inherited. Both males and females are equally at risk for Down syndrome. Most children with Down syndrome have mild to moderate mental retardation.

6. **Answer: d**

   RATIONALE: While obtaining the genetic history of the client, the nurse should find out if the members of the couple are related to each other or have blood ties, as this increases the risk of many genetic disorders. The socioeconomic status or the physical characteristics of family members do not have any significant bearing on the risk of genetic disorders. The nurse should ask questions about race or ethnic background because some races are more susceptible to certain disorders than others.

7. **Answer: c**

   RATIONALE: After the client has seen the specialist, the nurse should review what the specialist has discussed with the family and clarify any doubts the couple may have. The nurse should never make the decision for the client but rather should present all the relevant information and aid the couple in making an informed decision. There is no need for the nurse to refer the client to another specialist or for further diagnostic and screening tests unless instructed to do so by the specialist.

8. **Answer: a**

   RATIONALE: Tay-Sachs disease affects both male and female babies. The age of the client does not significantly increase the risk of Tay-Sachs disease. Even though the client and her husband are not related by blood, because of their background (Ashkenazi heritage), their baby is at a greater risk. There is a chance that the offspring may have Tay-Sachs disease even if both parents don't have it because they could be carriers.

9. **Answer: b, d, & e**

   RATIONALE: The nurse should explain to the client that individuals with hemophilia are usually males. Female carriers have a 50% chance of transmitting the disorder to their sons, and females are affected by the condition if it is a dominant X-linked disorder. Offspring of nonhemophilic parents may be hemophilic. Daughters of an affected male are usually carriers.

10. **Answer: a, b, & d**

    RATIONALE: The responsibilities of the nurse while counseling the client include knowing basic genetic terminology and inheritance patterns and explaining basic concepts of probability and disorder susceptibility. The nurse should also ensure complete informed consent to facilitate decisions about genetic testing. The nurse should explain ethical and legal issues related to genetics as well. The nurse should never instruct the client on which decision to make and should let the client make the decision.

11. **Answer: d**

    RATIONALE: The nurse should inform the client that her children will have a 50% chance of acquiring the disease. The client's children are at risk even if her husband has a normal matching gene. The presence of the gene mutation in an individual does not necessarily mean that the person will have the disease. Both male and female members are at risk for developing the disease.

12. **Answer: a & d**

    RATIONALE: The nurse should inform the client that fertilization or conception typically occurs around two weeks after the last normal menstrual period in a 28-day cycle. It requires a timely interaction between the release of the mature ovum at ovulation and the ejaculation of enough healthy, mobile sperm to survive the hostile vaginal environment through which they must travel to meet the ovum. This stage is referred to as the pre-embryonic, not embryonic, stage. It takes five, not 12, hours for the sperm to reach the ovum.

13. **Answer: d**

    RATIONALE: The hormone human chorionic gonadotropin (or hCG) is the basis for pregnancy tests. It preserves the corpus luteum and its progesterone production so that the endometrial lining of the uterus is maintained. Estrogen causes enlargement of a woman's breasts, uterus, and external genitalia and stimulates myometrial contractility. Progesterone maintains the endometrium, decreases the contractility of the uterus, stimulates maternal metabolism and breast development, and provides nourishment for the early conceptus. Human placental lactogen modulates fetal and maternal metabolism, participates in the development of maternal breasts for lactation, and decreases maternal insulin sensitivity to increase its availability for fetal nutrition.

14. Answer: a

RATIONALE: The ideal time for genetic counseling is before conception, not in the first week of pregnancy or in the second or third trimester. Preconception counseling allows couples the chance to identify and reduce potential pregnancy risks, plan for known risks, and establish early prenatal care.

15 Answer: b, a, e, d, & c

RATIONALE: The nurse first obtains the client's genetic history during the initial encounter. Then the nurse questions the client's family members to discover any additional details that may have been left out. After obtaining as much information about the client's genetic background as possible, the nurse identifies hereditary conditions, if there are any, prevalent in the family. Depending on the hereditary conditions identified, the nurse refers the client to the appropriate genetic specialist. The nurse also provides follow-up counseling support to the family to help review what has been discussed during the genetic counseling sessions and to answer any additional questions they might have.

CHAPTER 11

Activity A

1. cortisol
2. Ambivalence
3. Oxytocin
4. placenta
5. estrogen
6. sacroiliac
7. hemorrhoids
8. progesterone
9. Colostrum
10. leukorrhea

Activity B

1. The skin change is known as linea nigra, which develops during pregnancy in the middle of the abdomen, extending from the umbilicus to the pubic area.
2. **a.** Good food sources of folic acid include dark green vegetables, such as broccoli, romaine lettuce, and spinach; baked beans; black-eyed peas; citrus fruits; peanuts; and liver.
   b. The FDA has advised pregnant women and nursing mothers to avoid eating shark, swordfish, king mackerel, and tilefish because they contain traces of mercury that may harm a developing fetus.

Activity C

1. e   **2.** a   **3.** c   **4.** d   **5.** b

Activity D

1.

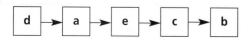

Activity E

1. Striae gravidarum, or stretch marks, are irregular reddish streaks that may appear on the abdomen, breasts, and buttocks in about half of pregnant women. Striae are most prominent by 6 to 7 months and occur in up to 90% of pregnant women. They are caused by reduced connective tissue strength resulting from elevated adrenal steroid levels and stretching of the structures secondary to growth. They are more common in younger women, women with larger infants, and women with higher body mass indices. Nonwhites and women with a history of breast or thigh striae or a family history of striae gravidarum are also at higher risk.

2. There is slight hypertrophy, or enlargement of the heart, during pregnancy to accommodate the increase in blood volume and cardiac output. The heart works harder and pumps more blood to supply the oxygen needs of the fetus as well as those of the mother. Both heart rate and venous return are increased in pregnancy, contributing to the increase in cardiac output seen throughout gestation.

3. Iron requirements during pregnancy increase because of the oxygen and nutrient demands of the growing fetus and the resulting increase in maternal blood volume. The fetal tissues take predominance over the mother's tissues with respect to use of iron stores. With the accelerated production of RBCs, iron is necessary for hemoglobin formation, the oxygen-carrying component of RBCs.

4. Pica is the compulsive ingestion of nonfood substances. The three main substances consumed by women with pica are soil or clay (geophagia), ice (pagophagia), and laundry starch (amylophagia). Nutritional implications of pica include iron-deficiency anemia, parasitic infection, and constipation.

5. Oxytocin is responsible for stimulating uterine contractions. After delivery, oxytocin secretion causes the myometrium to contract and helps constrict the uterine blood vessels, decreasing the amount of vaginal bleeding after delivery. Oxytocin is also responsible for milk ejection during breast-feeding. Stimulation of the breasts through sucking or touching stimulates the secretion of oxytocin from the posterior pituitary gland.

6. Varicose veins during pregnancy are the result of venous distention and instability, from poor circulation secondary to prolonged standing or sitting. Venous compression from the heavy gravid uterus places pressure on the pelvic veins, also preventing efficient venous return.

Activity F

1. **a.** The realization of a pregnancy can lead to fluctuating responses, possibly at opposite ends of the spectrum. For example, regardless of whether the pregnancy was planned, it is normal to be fearful and anxious of the implications. Your reaction may be influenced by several factors, including

the way you were raised by your family, your current family situation, the quality of the relationship with the expectant father, and your hopes for the future. It is common for some women to express concern over the timing of the pregnancy, wishing that goals and life objectives had been met before becoming pregnant. Other women may question how a newborn or infant will affect their careers or their relationships with friends and family. These feelings can cause conflict and confusion about the impending pregnancy.

Ambivalence, or having conflicting feelings at the same time, is a universal feeling and is considered normal when preparing for a lifestyle change and new role. Pregnant women commonly experience ambivalence during the first trimester. Usually ambivalence evolves into acceptance by the second trimester, when fetal movement is felt.

b. A pregnant woman may withdraw and become increasingly preoccupied with herself and her fetus. As a result, participation with the outside world may be less, and she may appear passive to her family and friends. This introspective behavior is a normal psychological adaptation to motherhood for most women. Introversion seems to heighten during the first and third trimesters, when the woman's focus is on behaviors that will ensure a safe and healthy pregnancy outcome. Women may also feel disinterested in certain activities because of nausea and fatigue experienced in the first trimester. Couples need to be aware of this behavior and be informed about measures to maintain and support the focus on the family.

c. During the second trimester, as the pregnancy progresses, the physical changes of the growing fetus, along with an enlarging abdomen and fetal movement, bring reality and validity to the pregnancy. The pregnant woman feels fetal movement and may hear the heartbeat. She may see the fetal image on an ultrasound screen and feel distinct parts, which allow her to identify the fetus as a separate individual. Many women will verbalize positive feelings of the pregnancy and will conceptualize the fetus. In addition, a reduction in physical discomfort will bring about an improvement in mood and physical well-being in the second trimester.

d. Frequently, pregnant women will start to cry without any apparent cause. Some feel as though they are riding an "emotional roller coaster." These extremes in emotion can make it difficult for partners and family members to communicate with the pregnant woman without placing blame on themselves for the woman's mood changes. Emotional lability is characteristic throughout most pregnancies. One moment a woman can feel great joy, and within a short time span feel shock and disbelief.

Activity G

1. **Answer: b**
RATIONALE: Absence of menstruation, or skipping a period, along with consistent nausea, fatigue, breast tenderness, and urinary frequency, are the presumptive signs of pregnancy. A positive home pregnancy test, abdominal enlargement, and softening of the cervix are the probable signs of pregnancy.

2. **Answer: c**
RATIONALE: During pregnancy, the vaginal secretions become more acidic, white, and thick. Most women experience an increase in a whitish vaginal discharge, called leukorrhea, during pregnancy. The nurse should inform the client that the vaginal discharge is normal except when it is accompanied by itching and irritation, possibly suggesting *Candida albicans* infection, a monilial vaginitis, which is a very common occurrence in this glycogen-rich environment. Monilial vaginitis is a benign fungal condition and is treated with local antifungal agents. The client need not refrain from sexual activity when there is an increase in a thick, whitish vaginal discharge.

3. **Answer: a**
RATIONALE: Estrogen aids in developing the ductal system of the breasts in preparation for lactation during pregnancy. Prolactin stimulates the glandular production of colostrum. During pregnancy, the ability of prolactin to produce milk is opposed by progesterone. Progesterone supports the endometrium of the uterus to provide an environment conducive to fetal survival. Oxytocin is responsible for uterine contractions, both before and after delivery. Oxytocin is also responsible for milk ejection during breastfeeding.

4. **Answer: d**
RATIONALE: The maternal emotional response experienced by the client is ambivalence. Ambivalence, or having conflicting feelings at the same time, is universal and is considered normal when preparing for a lifestyle change and new role. Pregnant women commonly experience ambivalence during the first trimester. The client is not experiencing introversion, acceptance, or mood swings. Introversion, or focusing on oneself, is common during the early part of pregnancy. The woman may withdraw and become increasingly preoccupied with herself and her fetus. Acceptance is the common maternal emotional response during the second trimester. As the pregnancy progresses, the physical changes of the growing fetus, along with an enlarging abdomen and fetal movement, bring reality and validity to the pregnancy. Although mood swings are common during pregnancy, this client is not experiencing mood swings.

5. **Answer: a, c, & e**
RATIONALE: Constipation during pregnancy is due to changes in the gastrointestinal system. Consti-

pation can result from decreased activity level, use of iron supplements, intestinal displacement secondary to a growing uterus, slow transition time of food throughout the GI tract, a low-fiber diet, and reduced fluid intake. Increase in progesterone, not estrogen levels, causes constipation during pregnancy. Reduced stomach acidity does not cause constipation. Morning sickness has been linked to stomach acidity.

6. **Answer: a, b, & d**

   RATIONALE: hCG levels in a normal pregnancy usually double every 48 to 72 hours, until they reach a peak at approximately 60 to 70 days after fertilization. This elevation of hCG corresponds to the morning sickness period of approximately 6 to 12 weeks during early pregnancy. Reduced stomach acidity and high levels of circulating estrogens are also believed to cause morning sickness. Elevation of hPL and RBC production do not cause morning sickness. hPL increases during the second half of pregnancy, and it helps in the preparation of mammary glands for lactation and is involved in the process of making glucose available for fetal growth by altering maternal carbohydrate, fat, and protein metabolism. The increase in RBCs is necessary to transport the additional oxygen required during pregnancy.

7. **Answer: c**

   RATIONALE: Spontaneous, irregular, painless contractions, called Braxton Hicks contractions, begin during the first trimester. These contractions are not the signs of preterm labor, infection of the GI tract, or acid indigestion. Acid indigestion causes heartburn. Acid indigestion or heartburn (pyrosis) is caused by regurgitation of the stomach contents into the upper esophagus and may be associated with the generalized relaxation of the entire digestive system.

8. **Answer: d**

   RATIONALE: The symptoms experienced by the client indicate supine hypotension syndrome. When the pregnant woman assumes a supine position, the expanding uterus exerts pressure on the inferior vena cava, causing a reduction in blood flow to the heart, most commonly during the third trimester. The nurse should place the client in the left lateral position to correct this syndrome and optimize cardiac output and uterine perfusion. Elevating the client's legs, placing the client in an orthopneic position, or keeping the head of the bed elevated will not help alleviate the client's condition.

9. **Answer: a**

   RATIONALE: The nurse should instruct the parents to provide constant reinforcement of love and care to reduce the sibling's fear of change and possible replacement by the new family member. The parents should neither avoid talking to the child about the new arrival nor pay less attention to the child. The nurse should urge parents to include siblings in this event and make them feel a part of the preparations for the new infant. The nurse should instruct the parents to continue to focus on the older sibling after the birth to reduce regressive or aggressive behavior that might manifest toward the newborn. The child is exhibiting sibling rivalry, which results from the child's fear of change in the security of his relationships with his parents. This behavior is common and does not require the intervention of a child psychologist.

10. **Answer: b**

    RATIONALE: Monilial vaginitis is a benign fungal condition that is uncomfortable for women; it can be transmitted from an infected mother to her newborn at birth. Neonates develop an oral infection known as thrush, which presents as white patches on the mucus membranes of the mouth. Although rubella, toxoplasmosis, and cytomegalovirus are infections transmitted to the newborn by the mother, this newborn is not experiencing any of these infections. Rubella causes fetal defects, known as congenital rubella syndrome; common defects of rubella are cataracts, deafness, congenital heart defects, cardiac disease, and mental retardation. Possible fetal effects due to toxoplasmosis include stillbirth, premature delivery, microcephaly, hydrocephaly, seizures, and mental retardation, whereas possible effects of cytomegalovirus infection include SGA, microcephaly, hydrocephaly, and mental retardation.

11. **Answer: a**

    RATIONALE: Between 38 and 40 weeks of gestation, the fundal height drops as the fetus begins to descend and engage into the pelvis. Because it pushes against the diaphragm, many women experience shortness of breath. By 40 weeks, the fetal head begins to descend and engage into the pelvis. Although breathing becomes easier because of this descent, the pressure on the urinary bladder now increases, and women experience urinary frequency. The fundus reaches its highest level at the xiphoid process at approximately 36, not 39, weeks. By 20 weeks' gestation, the fundus is at the level of the umbilicus and measures 20 cm. At between 6 and 8 weeks of gestation, the cervix begins to soften (Goodell's sign) and the lower uterine segment softens (Hegar's sign).

12. **Answer: c**

    RATIONALE: The skin and complexion of pregnant women undergo hyperpigmentation, primarily as a result of estrogen, progesterone, and melanocyte-stimulating hormone levels. The increased pigmentation that occurs on the breasts and genitalia also develops on the face to form the "mask of pregnancy," or facial melasma. This is a blotchy, brownish pigment that covers the forehead and cheeks in dark-haired women. The symptoms experienced by the client do not indicate linea nigra, striae gravidarum, or vascular spiders. The skin in the middle of the abdomen may develop a pig-

1. a. Th
   to
   th
   fo

   •
   •
   •
   •
   •
   •

   •

   •
   •

   •
   •

   •

b. T
   v
   •

   •

   •

c. T
   a
   ii
   •

   •
   •
   •

   •

mented line called the linea nigra, which extends from the umbilicus to the pubic area. Striae gravidarum, or stretch marks, are irregular reddish streaks that appear on the abdomen, breasts, and buttocks in about 50% of pregnant women after month 5 of gestation. Vascular spiders appear as small, spider-like blood vessels in the skin and are usually found above the waist and on the neck, thorax, face, and arms.

13. **Answer: c**
    RATIONALE: During pregnancy, there is an increase in the client's blood components. These changes, coupled with venous stasis secondary to venous pooling, which occurs during late pregnancy after standing long periods of time (with the pressure exerted by the uterus on the large pelvic veins), contribute to slowed venous return, pooling, and dependent edema. These factors also increase the woman's risk for venous thrombosis. The symptoms experienced by the client do not indicate that she is at risk for hemorrhoids, embolism, or supine hypotension syndrome. Supine hypotension syndrome occurs when the uterus expands and exerts pressure on the inferior vena cava, which causes a reduction in blood flow to the heart. A client with supine hypotension syndrome experiences dizziness, clamminess, and a marked decrease in blood pressure.

14. **Answer: a, c, & e**
    RATIONALE: Changes in the structures of the respiratory system take place to prepare the body for the enlarging uterus and increased lung volume. Increased vascularity of the respiratory tract is influenced by increased estrogen levels, leading to congestion. This congestion gives rise to nasal and sinus stuffiness and to epistaxis (nosebleed). As muscles and cartilage in the thoracic region relax, the chest broadens with a conversion from abdominal breathing to thoracic breathing. Persistent cough, Kussmaul's respirations, and dyspnea are not associated with the changes in the respiratory tract during pregnancy.

15 **Answer: d**
   RATIONALE: During the second trimester, many women will verbalize positive feelings about the pregnancy and will conceptualize the fetus. The woman may accept her new body image and talk about the new life within her. Generating a discussion about the woman's feelings and offering support and validation at prenatal visits are important nursing interventions. The nurse should encourage the client in her first trimester to focus on herself, not on the fetus; this is not required when the client is in her second trimester. The client's feelings are normal for the second trimester of pregnancy; hence, it is not necessary either to inform the primary health care provider about the client's feelings or to tell the client that it is too early to conceptualize the fetus.

16. **Answer: b**
    RATIONALE: The nurse should instruct the client to change sexual positions to increase comfort as the pregnancy progresses. Although the nurse should also encourage her to engage in alternative, non-coital modes of sexual expression, such as cuddling, caressing, and holding, the client need not restrict herself to such alternatives. It is not advisable to perform frequent douching, because this is believed to irritate the vaginal mucosa and predispose the client to infection. Using lubricants or performing stress-relieving and relaxation exercises will not alleviate discomfort during sexual activity.

17. **Answer: b**
    RATIONALE: During the second trimester of pregnancy, partners go through acceptance of their role of breadwinner, caretaker, and support person. They come to accept the reality of the fetus when movement is felt, and they experience confusion when dealing with the woman's mood swings and introspection. During the first trimester, the expectant partner may experience couvade syndrome—a sympathetic response to the partner's pregnancy—and may also experience ambivalence with extremes of emotions. During the third trimester, the expectant partner prepares for the reality of the new role and negotiates what his or her role will be during the labor and birthing process.

CHAPTER 12

Activity A

1. doula
2. primipara
3. Fundal
4. Montgomery's
5. Chadwick's
6. Pica
7. Amniocentesis
8. liver
9. nonstress
10. Hemorrhoids

Activity B

1. a. The figure shows the procedure for amniocentesis. Amniocentesis involves a transabdominal perforation of the amniotic sac to obtain a sample of amniotic fluid for analysis.
   b. The fluid contains fetal cells that are examined to detect chromosomal abnormalities and several hereditary metabolic defects in the fetus before birth. Amniocentesis is also used to confirm a fetal abnormality when other screening tests detect a possible problem.
2. a. The figure shows a pregnant client using pillows for support in the side-lying position.
   b. Using pillows for support in the side-lying position relieves pressure on major blood vessels that supply oxygen and nutrients to the fetus when resting.

ensiform cartilage when the client is in the 36th week of gestation; midway between symphysis and umbilicus in the 16th week of gestation; and at the umbilicus in the 20th week of gestation.

6. Answer: c

RATIONALE: While examining external genitalia, the nurse should assess for any infection due to hematomas, varicosities, inflammation, lesions, and discharge. The nurse assesses for a long, smooth, thick, and closed cervix when examining the internal genitalia. Other assessments when examining the internal genitalia include assessing for bluish coloration of cervix and vaginal mucosa and conducting a rectal examination to assess for lesions, masses, prolapse, or hemorrhoids.

7. Answer: b

RATIONALE: When assessing fetal well-being through abdominal ultrasonography, the nurse should instruct the client to refrain from emptying her bladder. The nurse must ensure that abdominal ultrasonography is conducted on a full bladder and should inform the client that she is likely to feel cold, not hot, initially in the test. The nurse should obtain the client's vital records and instruct the client to report the occurrence of fever when the client has to undergo amniocentesis, not ultrasonography.

8. Answer: a

RATIONALE: The nurse should inform the client that sexual activity is permissible during pregnancy unless there is a history of incompetent cervix, vaginal bleeding, placenta previa, risk of preterm labor, multiple gestation, premature rupture of membranes, or presence of any infection. Anemia and facial and hand edema would be contraindications to exercising but not intercourse. Freedom from anxieties and worries contributes to adequate sleep promotion.

9. Answer: a

RATIONALE: To help alleviate constipation, the nurse should instruct the client to ensure adequate hydration and bulk in the diet. The nurse should instruct the client to avoid spicy or greasy foods when a client complains of heartburn or indigestion. The nurse also should instruct the client to avoid lying down for two hours after meals if the client experiences heartburn or indigestion. The nurse should instruct the client to practice Kegel exercises when the client experiences urinary frequency.

10. Answer: d

RATIONALE: To promote easy and safe travel for the client, the nurse should instruct the client to always wear a three-point seat belt to prevent ejection or serious injury from collision. The nurse should instruct the client to deactivate the air bag if possible. The nurse should instruct the client to apply a nonpadded shoulder strap properly, ensuring that it crosses between the breasts and over the upper abdomen, above the uterus. The nurse should in-

struct the client to use a lap belt that crosses over the pelvis below—not over—the uterus.

11. Answer: b

RATIONALE: Nagele's rule can be used to establish the estimated date of birth. Using this rule, the nurse should subtract 3 months and then add 7 days to the first day of the last normal menstrual period. On the basis of Nagele's rule, the estimated date of birth (EDB) will be December 17, because the client started her last menstrual period on March 10. January 7, February 21, and January 30 are not the EDB according to Nagele's rule.

12. Answer: a

RATIONALE: Pica is characterized by a craving for substances that have no nutritional value. Consumption of these substances can be dangerous to the client and her developing fetus. The nurse should monitor the client for iron-deficiency anemia as a manifestation of the client's compulsion to consume soil. Consumption of ice due to pica is likely to lead to tooth fractures. The nurse should monitor for inefficient protein metabolism if the client has been consuming laundry starch as a result of pica. The nurse should monitor for constipation in the client if she has been consuming clay.

13. Answer: b, c, & e

RATIONALE: When caring for a pregnant client who follows a vegetarian diet, the nurse should monitor her for iron-deficiency anemia, decreased mineral absorption, and low gestational weight gain. Risk of epistaxis and increased risk of constipation are not reported to be associated with a vegetarian diet.

14. Answer: a

RATIONALE: In a client's second trimester of pregnancy, the nurse should educate the client to look for vaginal bleeding as a danger sign of pregnancy needing immediate attention from the physician. Generally, painful urination, severe/persistent vomiting, and lower abdominal and shoulder pain are the danger signs that the client has to monitor for during the first trimester of pregnancy.

15 Answer: c

RATIONALE: The nurse should instruct the client to serve the formula to her infant at room temperature. The nurse should instruct the client to follow the directions on the package when mixing the powder, because different formulas may have different instructions. The infant should be fed every 3 to 4 hours, not every 8 hours. The nurse should specifically instruct the client to avoid refrigerating the formula for subsequent feedings. Any leftover formula should be discarded.

16. Answer: d

RATIONALE: According to the Lamaze method of preparing for labor and childbirth, the nurse must remain quiet during the client's period of imagery and focal point visualization to avoid breaking her

concentration. The nurse should ensure deep ab-
dominopelvic breathing by the client according to
the Bradley method, along with ensuring the
client's concentration on pleasurable sensations.
The Bradley method emphasizes the pleasurable
sensations of childbirth and involves teaching
women to concentrate on these sensations when
"turning on" to their own bodies. The nurse
should ensure abdominal breathing during contractions when using the Dick-Read method.

17. **Answer: b**
    RATIONALE: To help the client alleviate varicosities
    of the legs, the nurse should instruct the client to
    refrain from crossing her legs when sitting for long
    periods. The nurse should instruct the client to
    avoid standing, not sitting, in one position for
    long periods. The nurse should instruct the client
    to wear support stockings to promote better circu-
    lation, though the client should stay away from
    constrictive stockings and socks. Applying heating
    pads on the extremities is not reported to alleviate
    varicosities of the legs.

18. **Answer: b, e, c, a, & d**
    RATIONALE: The client who is to undergo a nonstress
    test should have a meal before the procedure. The
    client is then placed in a lateral recumbent position
    to avoid supine hypotension syndrome. An external
    electronic fetal monitoring device is applied to her
    abdomen. The client is handed an "event marker"
    with a button that she pushes every time she per-
    ceives fetal movement. When the button is pushed,
    the fetal monitor strip is marked to identify that
    fetal movement has occurred.

CHAPTER 13

Activity A

1. gynecoid
2. effacement
3. sagittal
4. Zero
5. Lightening
6. contractions
7. decidua
8. passageway
9. nesting
10. molding

Activity B

1. **a.** The figure shows a frank breech presentation. In
   a frank breech, the buttocks present first, with
   both legs extended up toward the face.
   b. Breech presentations are associated with prematurity, placenta previa, multiparity, uterine abnormalities (fibroids), and some congenital
   anomalies such as hydrocephaly.
2. **a.** The figure shows a platypelloid, or flat, pelvis.
   This is the least common type of pelvic structure

among men and women, with an approximate
incidence of 5%.
b. The pelvic cavity in a platypelloid (flat) pelvis is
shallow but widens at the pelvic outlet, making
it difficult for the fetus to descend through the
mid-pelvis. It is not favorable for a vaginal birth
unless the fetal head can pass through the inlet.
Women with this type of pelvis usually require
cesarean birth.

Activity C

1. a   **2.** b   **3.** e   **4.** d   **5.** c

Activity D

1.

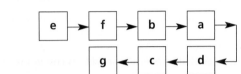

Activity E

1. Well-controlled research validates that nonmoving,
   back-lying positions during labor are not healthy.
   Despite this, most women lie flat on their backs.
   This position is preferred during labor mostly for
   the following reasons:
   • Laboring women need to conserve their energy
     and not tire themselves
   • Nurses can keep track of patients more easily if
     they are not ambulating
   • The supine position facilitates vaginal examina-
     tions and external belt adjustment
   • A bed is simply where one is usually supposed to
     be in a hospital setting
   • Blind routine practice is convenient for the deliv-
     ering health professional
   • Laboring women are "connected to things" that
     impede movement
2. The nurse should encourage the pregnant client to
   adopt the upright or lateral position because such a
   position
   • Reduces the duration of the second stage of labor
   • Reduces the number of assisted deliveries (vac-
     uum and forceps)
   • Reduces episiotomies and perineal tears
   • Contributes to fewer abnormal fetal heart rate
     patterns
   • Increases comfort and reduces requests for pain
     medication
   • Enhances a sense of control reported by mothers
   • Alters the shape and size of the pelvis, which as-
     sists descent
   • Assists gravity to move the fetus downward
   • Reduces the length of labor
3. Maternal physiologic responses that occur as a
   woman progresses through childbirth include:
   • Increase in heart rate, by 10 to 18 bpm
   • Increase in cardiac output, by 10% to 15% during
     the first stage of labor and by 30% to 50% during
     the second stage of labor

- Increase in blood pressure, by 10 to 30 mm Hg during uterine contractions in all labor stages
- Increase in white blood cell count, to 25,000 to 30,000 cells/mm^3, perhaps as a result of tissue trauma
- Increase in respiratory rate, along with greater oxygen consumption, related to the increase in metabolism
- Decrease in gastric motility and food absorption, which may increase the risk of nausea and vomiting during the transition stage of labor
- Decrease in gastric emptying and gastric pH, which increases the risk of vomiting with aspiration
- Slight elevation in temperature, possibly as a result of an increase in muscle activity
- Muscular aches/cramps, as a result of a stressed musculoskeletal system involved in the labor process
- Increase in BMR and decrease in blood glucose levels because of the stress of labor

4. The factors that influence the ability of a woman to cope with labor stress include these:
   - Previous birth experiences and their outcomes
   - Current pregnancy experience
   - Cultural considerations
   - Involvement of support system
   - Childbirth preparation
   - Expectations of the birthing experience
   - Anxiety level and fear of labor experience
   - Feelings of loss of control
   - Fatigue and weariness
   - Anxiety levels

5. The signs of separation that indicate the placenta is ready to deliver are the following:
   - Uterus rises upward
   - Umbilical cord lengthens
   - Blood trickles suddenly from the vaginal opening
   - Uterus changes its shape to globular

6. The following factors ensure a positive birth experience for the pregnant client:
   - Clear information on procedures
   - Positive support; not being alone
   - Sense of mastery, self-confidence
   - Trust in staff caring for her
   - Positive reaction to the pregnancy
   - Personal control over breathing
   - Preparation for the childbirth experience

Activity F

1. **a.** Many women fear being sent home from the hospital with "false labor." All women feel anxious when they feel contractions, but they should be informed that labor can be a long process, especially if it is their first pregnancy. With first pregnancies, the cervix can take up to 20 hours to dilate completely. False labor is a condition occurring during the latter weeks of some pregnancies, in which irregular uterine contractions are felt but the cervix is not affected. In contrast, true labor is characterized by contractions occurring at regular intervals that increase in frequency, duration, and intensity. True labor contractions bring about progressive cervical dilation and effacement.

   b. The client should be instructed to stay home until contractions are 5 minutes apart, lasting 45–60 seconds and strong enough so that a conversation during one is not possible. She should be instructed to drink fluids and walk to assess if there is any change in her contractions. In true labor, contractions are regular, become closer together, and become stronger with time. The contraction starts in the back and radiates around toward the front of the abdomen.

   c. Changing positions and moving around during labor and birth do offer several benefits. Maternal position can influence pelvic size and contours. Changing position and walking affect the pelvis joints, and they facilitate fetal descent and rotation. Squatting enlarges the pelvic outlet by approximately 25%, whereas a kneeling position removes pressure on the maternal vena cava and assists to rotate the fetus in the posterior position.

   The client should be encouraged to ask the nurse caring for her during labor if she can walk and have the nurse suggest positions to try.

   d. The second stage of labor begins with complete cervical dilation (10 cm) and effacement and ends with the birth of the newborn. Although the previous stage of labor primarily involved the thinning and opening of the cervix, this stage involves moving the fetus through the birth canal and out of the body. The cardinal movements of labor occur during the early phase of passive descent in the second stage of labor.

   Contractions occur every 2 to 3 minutes, last 60 to 90 seconds, and are described as strong by palpation. During this expulsive stage, the client may feel more in control and less irritable and agitated and be focused on the work of pushing. Traditionally, women have been taught to hold their breath to the count of 10, inhale again, push again, and repeat the process several times during a contraction. This sustained, strenuous style of pushing has been shown to lead to hemodynamic changes in the mother and interfere with oxygen exchange between the mother and the fetus. The newest protocol from the Association of Women's Health, Obstetric and Neonatal Nurses (AWHONN) recommends an open-glottis method in which air is released during pushing to prevent the buildup of intrathoracic pressure. During the second stage of labor, pushing can either follow a spontaneous urge or be directed by the nurse and/or health provider. The second stage of labor has two phases, related to the existence and quality of the maternal urge to push and to obstetric conditions related to fetal descent. The early phase of the second stage is called the pelvic phase, because it is during this phase that the fetal head is negotiating the pelvis, rotating, and advancing in descent. The later phase is called the perineal phase, because at this point the fetal head is lower in the pelvis and is distending the perineum. The occurrence of a strong urge to push characterizes the later phase of the second stage and has also been called the phase of active pushing. The perineum bulges and there is an increase in bloody show. The fetal head becomes apparent at the vaginal opening but disappears between contractions. When the top of the head no longer regresses between contractions, it is said to have crowned. The fetus rotates as it maneuvers out. The second stage commonly lasts up to 3 hours in a first labor.

Activity G

1. **Answer: b**
   RATIONALE: The nurse knows that the client is experiencing lightening. Lightening occurs when the fetal presenting part begins to descend into the maternal pelvis. The uterus lowers and moves into a more anterior position. The client may report increased respiratory capacity, decreased dyspnea, increased pelvic pressure, cramping, and low back pain. She also may note edema of the lower extremities as a result of the increased stasis of blood pooling, an increase in vaginal discharge, and more frequent urination. Some women report a sudden increase in energy before labor. This is sometimes referred to as nesting. Bloody show is a pink-tinged secretion that occurs when a small amount of blood released by cervical capillaries mixes with mucus. Braxton Hicks contractions are typically felt as a tightening or pulling sensation of the top of the uterus.

2. **Answer: a, b, & d**
   RATIONALE: Upon seeing the increased prostaglandin levels, the nurse should assess for myometrial contractions, leading to a reduction in cervical resistance and subsequent softening and thinning of the cervix. The uterus of the client will appear boggy during the fourth stage of delivery, after the completion of pregnancy and birth. Hypotonic character of the bladder is also marked during the fourth stage of pregnancy, not when the prostaglandin levels rise, marking the onset of labor.

3. **Answer: a**
   RATIONALE: Braxton Hicks contractions assist in labor by ripening and softening the cervix and moving the cervix from a posterior position to an anterior position. Prostaglandin levels increase late in pregnancy secondary to elevated estrogen levels; this is not due to the occurrence of Braxton Hicks contractions. Braxton Hicks contractions do not help in bringing about oxytocin sensitivity. Occurrence of lightening, not Braxton Hicks contractions, makes maternal breathing easier.

4. **Answer: c**
   RATIONALE: The labor of a first-time-pregnant woman lasts longer because during the first pregnancy the cervix takes between 12 and 16 hours to dilate completely. The intensity of the Braxton Hicks contractions stays the same during the first and second pregnancies. Spontaneous rupture of membranes occurs before the onset of labor during each delivery, not only during the first delivery.

5. **Answer: d**
   RATIONALE: The advantage of adopting a kneeling position during labor is that it helps to rotate the fetus in a posterior position. Facilitating vaginal examinations, facilitating external belt adjustment, and helping the woman in labor to save energy are advantages of the back-lying maternal position.

6. **Answer: a, b, & c**
   RATIONALE: When caring for a client in labor, the nurse should monitor for an increase in the heart rate by 10 to 18 bpm, an increase in blood pressure by 10 to 30 mm Hg, and an increase in respiratory rate. During labor, the nurse should monitor for a slight elevation in body temperature as a result of an increase in muscle activity. The nurse should also monitor for decreased gastric emptying and gastric pH, which increases the risk of vomiting with aspiration.

7. **Answer: d**
   RATIONALE: When monitoring fetal responses in a client experiencing labor, the nurse should monitor for a decrease in circulation and perfusion to the fetus secondary to uterine contractions. The nurse should monitor for an increase, not a decrease, in arterial carbon dioxide pressure. The nurse should also monitor for a decrease, not an increase, in fetal breathing movements throughout labor. The nurse should monitor for a decrease in fetal oxygen pressure with a decrease in the partial pressure of oxygen.

8. **Answer: c**
   RATIONALE: The nurse must massage the client's uterus briefly after placental expulsion to constrict the uterine blood vessels and minimize the possibility of hemorrhage. Massaging the client's uterus will not lessen the chances of conducting an episiotomy. In addition, an episiotomy, if required, is conducted in the second stage of labor, not the third. The client's uterus may appear boggy only in the fourth stage of labor—not in the third stage of labor. Ensuring that all sections of the placenta are present and that no piece is left attached to the uterine wall is confirmed through a placental examination after expulsion.

9. **Answer: d**
   RATIONALE: The first stage of labor terminates with the dilation of the cervix diameter to 10 cm. Diffused abdominal cramping and rupturing of the fetal membrane occurs during the first stage of labor. Regular contractions occur at the beginning

of the latent phase of the first stage; they do not mark the end of the first stage of labor.

10. **Answer: a, c, & e**
RATIONALE: The nurse knows that lower uterine segment distention, stretching and tearing of the structures, and dilation of the cervix cause pain in the first stage. The fetus moves along the birth canal during the second stage of labor, when the client is more in control and less agitated. Spontaneous expulsion of the placenta occurs in the third stage of labor, not the first.

11. **Answer: b**
RATIONALE: The nurse, along with the physician, has to assess for fetal anomalies, which are usually associated with a shoulder presentation during a vaginal birth. The other conditions include placenta previa and multiple gestations. Uterine abnormalities, congenital anomalies, and prematurity are conditions associated with a breech presentation of the fetus during a vaginal birth.

12. **Answer: a, b, & c**
RATIONALE: To ensure a positive childbirth experience for the client, the nurse should provide the client clear information on procedures involved, encourage the client to have a sense of mastery and self-control, and encourage the client to have a positive reaction to pregnancy. Instructing the client to spend some time alone is not an appropriate intervention; instead, the nurse should instruct the client to obtain positive support and avoid being alone. The client does not need to change the home environment; this does not ensure a positive childbirth experience.

13. **Answer: c**
RATIONALE: If the long axis of the fetus is perpendicular to that of the mother, then the client's fetus is in the transverse lie position. If the long axis of the fetus is parallel to that of the mother, the client's fetus is in the longitudinal lie position. The long axis of the fetus being at 45 or 60 degrees to that of the client does not indicate any specific position of the fetus.

14. **Answer: d**
RATIONALE: The pauses between contractions during labor are important because they allow the restoration of blood flow to the uterus and the placenta. Shortening of the upper uterine segment, reduction in length of the cervical canal, and effacement and dilation of the cervix are other processes that occur during uterine contractions.

15. **Answer: c**
RATIONALE: A shoulder presentation may be caused by anything that prevents the descent of the head or the breech into the lower pelvis. The condition that the nurse should try to observe during vaginal birth to identify a shoulder presentation is multiple gestations. The other conditions that should be observed are placenta previa and fetal anomalies. Multiparity, uterine abnormalities, and congenital

anomalies are factors associated with breech presentations.

16. **Answer: a, c, & d**
RATIONALE: To provide comfort to the pregnant client, the nurse should make use of massage, hand holding, and acupressure to bring comfort to the pregnant client during labor. It is not advisable to provide chewing gum to a client in labor; it may cause accidental asphyxiation. Pain killers are not prescribed for a client experiencing labor.

CHAPTER 14

Activity A

1. Nonpharmacologic
2. hypoglycemia
3. fern
4. uteroplacental
5. ischial
6. uterine
7. tocotransducer
8. Artifact
9. parasympathetic
10. accelerations

Activity B

1. **a.** The FHR pattern shown in the image indicates late decelerations.
   b. Late decelerations are associated with uteroplacental insufficiency, which occurs when blood flow within the intervillous space is decreased to the extent that fetal hypoxia occurs. Conditions that may decrease uteroplacental perfusion with resultant decelerations include maternal hypotension, gestational hypertension, placental aging secondary to diabetes and postmaturity, hyperstimulation via oxytocin infusion, maternal smoking, anemia, and cardiac disease.

Activity C

1. c   2. b   3. a   4. d

Activity D

1.

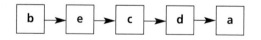

Activity E

1. The nurse should include biographical data such as the woman's name and age and the name of the delivering health care provider, prenatal record data, past health and family history, prenatal education, medications, risk factors, reason for admission, history of previous preterm births, allergies, the last time the client ate, method for infant feeding, name of birth attendant and pediatrician, and pain management plan.
2. The Apgar score assesses five parameters—heart rate (absent, slow, or fast), respiratory effort (absent,

weak cry, or good strong yell), muscle tone (limp, or lively and active), response to irritation stimulus, and color—that evaluate a newborn's cardiorespiratory adaptation after birth.

3. The purpose of vaginal examination is to assess the amount of cervical dilation, the percentage of cervical effacement, and the fetal membrane status, and to gather information about presentation, position, station, degree of fetal head flexion, and presence of fetal skull swelling or molding.

4. Advantage: Electronic fetal monitoring produces a continuous record of the fetal heart rate, unlike intermittent auscultation, when gaps are likely.

   Disadvantage: Continuous monitoring can limit maternal movement and encourages her to lie in the supine position, which reduces placental perfusion.

5. The typical signs of the second stage of labor are as follows:
   - Increase in apprehension or irritability
   - Spontaneous rupture of membranes
   - Sudden appearance of sweat on upper lip
   - Increase in blood-tinged show
   - Low grunting sounds from the woman
   - Complaints of rectal and perineal pressure
   - Beginning of involuntary bearing-down efforts

6. Ideal positions for the second stage of labor are as follows:
   - Lithotomy with feet up in stirrups: most convenient position for caregivers
   - Semi-sitting with pillows underneath knees, arms, and back
   - Lateral/side-lying with curved back and upper leg supported by partner
   - Sitting on birthing stool: opens pelvis, enhances the pull of gravity, and helps with pushing
   - Squatting/supported squatting: gives the woman a sense of control
   - Kneeling with hands on bed and knees comfortably apart

Activity F

1. **a.** If there was no vaginal bleeding on admission, the nurse should perform a vaginal examination to assess cervical dilation, after which it is monitored periodically as necessary to identify progress.

   b. The purpose of vaginal examination is to assess the amount of cervical dilation, the percentage of cervical effacement, and the fetal membrane status and to gather information about presentation, position, station, degree of fetal head flexion, and presence of fetal skull swelling or molding.

   c. Procedure for conducting vaginal examination:
   - Make the client comfortable
   - Put on sterile gloves
   - Use water as lubricant to check membrane status, if needed
   - Use antiseptic solution to prevent infection if the membrane has ruptured
   - Insert index and middle fingers into the vaginal introitus
   - Palpate cervix to assess dilation, effacement, and position

Activity G

1. **Answer: a**
   RATIONALE: When a nurse first comes in contact with a pregnant client during the admission assessment, it is important to first ascertain whether the woman is in true or false labor. Information regarding the number of pregnancies, addiction to drugs, or history of drug allergy is not important criteria for admitting the client.

2. **Answer: a, c, & d**
   RATIONALE: When conducting an admission assessment on the phone for a pregnant client, the nurse needs to obtain information regarding the estimated due date, characteristics of contractions, and appearance of vaginal blood to evaluate the need to admit her. History of drug abuse or a drug allergy is usually recorded as part of the client's medical history.

3. **Answer: b**
   RATIONALE: When a pregnant client is in the active phase of labor, the nurse should monitor the vital signs every 30 minutes. The nurse should monitor the vital signs every 30–60 minutes if the client is in the latent phase of labor and every 15–30 minutes during the transition phase of labor. Temperature is monitored every 4 hours in the active phase of labor.

4. **Answer: a**
   RATIONALE: In a cephalic presentation, the FHR is best heard in the lower quadrant of the maternal abdomen. In a breech presentation, it is heard at or above the level of the maternal umbilicus.

5. **Answer: c**
   RATIONALE: Fetal pulse oximetry measures fetal oxygen saturation directly and in real time. It is used with electronic fetal monitoring as an adjunct method of assessment when the FHR pattern is nonreassuring or inconclusive. Fetal scalp blood is obtained to measure the pH. The fetal position and weight can be determined through ultrasonography or abdominal palpation.

6. **Answer: a**
   RATIONALE: Increased sedation is an adverse effect of lorazepam. Diazepam and midazolam cause central nervous system depression for both the woman and the newborn. Opioids are associated with newborn respiratory depression and decreased alertness.

7. **Answer: d**
   RATIONALE: General anesthesia is administered in emergency cesarean births. Local anesthetic is injected into the superficial perineal nerves to numb the perineal area generally before an episiotomy. Although an epidural block is used in cesarean births, it is contraindicated in clients with spinal

injury. Regional anesthesia is contraindicated in cesarean births.

8. **Answer: b**
RATIONALE: During the latent phase of labor, the nurse should monitor the FHR every hour. FHR should be monitored every 30 minutes in the active phase and every 15–30 minutes in the transition phase of labor. Continuous monitoring is done when an electronic fetal monitor is used.

9. **Answer: b**
RATIONALE: If vaginal bleeding is absent during admission assessment, the nurse should perform vaginal examination to assess the amount of cervical dilation. Hydration status is monitored as part of the physical examination. A urine specimen is obtained for urinalysis to obtain a baseline. Vital signs are monitored frequently throughout the maternal assessment.

10. **Answer: c**
RATIONALE: The nitrazine tape shows a pH between 5 and 6, which indicates an acidic environment with the presence of vaginal fluid and less blood. If the membranes had ruptured, amniotic fluid was present, or there was excess blood, the nitrazine test tape would have indicated an alkaline environment.

11. **Answer: a, b, & e**
RATIONALE: The nurse should assess the frequency of contractions, intensity of contractions, and uterine resting tone to monitor uterine contractions. Monitoring changes in temperature and blood pressure is part of the general physical examination and does not help to monitor uterine contraction.

12. **Answer: a, b, & c**
RATIONALE: Leopold's maneuvers help the nurse to determine the presentation, position, and lie of the fetus. The approximate weight and size of the fetus can be determined with ultrasound sonography or abdominal palpation.

13. **Answer: a, c, & d**
RATIONALE: The nurse should turn the client on her left side to increase placental perfusion, administer oxygen by mask to increase fetal oxygenation, and assess the client for any underlying contributing causes. The client's questions should not be ignored; instead, the client should be reassured that interventions are to effect FHR pattern change. A reduced IV rate would decrease intravascular volume, affecting the FHR further.

14. **Answer: c**
RATIONALE: The client should be administered oxygen by mask, because the nonreassuring FHR pattern could be due to inadequate oxygen reserves in the fetus. Because the client is in preterm labor, it is not advisable to apply vibroacoustic stimulation, tactile stimulation, or fetal scalp stimulation.

15 **Answer: a**
RATIONALE: The nurse must monitor for respiratory depression. Accidental intrathecal blockade, inade-
quate or failed block, and postdural puncture headache are possible complications associated with combined spinal-epidural analgesia.

16. **Answer: b**
RATIONALE: The nurse should provide supplemental oxygen if a client who has been administered combined spinal-epidural analgesia exhibits signs of hypotension and associated FHR changes. The client should be assisted to a semi-Fowler's position; the client should not be kept in a supine position or be turned on her left side. Discontinuing IV fluid will cause dehydration.

17. **Answer: b**
RATIONALE: The nurse should monitor the client for uterine relaxation. Pruritus, inadequate or failed block, and maternal hypotension are associated with combined spinal-epidural analgesia.

18. **Answer: a**
RATIONALE: The recommendation for initiating hydrotherapy is that women be in active labor (>5 cm dilated), to prevent the slowing of labor contractions secondary to muscular relaxation. Women are encouraged to stay in the bath or shower as long as they feel they are comfortable. The water temperature should not exceed body temperature. The woman's membranes can be intact or ruptured.

19. **Answer: b**
RATIONALE: For slow-paced breathing, the nurse should instruct the woman to inhale slowly through her nose and exhale through pursed lips. In shallow or modified-pace breathing, the woman should inhale and exhale through her mouth at a rate of 4 breaths every 5 seconds. In pattern-paced breathing, the breathing is punctuated every few breaths by a forceful exhalation through pursed lips. Holding the breath for 5 seconds after every three breaths is not recommended in any of the three levels of patterned breathing.

20. **Answer: a, b, & d**
RATIONALE: The nurse should check for any abnormality of the spine, hypovolemia, or coagulation defects in the client. An epidural is contraindicated in women with these conditions. Varicose veins and skin rashes or bruises are not contraindications for an epidural block. They are contraindications for massage used for pain relief during labor.

CHAPTER 15

Activity A

1. pelvis
2. subinvolution
3. Afterpains
4. engorgement
5. uterus
6. Oxytocin
7. nonlactating
8. Lactation

9. Prolactin
10. diaphoresis

Activity B

1. d **2.** e **3.** a **4.** b **5.** c

Activity C

1.

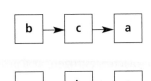

2.

c → b → a

Activity D

1. The timing of the first menses and ovulation after birth differs considerably in lactating and nonlactating women. In nonlactating women, menstruation resumes 7 to 9 weeks after giving birth; the first cycle is anovulatory. In lactating women, the return of menses depends on the frequency and duration of breastfeeding. It usually resumes anytime from 2 to 18 months after childbirth, and the first postpartum menses is usually heavier and frequently anovulatory. However, ovulation may occur before menstruation, so breastfeeding is not a reliable method of contraception.

2. Afterpains are more acute in multiparous women secondary to repeated stretching of the uterine muscles, which reduces muscle tone, allowing for alternate uterine contraction and relaxation.

3. Factors that facilitate uterine involution are
   • Complete expulsion of amniotic membranes and placenta at birth
   • Complication-free labor and birth process
   • Breastfeeding
   • Ambulation

4. Factors that inhibit involution include
   • Prolonged labor and difficult birth
   • Incomplete expulsion of amniotic membranes and placenta
   • Uterine infection
   • Overdistention of uterine muscles due to
     a. Multiple gestation, hydramnios, or large singleton fetus
     b. Full bladder, which displaces uterus and interferes with contractions
     c. Anesthesia, which relaxes uterine muscles
     d. Close childbirth spacing, leading to frequent and repeated distention and thus decreasing uterine tone and causing muscular relaxation

5. Women who have had cesarean births tend to have less flow because the uterine debris is removed manually with delivery of the placenta.

6. Afterpains are usually stronger during breastfeeding because oxytocin released by the sucking reflex strengthens uterine contractions. Mild analgesics can be used to reduce this discomfort.

Activity E

1. **a.** The nurse should suggest the following measures to resolve engorgement in the client who is breastfeeding:
   Empty the breasts frequently to minimize discomfort and resolve engorgement. Stand in a warm shower or apply warm compresses to the breasts to provide some relief.

   b. The nurse should suggest the following relief measures for the client with non-breastfeeding engorgement:
   • Wear a tight, supportive bra 24 hours daily.
   • Apply ice to the breasts for approximately 15 to 20 minutes every other hour.
   • Do not stimulate the breasts by squeezing or manually expressing milk from the nipples.
   • Avoid exposing the breasts to warmth.

Activity F

1. **Answer: a, c, & d**
   RATIONALE: Involution involves three retrogressive processes. The first of these is contraction of muscle fibers, which serves to reduce those previously stretched during pregnancy. Next, catabolism reduces enlarged, individual myometrial cells. Finally, there is regeneration of uterine epithelium from the lower layer of the decidua after the upper layers have been sloughed off and shed during lochia. The breasts do not return to their prepregnancy size as the uterus does. Urinary retention inhibits uterine involution.

2. **Answer: d**
   RATIONALE: Displacement of the uterus from the midline to the right and frequent voiding of small amounts suggests urinary retention with overflow. Catheterization may be necessary to empty the bladder to restore tone. A warm shower and warm compresses are recommended for clients with breastfeeding engorgement. Good body mechanics are recommended to prevent lower back and joint pains.

3. **Answer: b, c, & d**
   RATIONALE: The nurse should tell the client to use warm sitz baths, witch hazel pads, and anesthetic sprays to provide local comfort. Using good body mechanics and maintaining a correct position are important to prevent lower back pain and injury to the joints.

4. **Answer: a**
   RATIONALE: The nurse should recommend that the client practice Kegel exercises to improve pelvic floor tone, strengthen the perineal muscles, and promote healing. Witch hazel pads and sitz baths are useful in promoting local comfort in a client who had an episiotomy during the birth. Good body mechanics help to prevent lower back pain and injury to the joints.

5. Answer: a, b, & d

RATIONALE: Many women have difficulty with feeling the sensation to void after giving birth if they have received an anesthetic block during labor, which inhibits neural functioning of the bladder. This client will be at risk for incomplete emptying, bladder distention, difficulty voiding, and urinary retention. Ambulation difficulty and perineal lacerations are due to episiotomy.

6. Answer: c

RATIONALE: Postpartum diuresis is due to the buildup and retention of extra fluids during pregnancy. Bruising and swelling of the perineum, swelling of tissues surrounding the urinary meatus, and decreased bladder tone due to anesthesia cause urinary retention.

7. Answer: b

RATIONALE: The nurse should recommend that clients maintain correct position and good body mechanics to prevent pain in the lower back, hips, and joints. Anesthetic sprays are used to provide local comfort for clients with a bruised or swollen perineum. Kegel exercises are recommended to promote pelvic floor tone. Application of ice is suggested to help relieve breast engorgement in non-breastfeeding clients.

8. Answer: a

RATIONALE: The nurse should suggest that the father care for the newborn by holding and talking to the child. Reading up on parental care and speaking to his friends or the physician will not help the father resolve his fears about caring for the child.

9. Answer: c

RATIONALE: The nurse should encourage the client to change her gown to prevent chilling and reassure the client that it is normal to have postpartal diaphoresis. The use of good body mechanics is recommended to prevent lower back and joint injuries. Sitz baths are encouraged to promote local comfort in clients who had an episiotomy during the birth. Kegel exercises are recommended to promote pelvic floor tone.

10. Answer: c

RATIONALE: The nurse should tell the client that poor perineal muscular tone may cause urinary incontinence later in life. Kegel exercises are important to improve perineal muscular tone. Pain in the joints and lower back is due to improper body position. Postpartum diuresis is observed in the first week after birth.

11. Answer: c

RATIONALE: The nurse should tell the client to frequently empty the breasts to improve milk supply. Encouraging cold baths and applying ice on the breasts are recommended to relieve engorgement in non-breastfeeding clients. Kegel exercises are encouraged to promote pelvic floor tone.

12. Answer: a

RATIONALE: The nurse should explain to the client that lochia rubra is a deep red mixture of mucus, tissue debris, and blood. Discharge consisting of leukocytes, decidual tissue, RBCs, and serous fluid is called lochia serosa. Discharge consisting of only RBCs and leukocytes is blood. Discharge consisting of leukocytes and decidual tissue is called lochia alba.

13. Answer: d

RATIONALE: The nurse should explain to the client that the afterpains are due to oxytocin released by the sucking reflex, which strengthens uterine contractions. Prolactin, estrogen, and progesterone cause synthesis and secretion of colostrum.

CHAPTER 16

Activity A

1. peribottle
2. mastitis
3. hypertension
4. Pain
5. Orthostatic
6. fundus
7. cesarean
8. Reciprocity
9. Commitment
10. colostrum

Activity B

1. c   **2.** a   **3.** d   **4.** b

Activity C

1. Postpartum assessment of the mother typically includes vital signs, pain level, and a systematic head-to-toe review of the body systems: breasts, uterus, bladder, bowels, lochia, episiotomy/perineum, extremities, and emotional status.

2. The new mother might ignore her own needs for health and nutrition. She should be encouraged to take good care of herself and eat a healthy diet so that the nutrients lost during pregnancy can be replaced and she can return to a healthy weight. The nurse should provide nutritional recommendations, such as
   • Eating a wide variety of foods with high nutrient density
   • Using foods and recipes that require little or no preparation
   • Avoiding high-fat, fast foods and fad weight-reduction diets
   • Drinking plenty of fluids
   • Avoiding harmful substances such as alcohol, tobacco, and drugs
   • Avoiding excessive intake of fat, salt, sugar, and caffeine
   • Eating the recommended daily servings from each food group

3. The physical stress of pregnancy and birth, the required care-giving tasks associated with a newborn, meeting the needs of other family members, and fa-

tigue can cause the postpartum period to be quite stressful for the mother.

4. Postpartum danger signs include
   - Fever more than 38°C (100.4°F) after the first 24 hours following birth
   - Foul-smelling lochia or an unexpected change in color or amount
   - Visual changes, such as blurred vision or spots, or headaches
   - Calf pain experienced with dorsiflexion of the foot
   - Swelling, redness, or discharge at the episiotomy site
   - Dysuria, burning, or incomplete emptying of the bladder
   - Shortness of breath or difficulty breathing
   - Depression or extreme mood swings

5. The nurse should model behavior to family members as follows:
   - Holding the newborn close and speaking positively
   - Referring to the newborn by name in front of the parents
   - Speaking directly to the newborn in a calm voice
   - Encouraging both parents to pick up and hold the newborn
   - Monitoring newborn's response to parental stimulation
   - Pointing out positive physical features of the newborn

6. The nurse should suggest the following to the family to avoid sibling rivalry:
   - Expect and tolerate some regression
   - Discuss the new infant during relaxed family times
   - Teach safe handling of the newborn with a doll
   - Encourage older children to verbalize emotions about the newborn
   - Move the sibling from the crib to a youth bed months in advance of the birth of the newborn

Activity D

1. **a.** The nurse should perform the following assessments in a client intending to breastfeed her baby:
   - Inspect the breasts for size, contour, asymmetry, engorgement, or areas of erythema.
   - Check the nipples for cracks, redness, fissures, or bleeding.
   - Palpate the breasts to ascertain if they are soft, filling, or engorged, and document findings.
   - Palpate the breasts for any nodules, masses, or areas of warmth, which may indicate a plugged duct that may progress to mastitis if not treated promptly.
   - Describe and document any discharge from the nipple that is not creamy yellow or bluish white.

   b. The client is encouraged to offer frequent feedings, at least every 2 to 3 hours, using manual expression just before feeding to soften the breast so the newborn can latch on more effectively. The client should be told to allow the newborn to feed on the first breast until it softens before switching to the other side.

Activity E

1. **Answer: b**
   RATIONALE: Postpartum assessment typically is performed every 15 minutes for the first hour. After the second hour, assessment is performed every 30 minutes. The client has to be monitored closely during the first hour after delivery; assessment frequencies of 45 minutes or 60 minutes are too long.

2. **Answer: c**
   RATIONALE: Tachycardia in the postpartum woman can suggest anxiety, excitement, fatigue, pain, excessive blood loss, infection, or underlying cardiac problems. Pulmonary edema, atelectasis, and pulmonary embolism are associated with out–of–normal-range changes in respiratory rate.

3. **Answer: d**
   RATIONALE: A boggy or relaxed uterus is a sign of uterine atony. This can be the result of bladder distention, which displaces the uterus upward and to the right, or retained placental fragments. Foul-smelling urine and purulent drainage are signs of infections but are not related to uterine atony. The firm fundus is normal and not a sign of uterine atony.

4. **Answer: b**
   RATIONALE: "Scant" would describe a one- to two-inch lochia stain on the perineal pad, or an approximate 10-mL loss. "Light" or "small" would describe an approximate four-inch stain, or a 10- to 25-mL loss. "Moderate" lochia would describe a four- to six- inch stain, with an estimated loss of 25 to 50 mL. A large or heavy lochia loss would describe pad saturation within an hour after changing it.

5. **Answer: d**
   RATIONALE: The nurse should classify the laceration as fourth-degree, because it continues through the anterior rectal wall. First-degree laceration involves only skin and superficial structures above muscle; second-degree laceration extends through perineal muscles; and third-degree laceration extends through the anal sphincter muscle but not through the anterior rectal wall.

6. **Answer: c**
   RATIONALE: The nurse should ensure that the ice pack is changed frequently to promote good hygiene and to allow for periodic assessments. Ice packs are wrapped in a disposable covering or clean washcloth and then applied to the perineal area, not directly. The nurse should apply the ice pack for 20 minutes, not 40 minutes. Ice packs should be used for the first 24 hours, not for a week after delivery.

7. Answer: d
RATIONALE: Routine exercise should be resumed gradually, beginning with Kegel exercises on the first postpartum day. The client should be allowed to perform abdominal, buttock, and thigh-toning exercises only during the second week after delivery and not earlier.

8. Answer: a
RATIONALE: The nurse should reassure the mother that some newborns "latch on and catch on" right away, and some newborns take more time and patience; this information will help to reduce the feelings of frustration and uncertainty about their ability to breastfeed. The nurse should also explain that breastfeeding is a learned skill for both parties. It would not be correct to say that breastfeeding is a mechanical procedure. In fact, the nurse should encourage the mother to cuddle and caress the infant while feeding. The nurse should allow sufficient time to the mother and child to enjoy each other in an unhurried atmosphere. The nurse should teach the mother to burp the infant frequently. Different positions, such as cradle and football holds and side-lying positions, should be shown to the mother.

9. Answer: c
RATIONALE: The nurse should observe positioning and latching-on technique while breastfeeding so that she may offer suggestions based on observation to correct positioning/latching. This will help minimize trauma to the breast. The client should use only water, not soap, to clean the nipples to prevent dryness. Breast pads with plastic liners should be avoided. Leaving the nursing bra flaps down after feeding allows nipples to air dry.

10. Answer: b
RATIONALE: The nurse should inform the client that intercourse can be resumed if bright-red bleeding stops. Use of water-based gel lubricants can be helpful and should not be avoided. Pelvic floor exercises may enhance sensation and should not be avoided. Barrier methods such as a condom with spermicidal gel or foam should be used instead of oral contraceptives.

11. Answer: c
RATIONALE: The nurse should ensure that the follow-up appointment is fixed for within 2 weeks after hospital discharge. One week after hospital discharge is too early for a follow-up visit, whereas 3 weeks after discharge is too long because the client can develop complications that would go undiagnosed. For clients with an uncomplicated vaginal birth, an office visit is usually scheduled for between 4 and 6 weeks after childbirth.

12. Answer: a
RATIONALE: Mothers who are Rh-negative and have given birth to an infant who is Rh-positive should receive an injection of Rh immunoglobulin within 72 hours after birth; this prevents a sensitization reaction to Rh-positive blood cells received during the birthing process. It may be too late to administer Rh immunoglobulin after 72 hours.

13. Answer: a, b, & e
RATIONALE: Engorged breasts are hard, tender, and taut, and the nurse should assess for these signs. Improper positioning of the infant on the breast, not engorged breasts, results in cracked, blistered, fissured, bruised, or bleeding nipples in the breast-feeding woman.

14. Answer: b, d, & e
RATIONALE: Finding active bowel sounds, verification of passing gas, and a nondistended abdomen are normal assessment results. The abdomen should be non-tender and soft, not tender. Abdominal pain is not a normal assessment finding and should be immediately looked into.

15. Answer: b, c, & e
RATIONALE: The nurse should show mothers how to initiate breastfeeding within 30 minutes of birth. To ensure bonding, place the baby in uninterrupted skin-to-skin contact with the mother. Breastfeeding on demand should be encouraged. Pacifiers should not be used because they do not help fulfill nutritional requirements. The nurse should also ensure that no food or drink other than breast milk is given to newborns.

CHAPTER 17

Activity A
1. Habituation
2. reflex
3. acquired
4. Meconium
5. intestinal
6. amniotic
7. Jaundice
8. hemolysis
9. hemoglobin
10. hypothalamus

Activity B
1. d   2. a   3. c   4. b

Activity C
1. The newborn's response to auditory and visual stimuli is demonstrated by the following:
   • Moving the head and eyes to focus on stimulus
   • Staring at the object intently
   • Using sensory capacity to become familiar with people and objects
2. The expected neurobehavioral responses of the newborn include
   • Orientation
   • Habituation
   • Motor maturity
   • Self-quieting ability
   • Social behaviors

3. The following events must occur before the newborn's lungs can maintain respiratory function:
   - Initiation of respiratory movement
   - Expansion of the lungs
   - Establishment of functional residual capacity (ability to retain some air in the lungs on expiration)
   - Increased pulmonary blood flow
   - Redistribution of cardiac output

4. The amniotic fluid is removed from the lungs of a newborn by the following actions:
   - The passage through the birth canal squeezes the thorax, which helps eliminate the fluids in the lungs
   - The action of the pulmonary capillaries and lymphatics removes the remaining fluid

5. The nurse should look for the following signs of abnormality in the newborn's respiration:
   - Labored respiratory effort
   - Respiratory rate less than 30 breaths per minute or greater than 60 breaths per minute
   - Asymmetric chest movements
   - Periodic breathing
   - Apneic periods lasting more than 15 seconds with cyanosis and heart rate changes

6. The nursing interventions that may help minimize regurgitation are
   - Avoiding overfeeding
   - Stimulating frequent burping

Activity D

1. **a.** Normal factors that increase the heart rate and blood pressure in a newborn are
   - Wakefulness
   - Movement
   - Crying

   b. Normal factors affecting the hematologic values of a newborn are
   - Site of the blood sampling
   - Placental transfusion
   - Gestational age

   c. The benefits of delayed cord clamping after birth are
   - Improved cardiopulmonary adaptation and oxygen transport
   - Prevention of anemia
   - Increased blood pressures and RBC flow

Activity E

1. **Answer: b**
   RATIONALE: The nurse should instruct the mother to keep the newborn wrapped in a blanket, with a cap on its head. This ensures that the newborn is kept warm and helps prevent cold stress. Allowing cool air to circulate over the newborn's body leads to heat loss and is not desirable. Holding the newborn close to the body after taking a shower is not recommended, as the mother's body temperature will be lower than normal after a shower. The nurse need not instruct the client to refrain from using clothing and blankets in the crib. Using clothing and blankets in the crib is actually an effective means of reducing the newborn's exposed surface area and providing external insulation.

2. **Answer: a**
   RATIONALE: Breast milk is a major source of IgA, so breastfeeding is believed to have significant immunologic advantages over formula feeding. The newborn does not depend on IgD and IgE for defense mechanisms. IgM is found in blood and lymph fluid.

3. **Answer: a, c, & d**
   RATIONALE: Limited sweating ability, a crib that is too warm or one that is placed too close to a sunny window, and limited insulation are factors that predispose a newborn to overheating. The immaturity of the newborn's central nervous system makes it difficult to create and maintain balance between heat production, heat gain, and heat loss. Underdeveloped lungs do not increase the risk of overheating. Lack of brown fat will make the infant feel cold, because he or she will not have enough fat stores to burn in response to cold; it does not however, increase the risk of overheating.

4. **Answer: c**
   RATIONALE: The nurse should look for signs of lethargy and hypotonia in the newborn in order to confirm the occurrence of cold stress. Cold stress does not lead to any color change in the newborn's skin or urine. Cold stress leads to a decrease, not increase, in the newborn's body temperature.

5. **Answer: b**
   RATIONALE: Risk factors for the development of jaundice include drugs such as oxytocin, diazepam, and sulfisoxazole/erythromycin. Breastfeeding, not formula feeding, and male gender are other risk factors. Administering hepatitis A vaccine does not increase the risk of jaundice.

6. **Answer: d**
   RATIONALE: The possibility of fluid overload is increased and must be considered by a nurse when administering IV therapy to a newborn. IV therapy does not significantly increase heart rate or change blood pressure.

7. **Answer: b**
   RATIONALE: The nurse should tell the client not to worry, because it is perfectly normal for the stools of a formula-fed newborn to be greenish, loose, pasty, or formed in consistency, with an unpleasant odor. There is no need to administer vitamin K supplements, increase the newborn's fluid intake, or switch from formula to breast milk.

8. **Answer: b**
   RATIONALE: The ideal caloric intake for a term newborn to regain weight lost in the first week is 108 kcal/kg/day. Eighty kcal/kg/day is too little to meet the newborn's requirements, and 150 or 200 kcal/kg/day will be greater than the newborn's requirements.

9. Answer: a

RATIONALE: Preterm newborns are at a greater risk for cold stress than term or post-term newborns. Formula-fed newborns and larger-than-average newborns are not at a greater risk for cold stress than preterm newborns.

10. Answer: a

RATIONALE: The hand-to-mouth movement of the baby indicates the self-quieting ability of a newborn. Movement of the head and eyes, movements of the legs, and hyperactivity do not indicate the self-quieting ability of a newborn.

11. Answer: c

RATIONALE: Typically, a newborn's blood glucose levels are assessed with use of a heel stick sample of blood on admission to the nursery, not 5 or 24 hours after admission to the nursery. It is also not necessary or even reasonable to check the glucose level only after the newborn has been fed.

12. Answer: a

RATIONALE: The nurse should promote early breast-feeding to provide fuels for nonshivering thermogenesis. The nurse can bathe the newborn if he or she is medically stable. The nurse can also use a radiant heat source while bathing the newborn to maintain the temperature. Skin-to-skin contact with the mother should be encouraged, not discouraged, if the newborn is stable. The infant transporter should be kept fully charged and heated at all times.

13. Answer: c

RATIONALE: The nurse should place the temperature probe over the newborn's liver. Skin temperature probes should not be placed over a bony area like the forehead, or an area with brown fat such as the buttocks. The newborn should be in a supine or side-lying position.

14. Answer: a

RATIONALE: The nurse should monitor for yellow skin or mucous membranes in an infant at risk for developing jaundice. Pinkish appearance of the tongue and bluish skin discoloration are not consequences of increased bilirubin levels. A heart rate of 120 bpm is also normal for an infant.

15 Answer: d

RATIONALE: The stools of a breastfed newborn are yellowish gold in color. They are not firm in shape or solid. The smell is usually sour. A formula-fed infant's stools are formed in consistency, while a breastfed infant's stools are stringy to pasty in consistency.

CHAPTER 18

Activity A

1. Apgar
2. Lanugo
3. Postmature
4. large
5. prothrombin
6. acrocyanosis
7. Milia
8. Harlequin
9. anterior
10. Cephalhematoma

Activity B

1. The figure shows common skin variations found in newborns:
   - A. Stork bite
   - B. Milia
   - C. Mongolian spots
   - D. Erythema toxicum
   - E. Nevus flammeus (port-wine stain)
   - F. Strawberry hemangioma
2. The figure depicts molding in a newborn's head. Molding is the elongated shaping of the fetal head to accommodate passage through the birth canal.

Activity C

1. b   2. a   3. c   4. d

Activity D

1.

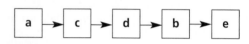

Activity E

1. The football hold is achieved by holding the infant's back and shoulders in the palm of the mother's hand and tucking the infant under the mother's arm. The infant's ear, shoulder, and hip should be in a straight line. The mother's hand should support the breast and bring it to the infant's lips to latch on until the infant begins to nurse. This position allows the mother to see the infant's mouth as she guides her infant to the nipple. Mothers who have had a cesarean birth can avoid pressure on the incision lines by adopting the football hold position for breastfeeding.
2. Colostrum is a thick, yellowish substance secreted during the first few days after birth. It is high in protein, minerals, and fat-soluble vitamins. It is rich in immunoglobulins (e.g., IgA), which help protect the newborn's GI tract against infections. It is a natural laxative to help rid the intestinal tract of meconium quickly.
3. Fiber optic pads (Biliblanket or Bilivest) are used for treatment of physiologic jaundice and can be wrapped around newborns or newborns can lie upon them. These pads consist of a light that is delivered from a tungsten–halogen bulb through a fiber optic cable and is emitted from the sides and ends of the fibers inside a plastic pad. They work on the premise that phototherapy can be improved by delivering higher-intensity therapeutic light to decrease bilirubin levels. The pads do not produce appreciable heat like banks of lights or spotlights do,

so insensible water loss is not increased. Eye patches also are not needed; thus, parents can feed and hold their newborns continuously to promote bonding.

4. The Moro reflex, or the embrace reflex, occurs when the neonate is startled. To elicit this reflex, the newborn is placed on his back. The upper body weight of the supine newborn is supported by the arms with use of a lifting motion, without lifting the newborn off the surface. When the arms are released suddenly, the newborn will throw the arms outward and flex the knees; arms then return to the chest. The fingers also spread to form a C. The newborn initially appears startled and then relaxes to a normal resting position.

5. Caput succedaneum is a localized edema on the scalp that occurs from the pressure of the birth process. It is commonly observed after prolonged labor. Clinically, it appears as a poorly demarcated soft tissue swelling that crosses suture lines. Pitting edema and overlying petechiae and ecchymosis are noted. The swelling will gradually dissipate in about 3 days without any treatment. Newborns who were delivered via vacuum extraction usually have a caput in the area where the cup was used.

6. Erythema toxicum is a benign, idiopathic, very common, generalized, transient rash occurring in as many as 70% of all newborns during the first week of life. It consists of small papules or pustules on the skin resembling flea bites. The rash is common on the face, chest, and back. One of the chief characteristics of this rash is its lack of pattern. It is caused by the newborn's eosinophils reacting to the environment as the immune system matures. It does not require any treatment, and it disappears in a few days.

Activity F

1. **a.** The nurse should inform the mother that newborns usually sleep for up to 20 hours daily, for periods of 2 to 4 hours at a time, but not through the night. This is because their stomach capacity is too small to go long periods of time without nourishment. All newborns develop their own sleep patterns and cycles.
   b. The nurse should ask the mother to place the newborn on her back to sleep; remove all fluffy bedding, quilts, sheepskins, stuffed animals, and pillows from the crib to prevent potential suffocation. Parents should avoid unsafe conditions such as placing the newborn in the prone position, using a crib that does not meet federal safety guidelines, allowing window cords to hang loose and in close proximity to the crib, or having the room temperature too high, causing overheating.
   c. The nurse should educate Karen about potential risks of bed-sharing. Bringing a newborn into bed to nurse or quiet her down and then falling asleep with the newborn is not a safe practice. Infants who sleep in adult beds are up to 40

times more likely to suffocate than those who sleep in cribs. Suffocation also can occur when the infant gets entangled in bedding or caught under pillows, or slips between the bed and the wall or the headboard and mattress. It can also happen when someone accidentally rolls against or on top of them. Therefore, the safest sleeping location for all newborns is in their crib, without any movable objects close.

Activity G

1. **Answer: b**
   RATIONALE: The nurse should complete the second assessment for the newborn within the first 2 to 4 hours, when the newborn is in the nursery. The nurse should complete the initial newborn assessment in the birthing area and the third assessment before the newborn is discharged.

2. **Answer: d**
   RATIONALE: The nurse should place the newborn skin-to-skin with mother. This would help to maintain baby's temperature as well as promote breastfeeding and bonding between the mother and baby. The nurse can weigh the infant as long as a warmed cover is placed on the scale. The stethoscope should be warmed before it makes contact with the infant's skin, rather than using the stethoscope over the garment, because it may obscure the reading. The newborn's crib should not be placed close to the outer walls in the room to prevent heat loss through radiation.

3. **Answer: a**
   RATIONALE: Skin turgor is checked by pinching the skin over chest or abdomen and noting the return to original position; if the skin remains "tented" after pinching, it denotes dehydration. Stork bites or salmon patches, unopened sebaceous glands, and blue or purple splotches on buttocks are common skin variations not related to skin turgor.

4. **Answer: c**
   RATIONALE: As per the recommendations of AAP, all infants should receive a daily supplement of vitamin D during the first two months of life to prevent rickets and vitamin D deficiency. There is no need to feed the infant water, as breast milk contains enough water to meet the newborn's needs. Iron supplements need not be given, as the infant is being breastfed. Infants over six months of age are given fluoride supplementation if they are not receiving fluoridated water.

5. **Answer: a**
   RATIONALE: The nurse should instruct the woman to use the sealed and chilled milk within 24 hours. The nurse should not instruct the woman to use frozen milk within 6 months of obtaining it, to use microwave ovens to warm chilled milk, or to refreeze the used milk and reuse it. Instead, the nurse should instruct the woman to use frozen milk within 3 months of obtaining it, to avoid using microwave

ovens to warm chilled milk, and to discard any used milk and never refreeze it.

6. **Answer: a**
RATIONALE: The nurse should ask the mother to hold the baby upright with the baby's head on her mother's shoulder. Alternatively, the nurse can also suggest the mother sit with the newborn on her lap with the newborn lying face down. Gently rubbing the baby's abdomen or giving frequent sips of warm water to the infant will not significantly induce burping; burping is induced by the newborn's position.

7. **Answer: b**
RATIONALE: The nurse should inform the client to introduce just one new single-ingredient food at a time to watch for allergies. The infant should not be coaxed to eat if he or she is not willing. Fruits should be introduced after cereals and before vegetables and eggs are introduced. A variety of solid foods should be introduced to provide a balanced diet.

8. **Answer: d**
RATIONALE: A concentration of immature blood vessels causes salmon patches. Mongolian spots are caused by a concentration of pigmented cells and usually disappear within the first 4 years of life. Erythema toxicum is caused by the newborn's eosinophils reacting to the environment as the immune system matures, and Harlequin sign is a result of immature autoregulation of blood flow and is commonly seen in low–birth-weight newborns.

9. **Answer: c**
RATIONALE: The nurse should obtain a newborn's temperature by placing an electronic temperature probe in the midaxillary area. The nurse should not tape an electronic thermistor probe to the abdominal skin, as this method is applied only when the newborn is placed under a radiant heat source. Rectal temperatures are no longer taken because of the risk of perforation. Oral temperature readings are not taken for newborns.

10. **Answer: c**
RATIONALE: The nurse should conclude that the newborn is facing moderate difficulty in adjusting to extrauterine life. The nurse need not conclude severe distress in adjusting to extrauterine life, better condition of the newborn, or abnormal central nervous system status. If the Apgar score is 8 points or higher, it indicates that the condition of the newborn is better. An Apgar score of 0 to 3 points represents severe distress in adjusting to extrauterine life.

11. **Answer: a**
RATIONALE: The nurse should instruct the parent to expose the newborn's bottom to air several times per day to prevent diaper rashes. Use of plastic pants and products such as powder and items with fragrance should be avoided. The parent should be instructed to place the newborn's buttocks in warm water after having had a diaper on all night.

12. **Answer: b, d, & e**
RATIONALE: The nurse should give the newborn oxygen, ensure the newborn's warmth, and observe the newborn's respiratory status frequently. The nurse need not give the infant warm water to drink or massage the infant's back.

13. **Answer: a, c, & e**
RATIONALE: The nurse should monitor the newborn for lethargy, cyanosis, and jitteriness. Low-pitched crying or rashes on the infant's skin are not signs generally associated with hypoglycemia.

14. **Answer: a, c, & e**
RATIONALE: To relieve breast engorgement in the client, the nurse should educate the client to take warm-to-hot showers to encourage milk release, express some milk manually before breastfeeding, and apply warm compresses to the breasts prior to nursing. The mother should be asked to feed the newborn in a variety of positions—sitting up and then lying down. The breasts should be massaged from under the axillary area, down toward the nipple.

15 **Answer: a, c, & e**
RATIONALE: Mongolian spots, swollen genitals in the female baby, and a short, creased neck are normal findings in a newborn. Mongolian spots are blue or purple splotches that appear on the lower back and buttocks of newborns. Female babies may have swollen genitals as a result of maternal estrogen. The newborn's neck will appear almost nonexistent because it is so short. Creases are usually noted. Enlarged fontanelles are associated with malnutrition; hydrocephaly; congenital hypothyroidism; trisomies 13, 18, and 21; and various bone disorders such as osteogenesis imperfecta. Low-set ears are characteristic of many syndromes and genetic abnormalities such as trisomies 13 and 18 and internal organ abnormalities involving the renal system.

CHAPTER 19

Activity A

1. Oligohydramnios
2. Clonus
3. latent
4. hyperreflexia
5. incompatibility
6. Monozygotic
7. infection
8. spontaneous
9. first
10. Gestational

Activity B

1. **a.** Partial abruption with concealed hemorrhage.
   b. Partial abruption with apparent hemorrhage.
   c. Complete abruption with concealed hemorrhage.

Activity C

1. c   **2.** e   **3.** a   **4.** b   **5.** d

Activity D

1.

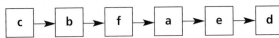

Activity E

1. Possible complications of hyperemesis gravidarum include persistent, uncontrollable nausea, dehydration, acid-base imbalances, electrolyte imbalances, and weight loss. If the condition is allowed to continue, it jeopardizes fetal well-being.

2. Conditions commonly associated with early bleeding (first half of pregnancy) include spontaneous abortion, ectopic pregnancy, and gestational trophoblastic disease (GTD).

3. Ectopic pregnancies usually result from conditions that obstruct or slow the passage of the fertilized ovum through the fallopian tube to the uterus. This may be a physical blockage in the tube or failure of the tubal epithelium to move the zygote (the cell formed after the egg is fertilized) down the tube into the uterus. In the general population, most cases are the result of tubal scarring secondary to pelvic inflammatory disease. Organisms such as *Neisseria gonorrhoeae* and *Chlamydia trachomatis* preferentially attack the fallopian tubes, producing silent infections.

4. Risk factors for hyperemesis gravidarum include young age, nausea and vomiting with previous pregnancy, history of intolerance of oral contraceptives, nulliparity, trophoblastic disease, multiple gestation, emotional or psychological stress, gastroesophageal reflux disease, primigravida status, obesity, hyperthyroidism, and *Helicobacter pylori* seropositivity.

5. A nurse should include the following in prevention education for ectopic pregnancies:
   - Reducing risk factors such as sexual intercourse with multiple partners or intercourse without a condom
   - Avoiding contracting STIs that lead to pelvic inflammatory disease (PID)
   - Obtaining early diagnosis and adequate treatment of STIs
   - Avoiding the use of an IUC as a contraceptive method to reduce the risk of repeat ascending infections responsible for tubal scarring
   - Using condoms to decrease the risk of infections that cause tubal scarring
   - Seeking prenatal care early if pregnant, to confirm location of pregnancy

6. The Kleihauer–Betke test detects fetal RBCs in the maternal circulation, determines the degree of fetal–maternal hemorrhage, and helps calculate the appropriate dosage of RhoGAM to give for Rh-negative clients.

Activity F

1. **a.** Recognizing preterm labor at an early stage requires that the expectant mother and her health care team identify the subtle symptoms of preterm labor. These may include
   - Change or increase in vaginal discharge
   - Pelvic pressure (pushing down sensation)
   - Low, dull backache
   - Menstrual-like cramps
   - Uterine contractions, with or without pain
   - Intestinal cramping, with or without diarrhea

   b. The nurse must teach Jenna how to palpate and time uterine contractions. Provide written materials to support this education at a level and in a language appropriate for her. Also, educate Jenna about the importance of prenatal care, risk reduction, and recognizing the signs and symptoms of preterm labor. The nurse may also include
   - Stressing good hydration and consumption of a nutritious diet
   - Advising against any activity, such as sexual activity or nipple stimulation, that might stimulate oxytocin release and initiate uterine contractions
   - Assessing stress levels of client and family, and making appropriate referrals
   - Providing emotional support and client empowerment throughout
   - Emphasizing the possible need for more frequent office visits and for notifying the health care provider if she has questions or concerns.

Activity G

1. **Answer: c**
   RATIONALE: The nurse should instruct the client with hyperemesis gravidarum to eat small, frequent meals throughout the day to minimize nausea and vomiting. The nurse should also instruct the client to avoid lying down or reclining for at least two hours after eating and to increase the intake of carbonated beverages. The nurse should instruct the client to try foods that settle the stomach such as dry crackers, toast, or soda.

2. **Answer: a**
   RATIONALE: A temperature elevation or an increase in the pulse of a client with PROM would indicate infection. Increase in the pulse does not indicate preterm labor or cord compression. The nurse should monitor fetal heart rate patterns continuously, reporting any variable decelerations suggesting cord compression. Respiratory distress syndrome is one of the perinatal risks associated with PROM.

3. **Answer: c**
   RATIONALE: The nurse should closely assess the woman for hemorrhage after giving birth by frequently assessing uterine involution. Assessing skin turgor and blood pressure and monitoring hCG titers will not help to determine hemorrhage.

4. Answer: b
RATIONALE: When meconium is present in the amniotic fluid, it typically indicates fetal distress related to hypoxia. Meconium stains the fluid yellow to greenish brown, depending on the amount present. A decreased amount of amniotic fluid reduces the cushioning effect, thereby making cord compression a possibility. A foul odor of amniotic fluid indicates infection. Meconium in the amniotic fluid does not indicate CNS involvement.

5. Answer: d
RATIONALE: The nurse should institute and maintain seizure precautions such as padding the side rails and having oxygen, suction equipment, and call light readily available to protect the client from injury. The nurse should provide a quiet, darkened room to stabilize the client. The nurse should maintain the client on complete bed rest in the left lateral lying position and not in a supine position. Keeping the head of the bed slightly elevated will not help maintain seizure precautions.

6. Answer: a
RATIONALE: If the client is receiving magnesium sulfate to suppress or control seizures, assess deep tendon reflexes to determine the effectiveness of therapy. Common sites utilized to assess DTRs are the biceps reflex, triceps reflex, patellar reflex, Achilles reflex, and plantar reflex. Assessing the mucous membranes for dryness and skin turgor for dehydration are the required interventions when caring for a client with hyperemesis gravidarum. Monitoring intake and output will not help to determine the effectiveness of therapy.

7. Answer: d
RATIONALE: A previous myomectomy to remove fibroids can be associated with the cause of placenta previa. Risk factors also include advanced maternal age (greater than 30 years old). A structurally defective cervix cannot be associated with the cause of placenta previa. However, it can be associated with the cause of cervical insufficiency. Alcohol ingestion is not a risk factor for developing placenta previa but is associated with abruptio placenta.

8. Answer: b
RATIONALE: The nurse should encourage a client with mild elevations in blood pressure to rest as much as possible in the lateral recumbent position to improve uteroplacental blood flow, reduce blood pressure, and promote diuresis. The nurse should maintain the client with severe preeclampsia on complete bed rest in the left lateral lying position. Keeping the head of the bed slightly elevated will not help to improve the condition of the client with mild elevations in blood pressure.

9. Answer: d
RATIONALE: The first choice for fluid replacement is generally 5% dextrose in lactated Ringer's solution with vitamins and electrolytes added. If the client does not improve after several days of bed rest, "gut rest," IV fluids, and antiemetics, then total parenteral nutrition (TPN) or percutaneous endoscopic gastrostomy (PEG) tube feeding is instituted to prevent malnutrition.

10. Answer: c
RATIONALE: The classic manifestations of abruptio placenta are painful dark red vaginal bleeding, "knife-like" abdominal pain, uterine tenderness, contractions, and decreased fetal movement. Painless bright red vaginal bleeding is the clinical manifestation of placenta previa. Generalized vasospasm is the clinical manifestation of preeclampsia and not of abruptio placenta.

11. Answer: a
RATIONALE: The symptoms if rupture or hemorrhaging occurs before successfully treating the pregnancy are lower abdomen pain, feelings of faintness, phrenic nerve irritation, hypotension, marked abdominal tenderness with distension, and hypovolemic shock. Painless bright red vaginal bleeding occurring during the second or third trimester is the clinical manifestation of placenta previa. Fetal distress and tetanic contractions are not the symptoms observed in a client if rupture or hemorrhaging occurs before successfully treating an ectopic pregnancy.

12. Answer: d
RATIONALE: When the woman arrives and is admitted, assessing her vital signs, the amount and color of the bleeding, and current pain rating on a scale of 1 to 10 are the priorities. Assessing the signs of shock, monitoring uterine contractility, and determining the amount of funneling are not priority assessments when a pregnant woman complaining of vaginal bleeding is admitted to the hospital.

13. Answer: c
RATIONALE: A nurse should closely monitor the client's vital signs, bleeding (peritoneal or vaginal) to identify hypovolemic shock that may occur with tubal rupture. Beta-hCG level is monitored to diagnose an ectopic pregnancy or impending abortion. Monitoring the mass with transvaginal ultrasound (TVS) and determining the size of the mass are done for diagnosing an ectopic pregnancy. Monitoring the fetal heart rate does not help to identify hypovolemic shock.

14. Answer: a
RATIONALE: The current recommendation is that every Rh-negative nonimmunized woman receives Rho-GAM at 28 weeks' gestation and again within 72 hours after giving birth. Consuming a well-balanced nutritional diet and avoiding sexual activity until after 28 weeks will not help to prevent complications of blood incompatibility. Transvaginal ultrasound helps to validate the position of the placenta and will not help to prevent complications of blood incompatibility.

15 Answer: c
RATIONALE: The nurse should know that coma usually follows an eclamptic seizure. Muscle rigidity occurs after facial twitching. Respirations do not

become rapid during the seizure; they cease. Coma usually follows the seizure activity, with respiration resuming.

16. **Answer: d**
    RATIONALE: The nurse should know that dependent edema may be seen in the sacral area if the client is on bed rest. Pitting edema leaves a small depression or pit after finger pressure is applied to a swollen area and can be measured. This is not possible in dependent edema. Dependent edema may occur in clients who are both ambulatory and on bed rest.

17. **Answer: a, c, & d**
    RATIONALE: Signs such as a change or increase in vaginal discharge, rupture of membranes, and uterine contractions should be further assessed as a possible sign of preterm labor. Phrenic nerve irritation and hypovolemic shock are the symptoms if rupture or hemorrhaging occurs before successfully treating the ectopic pregnancy.

18. **Answer: a, b, & e**
    RATIONALE: The associated conditions and complications of premature rupture of the membranes are infection, prolapsed cord, abruptio placenta, and preterm labor. Spontaneous abortion and placenta previa are not associated conditions or complications of premature rupture of the membranes.

19. **Answer: b, d, & e**
    RATIONALE: The signs and symptoms of HELLP syndrome are nausea, malaise, epigastric pain, upper right quadrant pain, demonstrable edema, and hyperbilirubinemia. Blood pressure higher than 160/110 and oliguria are the symptoms of severe preeclampsia rather than HELLP syndrome.

20. **Answer: b, d, & e**
    RATIONALE: Adverse effects commonly associated with misoprostol include dyspepsia, hypotension, tachycardia, diarrhea, abdominal pain, and vomiting. Constipation and headache are not adverse effects commonly associated with misoprostol.

CHAPTER 20

Activity A

1. somatotropin
2. Gestational
3. airway
4. lung
5. Anemia
6. bacterium
7. Toxoplasmosis
8. Adolescence
9. Nicotine
10. Cocaine

Activity B

1. **a.** This disorder is known as fetal alcohol spectrum disorder, which includes a full range of birth defects, such as structural anomalies and behavioral and neurocognitive disabilities caused by prenatal exposure to alcohol.

   b. Characteristics of fetal alcohol spectrum disorder include craniofacial dysmorphia (thin upper lip, small head circumference, and small eyes), intrauterine growth restriction, microcephaly, and congenital anomalies such as limb abnormalities and cardiac defects.

Activity C

1. f   2. e   3. d   4. c   5. b   6. a

Activity D

1. The most common complications in a pregnant client with hypertension are
   - Increased risk for developing preeclampsia
   - Fetal growth restriction during pregnancy
2. The nurse should include the following elements during the physical examination of pregnant clients with asthma:
   - Rate, rhythm, and depth of respirations
   - Skin color
   - Blood pressure
   - Pulse rate
   - Evaluation for signs of fatigue
3. The nurse should include the following factors in the teaching plan for a client with asthma:
   - Signs and symptoms of asthma progression and exacerbation
   - Importance and safety of medication to fetus and to herself
   - Warning signs; potential harm to fetus and self by undertreatment or delay in seeking help
   - Prevention and avoidance of known triggers
   - Home use of metered-dose inhalers
   - Adverse effects of medications
4. Assessment of tuberculosis in pregnant clients includes the following:
   - At antepartum visits, the nurse should be alert for clinical manifestations of tuberculosis such as fatigue, fever or night sweats, nonproductive cough, slow weight loss, anemia, hemoptysis, and anorexia
   - If tuberculosis is suspected or the woman is at risk for developing tuberculosis, the nurse should anticipate screening with purified protein derivative (PPD) administered by intradermal injection; if the client has been exposed to tuberculosis, a reddened induration will appear within 72 hours
   - A follow-up chest x-ray with a lead shield over the abdomen and sputum cultures will confirm the diagnosis
5. The developmental tasks associated with adolescent behavior are
   - Seeking economic and social stability
   - Developing a personal value system
   - Building meaningful relationships with others
   - Becoming comfortable with their changing bodies

- Working to become independent from their parents
- Learning to verbalize conceptually

6. The effects of sedatives by the mother on her infant are as follows:
   - Sedatives easily cross the placenta and cause birth defects and behavioral problems
   - Infants born to mothers who abuse sedatives may be physically dependent on the drugs and prone to respiratory problems, feeding difficulties, disturbed sleep, sweating, irritability, and fever

Activity E

1. **a.** The greatest increase in asthma attacks in the pregnant client usually occurs between 24 and 36 weeks' gestation; flare-ups are rare during the last four weeks of pregnancy and during labor.
   b. Successful management of asthma in pregnancy involves
   - Drug therapy
   - Client education
   - Elimination of environmental triggers
   c. The following are the nursing interventions involved when caring for the pregnant client with asthma during labor:
   - Monitor client's oxygen saturation by pulse oximetry
   - Provide pain management through epidural analgesia
   - Continuously monitor the fetus for distress during labor and assess fetal heart rate patterns for indications of hypoxia
   - Assess the newborn for signs and symptoms of hypoxia

Activity F

1. **Answer: b**
   RATIONALE: The nurse should identify postprandial hyperglycemia as the effect of insulin resistance in the client. Hypertension, hypercholesterolemia, and myocardial infarction are not the effects of insulin resistance in a diabetic client.

2. **Answer: a**
   RATIONALE: The nurse should identify respiratory distress syndrome as a major risk that can be faced by the offspring of a client with cardiovascular disease. Congenital varicella syndrome can occur in an offspring of a mother infected with varicella during early pregnancy. Sudden infant death syndrome can occur in an offspring of a mother who smokes during pregnancy. Prune belly syndrome is a fetal anomaly associated with cocaine use in early pregnancy.

3. **Answer: b**
   RATIONALE: The nurse should stress the positive benefits of a healthy lifestyle during the preconception counseling of a client with chronic hypertension. The client need not avoid dairy products or increase intake of vitamin D supplements. It may not be advisable for a client with chronic hypertension to exercise without consultation.

4. **Answer: a**
   RATIONALE: Swelling of the face is a symptom of cardiac decompensation, along with moist, frequent cough and rapid respirations. Dry, rasping cough; slow, labored respiration; and an elevated temperature are not symptoms of cardiac decompensation.

5. **Answer: d**
   RATIONALE: The nurse should assess the client with heart disease for cardiac decompensation, which is most common from 28 to 32 weeks of gestation and in the first 48 hours postpartum. Limiting sodium intake, inspecting the extremities for edema, and ensuring that the client consumes a high-fiber diet are interventions during pregnancy, not in the first 48 hours postpartum.

6. **Answer: b**
   RATIONALE: The nurse should evaluate for signs of fatigue during the physical examination of a client with asthma. The nurse need not monitor the client's temperature, frequency of headache, or feelings of nausea, because these conditions are not related to asthma.

7. **Answer: a**
   RATIONALE: The nurse should instruct the pregnant client with tuberculosis to maintain adequate hydration as a health-promoting activity. The client need not avoid direct sunlight or red meat, or wear light clothes; these have no impact on the client's condition.

8. **Answer: c**
   RATIONALE: The nurse should identify preterm birth as a risk associated with anemia during pregnancy. Anemia during pregnancy does not increase the risk of a newborn with heart problems, an enlarged liver, or fetal asphyxia.

9. **Answer: b**
   RATIONALE: The nurse should assess for possible fluid overload in a client with cardiovascular disease who has just delivered. The nurse need not assess for shortness of breath or edema or auscultate heart sounds for abnormalities. It is important for the nurse to assess for edema and note any pitting and auscultate heart sounds for abnormalities during the antepartum period to ensure early detection of cardiac decompensation.

10. **Answer: a**
    RATIONALE: The nurse should stress the importance of good handwashing and use of sound hygiene practices to reduce transmission of the virus to a client who could pass the virus on to her fetus. Drinking plenty of fluids will not help minimize this risk. The client need not take antibiotics if she has not been infected. It is not practical for the client to avoid interaction with children.

11. **Answer: d**
    RATIONALE: The nurse should address the client's knowledge of child development during assessment of the pregnant adolescent client. The nurse need not address the sexual development of the

client, whether sex was consensual, or the stress levels of the client.

12. Answer: a

RATIONALE: The nurse should inform the client that she could be at risk for coronary artery disease because medical conditions such as coronary artery disease and myocardial infarction may result in the older pregnant woman. The nurse need not ask the client to avoid excessive exposure to sunlight or consumption of poultry. The nurse should not ask the client to perform aerobic exercises if the client is not accustomed to exercising.

13. Answer: d

RATIONALE: The nurse should stress the avoidance of breastfeeding when counseling a pregnant client who is HIV-positive. The nurse need not discuss the client's relationship with the spouse. The client can be taught gradually about care to be taken during physical contact with the infant or when visiting crowded places.

14. Answer: b

RATIONALE: The nurse should caution the client about high levels of anxiety as a risk associated with substance abuse during pregnancy. Substance abuse does not increase the risk of post-term birth, stillbirth, or transient tachypnea of the newborn.

15 Answer: b

RATIONALE: The nurse should make the client aware of increased risk of anemia as a possible effect of maternal coffee consumption during pregnancy, as it decreases iron absorption. Maternal coffee consumption during pregnancy does not increase the risk of heart disease, rickets, or scurvy.

16. Answer: a, b, & e

RATIONALE: To minimize risk of toxoplasmosis, the nurse should instruct the client to eat meat that has been cooked to an internal temperature of 160°F throughout and to avoid cleaning the cat's litter box or performing activities such as gardening. The client should avoid feeding the cat raw or undercooked meat. The cat should be kept indoors to prevent it from hunting and eating birds or rodents.

17. Answer: c, d, & e

RATIONALE: Obesity, hypertension, and a previous infant weighing more than 9 pounds are risk factors for developing gestational diabetes. Maternal age less than 18 years and genitourinary tract abnormalities do not increase the risk of developing gestational diabetes.

18. Answer: a, d, & e

RATIONALE: The nurse caring for a pregnant client with sickle cell anemia should teach the client meticulous handwashing to prevent the risk of infection, assess the hydration status of the client at each visit, and urge the client to drink 8 to 10 glasses of fluid daily. The nurse need not assess serum electrolyte levels of the client at each visit or instruct the client to consume protein-rich food.

19. Answer: a

RATIONALE: The nurse should assess for small head circumference in a newborn being assessed for fetal alcohol spectrum disorder. Fetal alcohol spectrum disorder does not cause decreased blood glucose level, a poor breathing pattern, or wide eyes.

20. Answer: b

RATIONALE: The nurse should stress the inclusion of complex carbohydrates in the diet in the dietary plan for a pregnant woman with pregestational diabetes. The pregnant client with pregestational diabetes need not include more dairy products in the diet, eat only two meals per day, or eat at least one egg per day; these have no impact on the client's condition.

CHAPTER 21

Activity A

1. dystocia
2. Breech
3. Leopold's
4. Tocolytic
5. Steroids
6. fibronectin
7. Bishop
8. Hygroscopic
9. amniotomy
10. Oxytocin

Activity B

1. The figures depict various maneuvers to relieve shoulder dystocia. A. McRobert's maneuver. The mother's thighs are flexed and abducted as much as possible to straighten the pelvic curve. B. Suprapubic pressure. Pressure is applied just above the pubic bone, pushing the fetal anterior shoulder downward to displace it from above the mother's symphysis pubis. The newborn's head is depressed toward the maternal anus while suprapubic pressure is applied.
2. The figures depict prolapsed cord. A. Prolapse within the uterus. B. Prolapse with the cord visible at the vulva.

Activity C

1. c   2. a   3. e   4. b   5. d

Activity D

1.

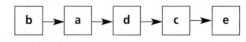

Activity E

1. The symptoms of preterm labor are
   • Change or increase in vaginal discharge
   • Pelvic pressure (pushing down sensation)
   • Low, dull backache
   • Menstrual-like cramps

- Heaviness or aching in the thighs
- Uterine contractions, with or without pain
- Intestinal cramping, with or without diarrhea

2. Cervical ripeness is an assessment of the readiness of the cervix to efface and dilate in response to uterine contractions. It is an important variable when labor induction is being considered. A ripe cervix is shortened, centered (anterior), softened, and partially dilated. An unripe cervix is long, closed, posterior, and firm. Cervical ripening usually begins prior to the onset of labor contractions and is necessary for cervical dilatation and the passage of the fetus.

3. Uterine rupture is a catastrophic tearing of the uterus at the site of a previous scar into the abdominal cavity. The onset is often marked only by sudden fetal bradycardia, and the obliteration of intrauterine pressure/cessation of contractions. Treatment requires rapid surgical attention. In uterine rupture, fetal morbidity occurs secondary to catastrophic hemorrhage, fetal anoxia, or both.

4. Indications of amnioinfusion are severe variable decelerations due to cord compression, oligohydramnios due to placental insufficiency, postmaturity or rupture of membranes, preterm labor with premature rupture of membranes, and thick meconium fluid. Vaginal bleeding of unknown origin, umbilical cord prolapse, amnionitis, uterine hypertonicity, and severe fetal distress are contraindications to amnioinfusion.

5. The nurse assesses each client to help predict her risk status. The nurse should be aware that cord prolapse is more common in pregnancies involving malpresentation, growth restriction, prematurity, ruptured membranes with a fetus at a high station, hydramnios, grand multiparity, and multifetal gestation. The client and fetus should be thoroughly assessed to detect changes and evaluate the effectiveness of any interventions performed.

6. Shoulder dystocia can cause postpartum hemorrhage, secondary to uterine atony or vaginal lacerations in the mother. In the fetus, shoulder dystocia can result in transient and/or permanent Erb or Duchenne brachial plexus palsies and clavicular or humeral fractures, as well as hypoxic encephalopathy.

Activity F

1. The nurse should perform the following interventions during amnioinfusion to prevent maternal and fetal complications:
   - Explain the need for the procedure, what it involves, and how it may solve the problem
   - Inform the mother that she will need to remain on bed rest during the procedure
   - Assess the mother's vital signs and associated discomfort level
   - Maintain adequate intake and output records
   - Assess the duration and intensity of uterine contractions frequently to identify overdistention or increased uterine tone

- Monitor FHR pattern to determine whether the amnioinfusion is improving the fetal status
- Prepare the mother for a possible cesarean birth if the FHR does not improve after the amnioinfusion

Activity G

1. **Answer: a**
   RATIONALE: A forceps and vacuum–assisted birth is required for the client having a prolonged second stage of labor. In cases of uterine rupture, the baby has to be immediately delivered by cesarean section. Oligohydramnios due to placental insufficiency and preterm labor with premature rupture of membranes are treated with amnioinfusion.

2. **Answer: d**
   RATIONALE: The nurse should know that gestational hypertension leads to placental abruption. Other factors leading to placental abruption include preeclampsia, seizure activity, uterine rupture, trauma, smoking, cocaine use, coagulation defects, previous history of abruption, domestic violence, and placental pathology. These conditions may force blood into the under layer of the placenta and cause it to detach. Gestational diabetes, cardiovascular disease, and excess weight gain during pregnancy, though dangerous conditions, are not known to specifically cause placental abruption.

3. **Answer: a**
   RATIONALE: The nurse should monitor cyanosis when caring for a client with amniotic fluid embolism. Other signs and symptoms of this condition include hypotension, cyanosis, seizures, tachycardia, coagulation failure, disseminated intravascular coagulation, pulmonary edema, uterine atony with subsequent hemorrhage, adult respiratory distress syndrome, and cardiac arrest. Arrhythmia, hematuria, and hyperglycemia are not known to occur in cases of amniotic fluid embolism. Hematuria is seen in clients having uterine rupture.

4. **Answer: a**
   RATIONALE: Chorioamnionitis is an indication for labor induction. Complete placenta previa, abruptio placenta, and transverse fetal lie are contraindications for labor induction.

5. **Answer: a**
   RATIONALE: The nurse should ensure that the client does not have uterine hypertonicity to confirm that amnioinfusion is not contraindicated. Other factors that enforce contraindication of amnioinfusion include vaginal bleeding of unknown origin, umbilical cord prolapse, amnionitis, and severe fetal distress. Active genital herpes infection, abruptio placentae, and invasive cervical cancer are conditions that enforce contraindication of labor induction rather than amnioinfusion.

6. **Answer: d**
   RATIONALE: The nurse should identify nerve damage as a risk to the fetus in cases of shoulder dystocia. Other fetal risks include asphyxia, clavicle

fracture, central nervous system (CNS) injury or dysfunction, and death. Bladder injury, infection, and extensive lacerations are poor maternal outcomes due to the occurrence of shoulder dystocia.

7. **Answer: a**
RATIONALE: A Bishop score of less than six indicates that a cervical ripening method should be used before inducing labor. A low Bishop score is not an indication for cesarean birth; there are several other factors that need to be considered for a cesarean birth. A Bishop score of less than six indicates that vaginal birth will be unsuccessful and prolonged, because the duration of labor is inversely correlated with the Bishop score.

8. **Answer: a**
RATIONALE: When caring for a client who has undergone a cesarean section, the nurse should assess the client's uterine tone to determine fundal firmness. The nurse should assist with breastfeeding initiation and offer continued support. The nurse can also suggest alternate positioning techniques to reduce incisional discomfort while breastfeeding. Delaying breastfeeding may not be required. The nurse should encourage the client to cough, perform deep-breathing exercises, and use the incentive spirometer every 2 hours. The nurse should assist the client with early ambulation to prevent respiratory and cardiovascular problems.

9. **Answer: d**
RATIONALE: Overdistended uterus is a contraindication for oxytocin administration. Post-term status, dysfunctional labor pattern, and prolonged ruptured membranes are indications for administration of oxytocin.

10. **Answer: a**
RATIONALE: The nurse caring for the client in labor with shoulder dystocia of the fetus should assist with positioning the client in squatting position. The client can also be helped into the hands and knees position or lateral recumbent position for birth, to free the shoulders. Assessing for complaints of intense back pain in first stage of labor, anticipating possible use of forceps to rotate to anterior position at birth, and assessing for prolonged second stage of labor with arrest of descent are important interventions when caring for a client with persistent occiput posterior position of fetus.

11. **Answer: a**
RATIONALE: The nurse should assess infertility treatment as a contributor to increased probability of multiple gestations. Multiple gestations do not occur with an adolescent delivery; instead, chances of multiple gestations are known to increase due to the increasing number of women giving birth at older ages. Medications and advanced maternal age are not known to cause multiple gestations.

12. **Answer: d**
RATIONALE: Cephalopelvic disproportion is associated with post-term pregnancy. Underdeveloped

suck reflex, congenital heart defects, and intraventricular hemorrhage are associated with preterm pregnancy.

13. **Answer: c**
RATIONALE: The nurse should assess for fetal complications such as head trauma associated with intracranial hemorrhage, nerve damage, and hypoxia in cases of precipitous labor. Facial and scalp lacerations, facial nerve injury, and cephalhematoma are all newborn traumas associated with the use of the forceps of vacuum extractors during birth. These conditions are not neonatal complications associated with precipitous labor.

14. **Answer: c**
RATIONALE: Prolonged pregnancy is the cause of intrauterine fetal demise in late pregnancy that the nurse should be aware of. Other factors resulting in intrauterine fetal demise include infection, hypertension, advanced maternal age, Rh disease, uterine rupture, diabetes, congenital anomalies, cord accident, abruption, premature rupture of membranes, or hemorrhage. Hydramnios, multifetal gestation, and malpresentation are not the causes of intrauterine fetal demise in late pregnancy; they are causes of umbilical cord prolapse.

15. **Answer: a**
RATIONALE: The nurse should monitor for fetal hypoxia in cases of umbilical cord prolapse. Because this is the fetus's only lifeline, fetal perfusion deteriorates rapidly. Complete occlusion renders the fetus helpless and oxygen-deprived. Preeclampsia, coagulation defects, and placental pathology are not risks associated with umbilical cord prolapse.

CHAPTER 22

Activity A

1. atony
2. Subinvolution
3. decrease
4. thrombus
5. thromboembolism
6. Metritis
7. mastitis
8. early
9. accreta
10. inversion

Activity B

1. The figure shows perineal hematoma with a bulging swollen mass.
2. The figure depicts postpartum wound infections: A, infected episiotomy site; B, infected cesarean birth incision.

Activity C

1. b   2. a   3. d   4. c

Activity D

1. Overdistention of the uterus can be caused by multifetal gestation, fetal macrosomia, polyhydramnios, fetal abnormality, or placental fragments. Other causes might include prolonged or rapid, forceful labor, especially if stimulated; bacterial toxins; use of anesthesia; and magnesium sulfate used in the treatment of preeclampsia. Overdistention of the uterus is a major risk factor for uterine atony, the most common cause of early postpartum hemorrhage, which can lead to hypovolemic shock.

2. Idiopathic thrombocytopenia purpura (ITP) is characterized by increased platelet destruction caused by the development of autoantibodies to platelet-membrane antigens. The incidence of ITP in adults is approximately 66 cases per 1 million per year. The characteristic features of the disorder are thrombocytopenia, capillary fragility, and increased bleeding time. Clients with ITP present with easy bruising, bleeding from mucous membranes, menorrhagia, epistaxis, bleeding gums, hematomas, and severe hemorrhage after a cesarean birth or lacerations.

3. Postpartum infections are usually polymicrobial and involve *Staphylococcus aureus, Escherichia coli, Klebsiella* species, *Gardnerella vaginalis,* gonococci, coliform bacteria, group A or B hemolytic streptococci, *Chlamydia trachomatis,* and the anaerobes that are common to bacterial vaginosis.

4. Most postpartum women experience baby blues. The woman exhibits mild depressive symptoms of anxiety, irritability, mood swings, tearfulness, and increased sensitivity, feelings of being overwhelmed, and fatigue after the birth of the baby. The condition typically peaks on postpartum days 4 and 5 and usually resolves by postpartum day 10. Baby blues are usually self-limiting and require no formal treatment other than reassurance and validation of the woman's experience, as well as assistance in caring for herself and the newborn.

5. Symptoms of postpartum psychosis surface within three weeks of giving birth. The main symptoms include sleep disturbances, fatigue, depression, and hypomania. The mother will be tearful, confused, and preoccupied with feelings of guilt and worthlessness. The symptoms may escalate to delirium, hallucinations, anger toward herself and her infant, bizarre behavior, manifestations of mania, and thoughts of hurting herself and the infant. The mother frequently loses touch with reality and experiences a severe regressive breakdown, associated with a high risk of suicide or infanticide.

6. A thrombosis refers to the development of a blood clot in the blood vessel. It can cause an inflammation of the blood vessel lining, which in turn can lead to a possible thromboembolism. Thrombi can involve the superficial or deep veins in the legs or pelvis:

- Superficial venous thrombosis usually involves the saphenous venous system and is confined to the lower leg. The lithotomy position during birth can cause superficial thrombophlebitis in some women.
- Deep venous thrombosis can involve deep veins from the foot to the calf, to the thighs, or to the pelvis.

In both locations, thrombi can dislodge and migrate to the lungs, causing a pulmonary embolism.

Activity E

1. a. The major causes of thrombus formation are venous stasis, injury to the innermost layer of the blood vessel, and hypercoagulation. Venous stasis and hypercoagulation are common in the postpartum period. The risk factors for thrombosis are
   - Prolonged bed rest
   - Diabetes
   - Obesity
   - Cesarean birth
   - Smoking
   - Severe anemia
   - History of previous thrombosis
   - Varicose veins
   - Advanced maternal age (greater than 35 years)
   - Multiparity
   - Use of oral contraceptives before pregnancy

   b. The nurse should perform the following nursing interventions to prevent thromboembolic complications in a client:
   - Educate the client on the need for early and frequent ambulation
   - Encourage activities that cause leg muscles to contract (leg exercises and walking) to promote venous return in order to prevent venous stasis
   - Use intermittent sequential compression devices, which cause passive leg contractions. until the client is ambulatory
   - Elevate the client's leg above heart level to promote venous return
   - Ensure stockings are applied and removed every day for inspections of the legs
   - Encourage the client to perform passive exercises on the bed
   - Ensure that the client is involved in postoperative deep-breathing exercises; this improves venous return
   - In order to prevent venous pooling, avoid placing pillows under the knees or keeping the legs in stirrups for a long time
   - Ensure the use of bed cradles; this helps in keeping linens and blankets off the extremity

   c. For clients with superficial venous thrombosis, the nurse should perform the following interventions:
   - Administer NSAIDs for analgesic effect
   - Provide rest and elevation of the affected leg

- Apply warm compresses over the affected area to promote healing
- Use anti-embolism stockings, which promote circulation to the extremities

Activity F

1. Answer: c
RATIONALE: The nurse should monitor the client for swelling in the calf. Swelling in the calf, erythema, and pedal edema are early manifestations of deep venous thrombosis, which may lead to pulmonary embolism if not prevented at an early stage. Sudden change in the mental status, difficulty in breathing, and sudden chest pain are manifestations of pulmonary embolism, beyond the stage of prevention.

2. Answer: d
RATIONALE: When caring for a client with deep vein thrombosis (DVT), the nurse should instruct the client to avoid using oral contraceptives. Cigarette smoking, use of oral contraceptives, a sedentary lifestyle, and obesity increase the risk for developing DVT. The nurse should encourage the client with deep vein thrombosis to wear compression stockings. The nurse should instruct the client to avoid using products containing aspirin when caring for clients with bleeding, but not for clients with DVT. Prolonged bed rest should be avoided. Prolonged bed rest involves staying motionless; this could lead to venous stasis, which needs to be avoided in cases of DVT.

3. Answer: b
RATIONALE: When caring for a client with idiopathic thrombocytopenic purpura, the nurse should administer platelet transfusions as ordered to control bleeding. Glucocorticoids, intravenous immunoglobulins, and intravenous anti-Rho D are also administered to the client. The nurse should not administer NSAIDs when caring for this client since nonsteroidal anti-inflammatory drugs cause platelet dysfunction. ITP is a disorder of increased platelet destruction due to the presence of autoantibodies to platelet-membrane antigens. As the client is bleeding, the nurse should continue with the administration of oxytocics, which helps to control the bleeding. Continuous firm uterine massage results in uterine exhaustion, leading to augmentation of bleeding.

4. Answer: a
RATIONALE: The nurse should monitor for foul-smelling vaginal discharge to verify the presence of an episiotomy infection. Sudden onset of shortness of breath, sudden change in mental status, and apprehension and diaphoresis are signs of pulmonary embolism and do not indicate episiotomy infection.

5. Answer: a
RATIONALE: The nurse should assess the client for prolonged bleeding time. von Willebrand disease (vWD) is a congenital bleeding disorder, inherited as an autosomal dominant trait, that is characterized by a prolonged bleeding time, a deficiency of von Willebrand factor, and impairment of platelet adhesion. A fever of 100.4°F after the first 24 hours after childbirth and presence of foul-smelling vaginal discharge indicate infection. A client with a postpartum fundal height that is higher than expected may have subinvolution of the uterus.

6. Answer: d
RATIONALE: The nurse should assess for calf tenderness in the client to verify the diagnosis of a deep vein thrombosis. Other signs and symptoms of deep vein thrombosis include calf swelling, erythema, warmth and tenderness, and pedal edema. Sudden chest pain, dyspnea, and tachypnea are signs and symptoms associated with pulmonary embolism and not deep vein thrombosis.

7. Answer: d
RATIONALE: The presence of a large uterus with painless dark-red blood mixed with clots indicates retained placental fragments in the uterus. This cause of hemorrhage can be prevented by carefully inspecting the placenta for intactness. A firm uterus with a trickle or steady stream of bright-red blood in the perineum indicates bleeding from trauma. A soft and boggy uterus that deviates from the midline indicates a full bladder, interfering with uterine involution.

8. Answer: a
RATIONALE: The nurse can identify if the bleeding is from lacerations by looking for a well-contracted uterus with bright-red vaginal bleeding. Lacerations commonly occur during forceps delivery. In subinvolution of the uterus, there is inadequate contraction, resulting in bleeding. A boggy uterus with vaginal bleeding is seen in uterine atony. An inverted uterus with vaginal bleeding is seen in uterine inversion.

9. Answer: c
RATIONALE: Early postpartal hemorrhage can be assessed within the first few hours following delivery. Postpartal infection may be noticed as a rise in temperature after the first 24 hours following childbirth. Postpartal blues and postpartum depression are emotional disorders noticed much later, in the weeks following delivery.

10. Answer: c
RATIONALE: To help prevent the occurrence of postpartum thromboembolic complications, the nurse should instruct the client to avoid sitting or standing in one position for long periods of time. This prevents venous pooling. The nurse should instruct the client to perform postoperative deep-breathing exercises to improve venous return by relieving the negative thoracic pressure on leg veins. The nurse should instruct the client to prevent venous pooling by avoiding the use of pillows under the knees. Elevating the legs above heart level promotes venous return, and therefore the nurse should encourage it.

11. **Answer: c**
    RATIONALE: A nurse should monitor for decreased blood pressure when evaluating the client for signs of hemorrhage. A falling blood pressure along with increased heart rate and decreased urinary output are the typical signs of severe hemorrhage. The client will also experience reduced, not increased, body temperature during hemorrhage.

12. **Answer: b**
    RATIONALE: The nurse should educate the client to perform hand-washing before and after breastfeeding to prevent mastitis. Discontinuing breastfeeding to allow time for healing, avoiding hot or cold compresses on the breast, and discouraging manual compression of breast for expressing milk are inappropriate interventions. The nurse should educate the client to continue breastfeeding, because it reverses milk stasis, and to manually compress the breast to express excess milk. Hot and cold compresses can be applied for comfort.

13. **Answer: b, c, & d**
    RATIONALE: The nurse should monitor for bleeding gums, tachycardia, and acute renal failure to assess for an increased risk of disseminated intravascular coagulation in the client. The other clinical manifestations of this condition include petechiae, ecchymosis, and uncontrolled bleeding during birth. Hypotension and amount of lochia greater than usual are findings that might suggest a coagulopathy.

14. **Answer: a, b, & d**
    RATIONALE: The nurse should monitor the client for symptoms such as inability to concentrate, loss of confidence, and decreased interest in life to verify the presence of postpartum depression. Manifestations of mania and bizarre behavior are noted in clients with postpartum psychosis.

15. **Answer: a, b, & d**
    RATIONALE: A nurse should evaluate the efficacy of IV oxytocin therapy by assessing the uterine tone, monitoring vital signs, and getting a pad count. Assessing the skin turgor and assessing deep tendon reflexes are inappropriate interventions and are not applicable when administering oxytocin to the client.

CHAPTER 23

Activity A

1. Polycythemia
2. Gavage
3. asphyxia
4. preterm
5. atelectasis
6. term
7. Retinopathy
8. Pain
9. inversely
10. genetic

Activity B

1. **a.** The figure displays a low–birth-weight newborn in an Isolette.
   b. An Isolette keeps the newborn warm to conserve energy and prevent cold stress. The Isolette may be warmed or may have an overhead radiant warmer.

Activity C

1. c   2. a   3. b   4. d

Activity D

1.

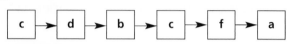

Activity E

1. The common physical characteristics of preterm newborns include
   - Birth weight of less than 5.5 lb
   - Scrawny appearance
   - Head disproportionately larger than chest circumference
   - Poor muscle tone
   - Minimal subcutaneous fat
   - Undescended testes
   - Plentiful lanugo (a soft downy hair), especially over the face and back
   - Poorly formed ear pinna with soft, pliable cartilage
   - Fused eyelids
   - Soft and spongy skull bones, especially along suture lines
   - Matted scalp hair, wooly in appearance
   - Absent or only a few creases in the soles and palms
   - Minimal scrotal rugae in male infants; prominent labia and clitoris in female infants
   - Thin, transparent skin with visible veins
   - Breast and nipples not clearly delineated
   - Abundant vernix caseosa

2. The clinical signs of hypoglycemia in the newborn are often subtle and include lethargy, apathy, drowsiness, irritability, tachypnea, weak cry, temperature instability, jitteriness, seizures, apnea, bradycardia, cyanosis or pallor, feeble suck and poor feeding, hypotonia, and coma. Blood glucose level below 40mg/dL in term newborns and below 20 mg/dL in preterm newborns is indicative of hypoglycemia in the newborn.

3. Developmentally supportive care is defined as care of a newborn or infant to support growth and development. Developmental care focuses on what newborns or infants can do at that stage of development; it uses therapeutic interventions only to the point that they are beneficial; and it provides for the development of the newborn–family unit.

4. Preterm infants are at a high risk for neurodevelopmental disorders such as cerebral palsy or mental

retardation, intraventricular hemorrhage, congenital anomalies, neurosensory impairment, behavioral disadaptation, and chronic lung disease.
5. The characteristics of large-for-gestational-age newborns are
   • Large body; appears plump and full-faced
   • Increase in body size is proportional
   • Head circumference and body length in upper limits of intrauterine growth
   • Poor motor skills
   • Difficulty in regulating behavioral states
   • More difficult to arouse to a quiet alert state
6. Post-term newborns typically exhibit the following characteristics:
   • Dry, cracked, wrinkled skin
   • Long, thin extremities
   • Creases that cover the entire soles of the feet
   • Wide-eyed, alert expression
   • Abundant hair on scalp
   • Thin umbilical cord
   • Limited vernix and lanugo
   • Meconium-stained skin
   • Long nails

Activity F

1. a. A nurse can help the parents in the detachment process in the following ways:
      • To see their newborn through the maze of equipment
      • Explain the various procedures and equipment
      • Encourage them to express their feelings about the fragile newborn's status
      • Provide the parents time to spend with their dying newborn
   b. The nursing interventions when caring for a family experiencing a perinatal loss are as follows:
      • Help the family to accept the reality of death by using the word "died"
      • Acknowledge their grief and the fact that their newborn has died
      • Help the family to work through their grief by validating and listening
      • Provide the family with realistic information about the causes of death
      • Offer condolences to the family in a sincere manner
      • Initiate spiritual comfort by calling the hospital clergy if needed
      • Acknowledge variations in spiritual needs and readiness
      • Encourage the parents to have a funeral or memorial service to bring closure
      • Encourage the parents to take photographs, make memory boxes, and record their thoughts in a journal
      • Suggest that the parents plant a tree or flowers to remember the infant
      • Explore with family members how they dealt with previous losses

• Discuss meditation and relaxation techniques to reduce stress
• Provide opportunities for the family to hold the newborn if they choose to do so
• Assess the family's support network
• Address attachment issues concerning subsequent pregnancies
• Reassure the family that their feelings and grieving responses are normal
• Provide information about local support groups
• Provide nticipatory guidance regarding the grieving process
• Recommend that family members maintain a healthy diet and get adequate rest and exercise to preserve their health

Activity G

1. **Answer: a**
   RATIONALE: The nurse should focus on decreasing blood viscosity by increasing fluid volume in the newborn with polycythemia. Checking blood glucose within two hours of birth by a reagent test strip and screening every two to three hours or before feeds are not interventions that will alleviate the condition of an infant with polycythemia. The nurse should monitor and maintain blood glucose levels when caring for a newborn with hypoglycemia, not polycythemia.
2. **Answer: a, c, & e**
   RATIONALE: To minimize the risk of infections, the nurse should avoid coming to work when ill, use sterile gloves for an invasive procedure, and monitor laboratory test results for changes. The nurse should remove all jewelry prior to washing hands, not cover the jewelry. The nurse should use disposable equipment rather than avoid it.
3. **Answer: a**
   RATIONALE: When preterm infants receive sensorimotor interventions such as rocking, massaging, holding, or sleeping on waterbeds, they gain weight faster, progress in feeding abilities more quickly, and show improved interactive behavior. Interventions such as swaddling and positioning, use of minimal amount of tape, and use of distraction through objects are related to pain management.
4. **Answer: c**
   RATIONALE: The nurse should identify acute respiratory complication as the risk to the newborn that results from meconium in the amniotic fluid. Bradycardia, perinatal asphyxia, and polycythemia are some of the common problems faced by an SGA newborn but are not related to meconium in the amniotic fluid.
5. **Answer: d**
   RATIONALE: A good cry or good breathing efforts are signs that the resuscitation has been successful. A pulse above 100 bpm, not 80 bpm, is an indication

of a successful resuscitation. Pink tongue, not blue, indicates a good oxygen supply to the brain. Tremors are associated with the signs of hypothermia; this is not a sign of successful resuscitation.

6. **Answer: c**
   RATIONALE: The nurse should observe for clinical signs of cold stress, such as respiratory distress, central cyanosis, hypoglycemia, lethargy, weak cry, abdominal distention, apnea, bradycardia, and acidosis. The temperature of the radiant warmer should not be set at a fixed level and should be adjusted to the newborn's temperature. The nurse need not check the blood pressure of the infant every two hours. The infant's temperature should be measured more often than every five hours.

7. **Answer: b**
   RATIONALE: The nurse should administer 0.5 to 1 mL/kg/h of breast milk enterally to induce surges in gut hormones that enhance maturation of the intestine. Administering vitamin D supplements, iron supplements, or intravenous dextrose will not significantly help the preterm newborn's gut overcome the many feeding difficulties.

8. **Answer: a**
   RATIONALE: The nurse should maintain the fluid and electrolyte balance of an infant born with hypoglycemia. Dextrose should be given intravenously only if the infant refuses oral feedings, not before offering the infant oral feedings. Placing the infant on a radiant warmer will not help maintain blood glucose levels. The nurse should focus on decreasing blood viscosity in an infant who is at risk for polycythemia, not hypoglycemia.

9. **Answer: c**
   RATIONALE: The nurse should assess for a decrease in urinary output and fluid balance in the preterm or post-term newborn. Weight of the newborn should be measured daily, not once every two days. Increased muscle tone does not indicate nutrition and fluid imbalance. A rise, not fall, in temperature indicates dehydration.

10. **Answer: a, b, & d**
    RATIONALE: Diabetes mellitus, postdates gestation, and glucose intolerance are the maternal factors the nurse should consider that could lead to a newborn being large for gestational age. Renal condition and maternal alcohol use are not factors associated with a newborn's being large for gestational age.

11. **Answer: a**
    RATIONALE: Jaundice is a sign of polycythemia. Restlessness, temperature instability, and wheezing are not fetal distress signs; they are the signs of a newborn with hypothermia.

12. **Answer: c**
    RATIONALE: The nurse should administer glucose intravenously to the newborn immediately when the blood glucose level is less than 23 mg/dL. Administering dextrose intravenously or placing the infant on a radiant warmer will not help maintain the glu-

cose level. Monitoring the infant's pulse is not a priority.

13. **Answer: a, c, & e**
    RATIONALE: Hydration, early feedings, and phototherapy are measures that the nurse should take to reduce bilirubin levels in the newborn. Increasing the infant's water intake or administering vitamin supplements will not help reduce bilirubin levels in the infant.

14. **Answer: c**
    RATIONALE: A stained umbilical cord indicates a possibility of meconium aspiration, and the nurse should inform the primary care provider immediately. Listlessness or lethargy by themselves do not indicate meconium aspiration. Bluish skin discoloration is normal in infants, and so is pink discoloration of the tongue.

CHAPTER 24

Activity A

1. omphalocele
2. Cephalhematoma
3. Hyperbilirubinemia
4. sepsis
5. Methadone
6. hemolytic
7. phototherapy
8. Gastroschisis
9. asphyxia
10. Kernicterus

Activity B

1. The congenital condition is known as esophageal atresia. It is the most common type of esophageal atresia, in which the esophagus ends in a blind pouch and a fistula connects the trachea with the distal portion of the esophagus.

Activity C

1. a   2. b   3. d   4. c

Activity D

1. The characteristics of infants born to diabetic mothers are
   - Full, rosy cheeks with a ruddy skin color
   - Short neck with a buffalo hump over the nape of the neck
   - Massive shoulders showing full intrascapular area
   - Distended upper abdomen due to organ overgrowth
   - Excessive subcutaneous fat tissue, producing fat extremities
2. The most common types of malformations in infants of diabetic mothers involve anomalies in the
   - Cardiovascular system
   - Skeletal system
   - Central nervous system
   - Gastrointestinal system
   - Genitourinary systems

3. The treatment of infants born to diabetic mothers focuses on correcting hypoglycemia, hypocalcemia, hypomagnesemia, dehydration, and jaundice. Oxygenation and ventilation for the newborn are supported as necessary.

4. Birth trauma may result from the pressure of birth, especially in a prolonged or abrupt labor, abnormal or difficult presentation, cephalopelvic disproportion, or mechanical forces, such as forceps or vacuum used during delivery.

5. Meconium aspiration syndrome occurs when the newborn inhales particulate meconium mixed with amniotic fluid into the lungs while still in utero or on taking the first breath after birth. It is a common cause of newborn respiratory distress and can lead to severe illness.

6. Periventricular–intraventricular hemorrhage (PVH/IVH) is defined as bleeding that usually originates in the subependymal germinal matrix region of the brain, with extension into the ventricular system. It is a common problem of preterm infants, especially in those born before 32 weeks.

Activity E

1. **a.** The role of the nurse in handling substance-abusing mothers includes
   - Being knowledgeable about issues of substance abuse
   - Being alert for opportunities to identify, prevent, manage, and educate clients and families about this key public health issue

   b. The nurse can use the "5 A's" approach in the following way:
   - Ask: Ask the client if she smokes and if she would like to quit.
   - Advise: Encourage the use of clinically proven treatment plans.
   - Assess: Provide motivation by discussing the 5 R's:
     - Relevance of quitting to the client
     - Risk of continued smoking to the fetus
     - Rewards of quitting for both
     - Roadblocks to quitting
     - Repeat at every visit
   - Assist: Help the client to protect her fetus and newborn from the negative effects of smoking.
   - Arrange: Schedule follow-up visits to reinforce the client's commitment to quit.

Activity F

1. **Answer: d**
   RATIONALE: The nurse should assess for end-expiratory grunting, barrel-shaped chest with an increased anterior-posterior (AP) chest diameter, prolonged tachypnea, progression from mild to severe respiratory distress, intercostal retractions, cyanosis, surfactant dysfunction, airway obstruction, hypoxia, and chemical pneumonitis with inflammation of pulmonary tissues in a newborn with meconium aspiration syndrome. A high-

pitched cry may be noted in periventricular–intraventricular hemorrhage. Bile-stained emesis occurs in necrotizing enterocolitis. Increased intracranial pressure occurs in cases of hydrocephalus.

2. **Answer: a**
   RATIONALE: The nurse should assess for systolic ejection murmur. Respiratory alkalosis, rhinorrhea, and lacrimation may be symptoms of neonatal abstinence syndrome.

3. **Answer: d**
   RATIONALE: Noting any absence of or decrease in deep tendon reflexes is a nursing intervention when assessing a newborn with a risk for trauma. The nurse should examine the skin for cyanosis, should be alert for signs of apathy and listlessness, and should assess for any temperature instability when caring for a newborn born to a diabetic mother. These interventions are not required to assess for trauma or birth injuries in a newborn.

4. **Answer: b**
   RATIONALE: The nurse should know that the infant's mother must have been a diabetic. The large size of the infant born to a diabetic mother is secondary to exposure to high levels of maternal glucose crossing the placenta into the fetal circulation. Common problems among infants of diabetic mothers include macrosomia, RDS, birth trauma, hypoglycemia, hypocalcemia and hypomagnesemia, polycythemia, hyperbilirubinemia, and congenital anomalies. Listlessness is also a common symptom noted in these infants. Infants born to clients who have abused alcohol, infants who have experienced birth traumas, or infants whose mothers had a low birth weight are not known to exhibit these particular characteristics, though these conditions do not produce very positive pregnancy outcomes.

5. **Answer: a, d, & e**
   RATIONALE: A nurse should associate obstructive hydrocephalus, vision or hearing defects, and cerebral palsy with the occurrence of periventricular–intraventricular hemorrhage in a newborn. Acid–base imbalances are a complication occurring during exchange transfusion for lowering serum bilirubin levels. Pneumonitis is a complication associated with esophageal atresia.

6. **Answer: c**
   RATIONALE: The nurse should assess for meconium aspiration syndrome in the newborn. Meconium aspiration involves patchy, fluffy infiltrates unevenly distributed throughout the lungs and marked hyperaeration mixed with areas of atelectasis that can be seen through chest x-rays. Direct visualization of the vocal cords for meconium staining by means of a laryngoscope can confirm aspiration. Lung auscultation typically reveals coarse crackles and rhonchi. Arterial blood gas analysis will indicate metabolic acidosis with a low blood pH, decreased PaO_2, and increased $PaCO_2$.

Newborns with choanal atresia, necrotizing enterocolitis, and hyperbilirubinemia are not known to exhibit these manifestations.

7. **Answer: a**

    RATIONALE: When caring for a newborn with transient tachypnea, the nurse should administer IV fluids and gavage feedings until the respiratory rate decreases enough to allow oral feedings. Maintaining adequate hydration and performing gentle suctioning are relevant nursing interventions when caring for a newborn with respiratory distress syndrome. The nurse need not monitor the newborn for signs and symptoms of hypotonia, because hypotonia is not known to occur as a result of transient tachypnea. Hypotonia is observed in newborns with inborn errors of metabolism or in cases of periventricular-intraventricular hemorrhage.

8. **Answer: b**

    RATIONALE: Ensuring effective resuscitation measures is the nursing intervention involved when treating a newborn for asphyxia. Ensuring adequate tissue perfusion and administering surfactant are nursing interventions involved in the care of newborns with meconium aspiration syndrome. Similarly, administering intravenous (IV) fluids is a nursing intervention involved in the care of newborns with transient tachypnea.

9. **Answer: c**

    RATIONALE: The preoperative nursing care focuses on preventing aspiration by elevating the head of the bed 30 to 45 degrees to prevent reflux. Providing colostomy care is a part of postoperative nursing care for the newborn. Documenting the amount and color of drainage is the postoperative nursing care for the newborn with omphalocele. Administering antibiotics and total parenteral nutrition is a postoperative nursing intervention when caring for a newborn with esophageal atresia.

10. **Answer: d**

    RATIONALE: When caring for a substance-exposed newborn, the nurse should check the newborn's skin turgor and fontanels. Encouraging early initiation of feedings and monitoring the newborn's cardiovascular status are nursing interventions involved when caring for a newborn with pathologic jaundice. In case of pathologic jaundice, the nurse also encourages supplementing breast milk with formula to supply protein if bilirubin levels continue to increase with breastfeeding only.

11. **Answer: b**

    RATIONALE: The nurse should shield the newborn's eyes and cover the genitals to protect these areas from becoming irritated or burned when using direct lights and to ensure exposure of the greatest surface area. The nurse should place the newborn under the lights or on the fiberoptic blanket, exposing as much skin as possible. Breast or bottle feedings should be encouraged every two to three

hours. Loose, green and frequent stools indicate the presence of unconjugated bilirubin excreted in the feces. This is normal; therefore, there is no need for therapy to be discontinued. Lack of frequent green stools is a cause for concern.

12. **Answer: b, d, & e**

    RATIONALE: When caring for a newborn with meconium aspiration syndrome, the nurse should place the newborn under a radiant warmer or in a warmed incubator, administer oxygen therapy as ordered via a nasal cannula or with positive pressure ventilation, and administer broad-spectrum antibiotics to treat bacterial pneumonia. Repeated suctioning and stimulation should be limited to prevent overstimulation and further depression in the newborn. The nurse should also ensure minimal handling to reduce energy expenditure and oxygen consumption that could lead to further hypoxemia and acidosis. Handling and rubbing the newborn with a dry towel are needed to stimulate the onset of breathing in a newborn with asphyxia.

13. **Answer: a**

    RATIONALE: The nurse should know that gastroschisis is a herniation of abdominal contents in which there is no peritoneal sac protecting herniated organs. A peritoneal sac is present in omphalocele. In gastroschisis, the herniated organs are not normal; they are unprotected and become thickened, edematous, and inflamed due to exposure to amniotic fluid. Gastroschisis is not a defect of the umbilical ring; it is a herniation of abdominal contents through an abdominal wall defect. Despite surgical correction, feeding intolerance, failure to thrive, and prolonged hospital stays occur in nearly all newborns with gastroschisis.

14. **Answer: c**

    RATIONALE: The nurse should inform the parents that surgery for necrotizing enterocolitis requires the placement of a proximal enterostomy and ostomy care. Surgically treating NEC is a lengthy process, and the amount of bowel that has necrosed, as determined during the bowel resection, significantly increases the likelihood that infants requiring surgery for NEC may have long-term medical problems. If surgery for NEC is required, antibiotics may be needed for an extended period of time.

CHAPTER 25

Activity A

1. Colic
2. anticipatory
3. solitary
4. Development
5. Maturation
6. Acrocyanosis
7. binocularity

8. Stranger
9. Temperament
10. prone

Activity B

1. **a.** The figure shows a significant head lag in the newborn when pulled to sit.
   b. Gross motor skills develop in a cephalocaudal fashion. The baby learns to lift the head before learning to roll over and sit.

Activity C

1. e   2. b   3. c   4. a   5. d   6. f

Activity D

1.

| c | → | e | → | a | → | d | → | b |

2.

| e | → | a | → | b | → | d | → | c |

Activity E

1. The nursing interventions that will help achieve the Healthy People 2010 objective of increasing the proportion of mothers who breastfeed include:
   - Encouraging breastfeeding in all mothers, beginning with the prenatal visit if applicable
   - Providing accurate education related to breastfeeding
   - Being available for questions or problems related to initiation and continuation of breastfeeding; consulting a lactation consultant as needed
   - Encouraging pumping of breast milk when the mother returns to work in order to continue breastfeeding
   - Referring the mother to local breastfeeding support groups such as La Leche League
2. Spitting up once or twice a day after feedings is normal. Overfed babies or those who do not burp well are more likely to spit up. Very frequent spitting up may be caused by gastroesophageal reflux. Feeding the child smaller amounts or on a more frequent basis helps reduce spitting up. If the infant vomits one third or more of most feedings, chokes when vomiting, or experiences forceful emesis, the primary care provider should be notified.
3. Teach them that some infants are slower to warm up than others. These infants should be approached slowly and calmly. Some infants are considerably more active than others and will require more direct play with the parent. These infants may be the type who are in constant motion. The quiet infant may become overwhelmed with excess stimulation, whereas the very active baby may demonstrate a need for additional stimulation in order to be satisfied. Once parents are familiar with the infant's temperament, they can describe the best way for others

to approach the infant (such as childcare workers or health care professionals).

4. A normal newborn will ordinarily move through six states of consciousness:
   - Deep sleep: The infant lies quietly without movement.
   - Light sleep: The infant may move a little while sleeping and may startle from noises.
   - Drowsiness: Eyes may close and the infant may be dozing.
   - Quiet alert state: The infant's eyes are open wide and the body is calm.
   - Active alert state: The infant's face and body move actively.
   - Crying: The infant cries or screams and the body moves in a disorganized fashion.
5. The following anatomic differences are observed on comparison with the respiratory system in an adult:
   - The nasal passages are narrower
   - The trachea and chest wall are more compliant
   - The bronchi and bronchioles are shorter and narrower
   - The larynx is more funnel-shaped
   - The tongue is larger
   - There are significantly fewer alveoli
6. Occasionally, an infant is born with one or more teeth—termed natal teeth—or develops teeth in the first 28 days of life—termed neonatal teeth. On average, the first primary teeth begin to erupt between the ages of six and eight months. The lower central incisor teeth are usually the first to appear, followed by the upper central incisors when the infant is 8 to 12 months old. The lateral incisors appear when the infant is 9 to 13 months. The first molar teeth appear between 13 and 19 months of age, the cuspids appear between 16 and 22 months, and the second molars develop between 25 and 33 months.

Activity F

1. **a.** The nurse should explain to Carla's parents about stranger anxiety that may develop in infants around the age of eight months. The previously happy and friendly infant may become clingy and whiny when approached by strangers or people not well known. Stranger anxiety is an indicator that the infant is recognizing herself as separate from others. As the infant becomes more aware of new people and new places, she may view an interaction with a stranger as threatening and may start crying, even if the parent is right there. Family members whom the child sees infrequently, as well as others the child does not spend a lot of time with, should approach the infant calmly and slowly, with the parent in sight. Sometimes this will prevent a sudden crying spell.
   b. Generally, by eight months of age the infant is ready for more texture in his or her foods. The nurse can suggest that Carla's mother feed her

soft, mashed table food, avoiding large chunks. Finger foods such as Cheerios, soft green bean pieces, or soft peas may also be offered. The nurse should inform the mother to avoid hard foods that the infant may choke on.

Activity G

1. Answer: c
RATIONALE: The child's head size is large for her adjusted age of four months, which would be cause for concern. Normal growth would be 3.6 inches. At 10 pounds 2 ounces, the child is the right weight for a four months adjusted age. Palmar grasp reflex disappears between four and six months adjusted age, so this would not be a concern yet. The child is average weight for a four months adjusted age.

2. Answer: a
RATIONALE: Urging the parents to get time away from the child would be most helpful in the short term, particularly if the parents are very stressed. Educating the parents about when colic stops would help them see that there is an end to the stress. Watching how the parents respond to the child would help determine if the parent–child relationship was altered. Assessing the parents' care and feeding skills may identify other causes for the crying.

3. Answer: d
RATIONALE: Saying "no" in appropriate instances is a far more effective method of disciplining the child than threatening the child with punishment. Child curiosity can raise safety concerns, but establishing the coffee table as off limits and keeping the child in a child-safe room are poor substitutes for child-proofing the house and using a calm, rapid response to unforeseen dangers.

4. Answer: b
RATIONALE: The nurse should warn against putting the child to bed with a bottle of milk or juice because this allows the sugar content of these fluids to pool around the child's teeth at night. Not cleaning a neonate's gums when he has finished feeding will have little effect on dental caries, as will using a cloth instead of a brush for cleaning teeth when they erupt. Failure to clean the teeth with fluoridated toothpaste is not a problem if the water in the family's town is fluoridated.

5. Answer: b
RATIONALE: If the parents are keeping the child up until she falls asleep, they are not creating a bedtime routine for her. Infants need a transition to sleep at this age. If the parents are singing to her before she goes to bed, if she has a regular, scheduled bedtime, and if they check on her safety when she wakes at night and then lay her down and leave, they are using good sleep practices.

6. Answer: c
RATIONALE: The nurse would advise the mother to watch for increased biting and sucking. Running a mild fever, vomiting, and diarrhea are signs of infection. The child would more likely seek out hard foods or objects to teethe on.

7. Answer: d
RATIONALE: When introducing a new food to an infant, it may take 20 or more times before the child will accept it. Parents must be patient. Letting the child eat only the foods she prefers, forcing her to eat foods she does not want, or actively urging the child to eat new foods can negatively affect eating patterns.

8. Answer: a
RATIONALE: The best way to ensure effective feeding is by maintaining a feed-on-demand approach rather than a set schedule. Applying warm compresses to the breast helps engorgement. Encouraging the infant to latch on properly helps prevent sore nipples. Maintaining proper diet and fluid intake for the mother helps ensure an adequate milk supply.

9. Answer: b
RATIONALE: If the child's rectal temperature is greater than 100.4°F, the parents should call their care provider. Infants are very susceptible to infection. If the dried umbilical cord stump falls off or the child wets her diaper eight times per day, this is normal. In the first five to ten days of life, it is also normal for the child to eat but still lose weight.

10. Answer: c
RATIONALE: At six months of age, the child is able to put down one toy to pick up another. He will be able to shift a toy to his left hand to reach for another with his right hand by seven months. He will pick up an object with his thumb and fingertips at eight months, and he will enjoy hitting a plastic bowl with a large spoon at nine months.

11. Answer: a
RATIONALE: The infant is exhibiting Babinski reflex, which appears at birth and disappears by 12 months of age. On holding the infant such that one foot touches a flat surface, he exhibits a step reflex by putting the other foot down as if to "step." With sudden extension of the head, the arms abduct and move upward and the hands form a "C"; this is called a Moro reflex. The infant exhibits a plantar grasp by reflexively grasping with the bottom of the foot when pressure is applied to the plantar surface.

12. Answer: d
RATIONALE: Mucus-like or frothy stool is a cause for concern and should be reported to the primary care provider. The newborn's first stools or meconium are the result of digestion of amniotic fluid swallowed in utero; it is dark green to black and sticky. It gradually changes to yellowish or tan. The stool of a breastfed infant has a loose and seedy texture.

13. Answer: c
RATIONALE: A three-month-old child not smiling at people is a warning sign of possible problems with

social or emotional development. An infant who does not make sounds at four months of age, does not laugh or squeal by six months of age, or does not babble by eight months of age may have problems in language development.

14. **Answer: b**
    RATIONALE: The nurse should inform the mother that formula should not be sweetened with honey. Formula should not be heated in a microwave; it can be warmed by placing the bottle in a container of hot water. Cereal should not be added to the formula in the bottle. Any unused portion should be thrown away after each feeding.

CHAPTER 26

Activity A

1. Myelinization
2. primary
3. Receptive
4. urethra
5. weak
6. Erikson
7. parallel
8. autonomy
9. calcium
10. Extinction

Activity B

1. c   **2.** d   **3.** a   **4.** b   **5.** e

Activity C

1.

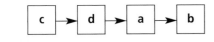

2.

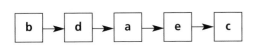

Activity D

1. Temper tantrums are a natural result of the frustration that toddlers experience. Toddlers are eager to explore new things, but they need time and maturity to learn the rules and regulations. They may be frustrated because of lack of language skills to express themselves. Fatigue or hunger may limit the toddler's coping abilities and promote negative behavior and temper tantrums. Temper tantrums are a normal part of the toddler's quest for independence. As toddlers mature, they become better able to express themselves and to understand their environment.

2. The "toddler gait" is characteristic of new walkers. The toddler does not walk smoothly and maturely. The legs are planted widely apart, toes are pointed forward, and the toddler seems to sway from side to side while moving forward. Often the toddler seems to speed along, pitching forward, appearing ready to topple over at any moment.

3. Telegraphic speech is common in the three-year-old. This type of speech contains only the essential words to get the point across, much like a telegram. A toddler who wants a cookie and milk might say, "Want cookie milk." In telegraphic speech, the nouns and verbs are present and are verbalized in the appropriate order.

4. Play is the major socializing medium for toddlers. Toddlers are egocentric; this makes it difficult for them to share. They usually play alongside another child rather than cooperatively. The short attention span makes the toddler change toys and types of play. Toddlers like dramatic play and play that recreates familiar activities in the home. They enjoy music and musical instruments and will often dance to whatever they hear on the radio. Adequate physical activity is necessary for the development and refinement of movement skills.

5. When choosing a preschool, the parent or caregiver should look for an environment that has the following qualities:
   - Goals and an overall philosophy with which the parents agree
   - Teachers and assistants trained in early childhood development as well as child cardiopulmonary resuscitation
   - Small class sizes and an adult-to-child ratio with which the parent feels comfortable
   - Disciplinary procedures consistent with the parents' values
   - An open-door policy allowing parents to visit at any time
   - Childproofing inside and outside the school
   - Appropriate hygiene procedures, including prohibiting sick children from attending

6. Parents should note that poor oral hygiene, prolonged use of a bottle or no-spill sippy cup, lack of fluoride intake, and delayed or absent professional dental care may all contribute to the development of dental caries. Cleaning of the toddler's teeth should progress from brushing with simply water to using a pea-sized amount of fluoridated toothpaste with brushing, beginning at two years of age. The toddler should be weaned from the bottle no later than 15 months of age. The use of a no-spill sippy cup should be severely restricted. The toddler's first dental visit should be at the age of one.

Activity E

1. **a.** The potentially bilingual child may blend two languages (parts of the word in both languages are blended into one word) or may mix language within a sentence (combine languages or grammar within a sentence). The assessment of adequate language development is more complicated in bilingual children. Due to possible language mixing, the bilingual child may be more difficult to assess for speech delay. The

bilingual child should have command of 20 words (between both languages) by 20 months of age and should be making word combinations. If this is not the case, then further investigation may be warranted.

b. Talking and singing to the toddler during routine activities such as feeding and dressing provides an environment that encourages conversation. Frequent, repetitive naming helps the toddler learn appropriate words for objects. Be attentive to what the toddler is saying, as well as to her moods. Listen to and answer the toddler's questions. Encouragement and elaboration convey confidence and interest to the toddler. Give the toddler time to complete her thoughts without interrupting or rushing. Remember that the toddler is just starting to be able to make the connections necessary to transfer thoughts and feelings into language. Do not overreact to the child's use of the word "no." Give the toddler opportunities to appropriately use the word "no" with silly questions such as "Can a cat drive a car?" Teach the toddler appropriate words for body parts and objects. Help the toddler choose appropriate words to label feelings and emotions. Toddlers' receptive language and interpretation of body language and subtle signs far surpass their expressive language, especially at a younger age. Encourage the use of both English and German in the home. Reading to the toddler every day is one of the best ways to promote language and cognitive development. Toddlers particularly enjoy books about feelings, family, friends, everyday life, animals and nature, and fun and fantasy. Board books have thick pages that are easier for young toddlers to turn. The toddler may also enjoy "reading" the story to the parent.

c. Erikson defines the toddler period as a time of autonomy versus shame and doubt. It is a time of exerting independence. Exertion of independence often results in the toddler's favorite response, "no." The toddler will often answer "no" even when she really means "yes." Always saying "no," referred to as negativism, is a normal part of healthy development. It occurs as a result of the toddler's attempt to assert her independence. Avoid asking closed-ended yes/no questions, as the toddler's usual response is "no" whether she means it or not. Offer the child simple choices such as, "Do you want to use the red cup or the blue cup?" This helps give the toddler a sense of control. Do not ask toddlers if they "want" to do something if not doing it is not an option. For instance, when getting ready to leave, do not ask the child if she "wants" to put her shoes on. Simply state in a matter-of-fact tone that shoes must be worn outside, and give the toddler a choice on the type of shoe or the color of socks. If the child continues with nega-

tive answers, then the parent should remain calm and make the decision for the child.

d. The nurse should assess Alena to find out if she uses two-word sentences, imitates actions, follows basic instructions, and is capable of pushing a toy with wheels.

Activity F

1. **Answer: c**
RATIONALE: Suggesting that the parents encourage the child to eat a healthier diet by serving him healthier choices along with smaller portions of junk food will reassure them that they are not starving their child. The parents would have less success with an abrupt change to healthy foods. Explaining calorie requirements and the timeline for acceptance of a new food does not offer a practical reason for making a change in diet.

2. **Answer: a**
RATIONALE: This child has most recently acquired the ability to undress himself. Pushing a toy lawnmower and kicking a ball are motor skills that the boy has learned at about 24 months. At about 18 months of age, the boy should be capable of pulling a toy while walking around.

3. **Answer: d**
RATIONALE: Stopping the child when she is misbehaving and describing proper behavior sets limits and models good behavior and will be the most helpful advice to the parents. The child is too young to use time out or extinction as discipline. Slapping her hand, even done carefully with two fingers, is corporal punishment, which has been found to have negative effects on child development.

4. **Answer: b**
RATIONALE: The most effective overall safety information is never to let the child out of sight. Toddlers are curious and mobile; therefore, they require direct observation and cannot be trusted to be left alone. Gating stairways, locking up chemicals, and not smoking around the child are excellent, but specific, safety interventions.

5. **Answer: b**
RATIONALE: The nurse would be concerned if the child is babbling to herself rather than using real words. By the age of two, the child should be using simple sentences with a vocabulary of 150 to 300 words. Being unwilling to share toys, playing parallel with other children, and changing toys frequently are typical toddler behaviors.

6. **Answer: c**
RATIONALE: The fact that the child does not respond when the mother waves to him suggests he may have a vision problem. The toddler's sense of smell is still developing, so he may not be affected by odors. The sense of taste is not well developed either, so he may eat or drink poisons without concern. The child's crying at a sudden noise assures the nurse that his hearing is adequate.

7. **Answer: a**
   RATIONALE: If the child is still speaking telegraphically in only two- to three-word sentences, it suggests she has a language development problem. If the child makes simple conversation, tells about something that happened in the past, or tells the nurse her name, she is meeting developmental milestones for language.

8. **Answer: a**
   RATIONALE: Separation anxiety should have disappeared or be subsiding by 3 years of age. The fact that it is persistent suggests that there might be an emotional problem. Emotional lability, self-soothing by thumb sucking, and the inability to share are common for this age.

9. **Answer: d**
   RATIONALE: The nurse should tell the mother to feed her child iron-fortified cereal and other iron-rich foods when she weans her child off the breast or formula. Weaning from the breast depends on the mother's need and desires, with no set time. It is important that the child is weaned from the bottle by the age of one, and the use of a no-spill sippy cup is severely restricted to prevent dental caries.

10. **Answer: a, b, & e**
    RATIONALE: The nurse should ask the parents to limit the use of a pacifier to stressful situations only. To ensure safety with pacifier use, the nurse should inform the parents that only one-piece pacifiers should be used, and worn pacifiers should be replaced with new ones. Additionally, pacifiers should never be tied around the toddler's neck. For most children there is no need to worry about a sucking habit until it is time for permanent teeth to erupt, but prolonged and frequent sucking could cause changes to the tooth and jaw structure.

11. **Answer: c**
    RATIONALE: The nurse should tell the parents to involve the toddler as much as possible in the care of the baby. The parents should treat the toddler as capable of helping with small tasks such as fetching a diaper or singing to the baby. Parents should attempt to keep the toddler's routine as close to normal as possible, rather than modifying the toddler's routine to suit the baby's schedule. Parents need to spend individual time with the toddler on a daily basis.

12. **Answer: b, d, & e**
    RATIONALE: Parents should limit the toddler's intake of milk to 16 to 24 ounces per day, provide foods rich in iron and vitamin C, and offer three full meals and two snacks daily. High fat, high-sugar, processed food should not be a substitute for healthy food choices at meal or snack time. Juice intake should be limited to 4 to 6 ounces per day.

13. **Answer: b**
    RATIONALE: The nurse should tell the parents to supervise the toddler when he is eating to ensure that the child does not choke on food. Foods such as nuts, raw carrots, and popcorn should be avoided, as they are hard to chew and may become lodged in the airway. Child-sized spoons and forks with dull tines are used to assist the toddler in eating; it may not help in preventing the child from choking. Grapes and hotdogs should be cut into quarters, not halves.

CHAPTER 27

Activity A

1. iron
2. concrete
3. urethra
4. Psychosocial
5. magical
6. transduction
7. musculoskeletal
8. telegraphic
9. physical
10. caries

Activity B

1. b   2. d   3. c   4. a   5. e

Activity C

1.

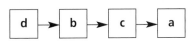

Activity D

1. The child in the intuitive phase can count ten or more objects, can correctly name at least four colors, can understand the concept of time, and knows about things that are used in everyday life, such as appliances, money, and food.

2. Store potentially dangerous fluids in their original containers and keep them out of reach of preschoolers. Do not pour dangerous fluids into containers that look like ordinary drinking glasses or cups. Ensure that medications have childproof caps and keep them in a locked cabinet. Post the poison control telephone number on or near the home phone.

3. The preschooler should have his or her teeth brushed and flossed daily with a pea-sized amount of toothpaste. Cariogenic foods should be avoided. If sugary foods are consumed, the mouth should be rinsed with water if it is not possible to brush the teeth directly after their consumption. The preschool child should visit the dentist every six months.

4. Exposure to tobacco smoke is associated with increased incidence of otitis media and respiratory infections. It can also lead to increased symptoms and medication use in children with asthma. Other effects include decreased lung function and behav-

ioral difficulties. Therefore, it is important that preschoolers be protected from second-hand tobacco smoke.

5. A three- to five-year-old requires 500 to 800 mg calcium and 10 mg iron daily. A three-year-old should consume 19 mg dietary fiber daily, while the four- to eight-year-old requires 25 mg dietary fiber per day. The typical preschooler requires about 85 kcal per kilogram of body weight. Saturated fats should account for less than 10% of total calories. Preschool children's diets should include a daily total fat intake of no less than 20% and not more than 30% of total calories to promote and maintain healthy cholesterol levels.

6. A preschooler should be agile while standing, walking, running, and jumping. He or she can go up and down stairs and walk forward and backward easily. Standing on tiptoes or on one foot still requires extra concentration. He or she also uses the body to understand new concepts or describe them.

Activity E

1. **a.** Magical thinking and playing make-believe are a normal part of preschool development. The preschool child believes her thoughts to be all-powerful. The fantasy experienced through magical thinking and make-believe allows the preschooler to make room in her world for the actual or the real and to satisfy her curiosity about differences in the world around her. Encouraging pretend play and providing props for dress-up stimulate and develop curiosity and creativity. Fantasy play is usually cooperative in nature and encourages the preschooler to develop social skills like taking turns, communicating, paying attention, and responding to another's words and actions. Fantasy play also allows preschoolers to explore complex social ideas such as power, compassion, and cruelty.

   b. Kindergarten may be a significant change for children. The hours are usually longer than preschool and it is usually held 5 days per week. The setting and personnel are new, and rules and expectations are often very different. The nurse should make these suggestions: When talking about starting kindergarten with Sonia, use an enthusiastic approach and keep the conversation light and positive. Meet with Sonia's teacher prior to the start of school and discuss any specific needs or concerns you may have. A tour of the school and attending the school's open house can also help ease the transition. Incorporate and practice the new daily routine before school starts. This can help the child adjust to the changes that are occurring.

   c. The following findings are developmental warning signs that would be of concern to the nurse: inability of the child to jump in place or ride a tricycle, stack four blocks, throw a ball overhand, or grasp a crayon with thumb and fingers;

difficulty with scribbling; inability to copy a circle; not using sentences with three or more words; not using the words "me" and "you" appropriately; ignoring other children or not showing interest in interactive games; not responding to people outside the family and still clinging or crying when parents leave; resisting use of toilet, dressing, sleeping; and not engaging in fantasy play.

Activity F

1. **Answer: b**
   RATIONALE: The presence of only 10 deciduous teeth would warrant further investigation. The preschooler should have 20 deciduous teeth present. The absence of dental caries or the presence of 19 teeth does not warrant further investigation.

2. **Answer: d**
   RATIONALE: The nurse should encourage the mother to schedule a meeting with the teacher before school starts and set up a time to tour the classroom and school so the boy knows what to expect. The other statements are not helpful and do not address the mother's or boy's concerns.

3. **Answer: c**
   RATIONALE: The average preschool child grows 2.5 to 3 inches per year.

4. **Answer: a**
   RATIONALE: By age five, persons outside of the family should be able to understand most of the child's speech without the parents' "translation." The other statements would not warrant additional referral or follow-up. A child of five should be able to count to at least ten, should know his or her address, and should be able to participate in long, detailed conversations.

5. **Answer: c**
   RATIONALE: During a night terror, the child is typically unaware of a parent's presence and may scream and thrash more if restrained. During a nightmare, the child is responsive to a parent's soothing and reassurances. The other statements describe a nightmare.

6. **Answer: d**
   RATIONALE: The preschooler is not mature enough to ride a bicycle in the street, even if riding with an adult, so the nurse should emphasize that the girl should always ride on the sidewalk even if the mother is riding with her daughter. The other statements do not indicate a need for further teaching.

7. **Answer: c**
   RATIONALE: The nurse needs to emphasize that there are number of reasons that a parent should not choose a preschool that uses corporal punishment. It may hurt a child's self-esteem as well as his ability to achieve in school. It may also lead to disruptive and violent behavior in the classroom and should be discouraged. The other statements would not warrant further discussion or intervention.

8. **Answer: b**
RATIONALE: The nurse should explain to the parents that attributing life-like qualities to inanimate objects is quite normal. Telling the parents that their daughter is demonstrating animism is correct, but it would be better to explain what animism is and then remind them that it is developmentally appropriate. Asking whether they think their daughter is hallucinating or whether there is a family history of mental illness is inappropriate and does not teach.

9. **Answer: a**
RATIONALE: The nurse needs to remind the parents that the girl should use a helmet when riding any wheeled toy, not just her bicycle. The other statements by the parents do not indicate a need for further teaching.

10. **Answer: b**
RATIONALE: The parents should perform flossing in the preschool period because the child cannot perform this task. The other statements by the parents do not indicate a need for further teaching.

11. **Answer: a**
RATIONALE: A preschool child who sleeps for about eight hours a day needs an additional referral or follow-up. The preschool child needs about 12 hours of sleep each day. The other statements do not warrant further discussion or intervention.

12. **Answer: b**
RATIONALE: Since preschool children have vivid imaginations, it is important to be careful about what television they watch. The violence in some television programs may scare the preschool child or inspire him or her to act out violent behavior. Five years of age is an appropriate time for a child to learn to swim. Preschool children may be picky eaters; coaxing could lead to a negative relationship between the parent and child relating to mealtime. Spanking is the least effective discipline practice. Therefore, the other statements do not call for any intervention.

13. **Answer: a**
RATIONALE: Preschoolers should use a glass or a cup for fluids, but the main reason why they should be discouraged from using no-spill cups is that they contribute to dental caries. They also allow unlimited access to fluids, possibly decreasing appetite for appropriate solid foods.

14. **Answer: c**
RATIONALE: The nurse should teach parents to limit the preschooler's television viewing to 1 to 2 hours per day and encourage participation in physical activities. The other listed behaviors are common and even normal for a preschooler.

15. **Answer: b**
RATIONALE: Lying is a very wrong habit; the nurse should help the parents ascertain why the child lies and help them remedy the problem. Some preschoolers can be afraid of loud noises, and it is

not a matter of concern. About 8 ounces of milk a day is sufficient for a three-year old. Standing on one foot is a gross motor skill expected generally from a five-year-old. Therefore, the other statements do not call for further discussion.

CHAPTER 28

Activity A
1. Prepubescence
2. bruxism
3. strabismus
4. latchkey
5. conservation
6. deciduous
7. metalinguistic
8. peer
9. lower
10. decreases

Activity B
1. a   2. c   3. d   4. b

Activity C
1.

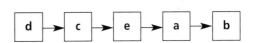

d → c → e → a → b

Activity D
1. Children aged six to eight enjoy bicycling, skating, and swimming. Children between eight and ten years of age have greater rhythm and gracefulness of muscular movements; they enjoy activities such as sports. Those aged 10 to 12 years, especially girls, are more controlled and focused, similar to adults.
2. The child typically feels discomfort in new situations, requires additional time to adjust, and exhibits frustration with tears or somatic complaints. Also described as irritable and moody, the child could benefit from patience, firmness, and understanding when faced with new situations.
3. Children between ages six and eight years require approximately 12 hours of sleep per night; those between eight and ten years of age require 10 to 12 hours of sleep per night. Children between 10 and 12 years of age require 9 to 10 hours of sleep per night. Some children, regardless of their age group, may need an occasional nap.
4. School refusal or school phobia has been defined as frequent absences, dropping out of school, or academic disengagement or disruption. Children with school phobia may refuse to attend school or create reasons why they cannot go to school.
5. Latchkey kids have both parents in the workforce and are usually home alone without any adult supervision for a number of hours. These latchkey kids are more prone to misbehave and to take risks.

6. The sense of smell can be tested in the school-age child by using scents that children are familiar with, such as chocolate or other familiar odors. In addition, the sense of touch may be tested with objects to discriminate cold from hot, soft from hard, and blunt from sharp.

Activity E

1. a. The role of the family in promoting healthy growth and development is critical. Respectful communication between the parent and child will foster self-esteem and self-confidence. This respect will give the child confidence in achieving personal, educational, and social goals appropriate for his or her age. During your exam, model appropriate behaviors by listening to the child and making appropriate responses. Serve as a resource for parents and as an advocate for the child in promoting healthy growth and development.

   b. The school-age child is able to see how her actions affect others and to realize that her behaviors can have consequences. Therefore, discipline techniques with consequences often work well. For example, if the child refuses to put away toys, the parent forbids playing with those toys. Parents need to teach children the rules established by the family, values, and social rules of conduct. This will help give the child guidelines as to which behaviors are acceptable and which are unacceptable. Parents need to be role models and demonstrate appropriate expressions of feelings and emotions, and allow the child to express emotions and feelings. They should never belittle the child, and they need to preserve the child's self-esteem and dignity. Parents should be encouraged to discipline with praise. This positive acknowledgement can encourage appropriate behavior. When misbehaviors occur, the type and amount of discipline should be based on the developmental level of the child and the parents, severity of misbehavior, established roles of the family, temperament of the child, and response of the child to rewards. The child should participate in developing a plan of action for his or her misbehavior. Consistency in discipline, along with providing it in a nurturing environment, is essential.

   c. Although some television shows and video games can have positive influences on children, guidelines on the use of television and video games are important. Research has shown that an excessive amount of time watching television or playing video games can lead to aggressive behavior, less physical activity, and altered body image. Parents should set limits on how much television the child is allowed to watch. The Academy of Pediatrics recommends 2 hours or less of television viewing per day. The parent should establish guidelines on when the child can watch television, and television watching should not be used as a reward. The parents should monitor what the child is watching, and they should watch the programs together and use that opportunity to discuss the subject matter with the child. Parents should also prohibit television shows or video games with violence. There should be no television during dinner and no television in the child's room. The parents need to set examples for the child and encourage sports, interactive play, and reading. They should encourage their child to read instead of watching television or to do a physical activity together as a family. If the television causes fights or arguments, it should be turned off for a period of time.

Activity F

1. Answer: a
RATIONALE: The child will be able to classify or group objects by their common elements in Piaget's period of concrete operational thought. According to Kohlberg's conventional stage 3, the child does not understand the reason behind rules. Development of social skills in relating to same-sex friends takes place in the Freud's latency stage. The child develops a sense of inferiority with failures and lack of support according to Erikson's sense of industry vs. inferiority as a task of the school-age years.

2. Answer: b
RATIONALE: The child with an easy temperament will adapt to school with only minor stresses. The slow-to-warm child will experience frustration. The difficult child will be moody and irritable and may benefit from a school visit.

3. Answer: b
RATIONALE: It is very important to get a bike of the proper size for the child. Getting a bike that the child can "grow into" is dangerous. Using training wheels and learning to fall on the grass are not acceptable substitutes for using the proper protective gear. The child should already demonstrate good coordination in other playing skills before attempting to ride a bike.

4. Answer: c
RATIONALE: Asking how often the family eats together is an appropriate question for the girl. All the others should be directed to the parents.

5. Answer: c
RATIONALE: The nurse would probably have found that the child still has a leaner body mass than girls at this age. Both boys and girls increase body fat at this age. Food preferences will be highly influenced by those of the parents. Although caloric intake may diminish, appetite will increase.

6. Answer: d
RATIONALE: Parents are major influences on school-age children and should discuss the dangers of tobacco and alcohol use with the child. Not smoking

in the house and hiding alcohol send mixed messages to the child. An open and honest discussion is the best approach rather than forbidding the child to make friends with kids who use tobacco or alcohol.

7. Answer: b
RATIONALE: The girl would need approximately 2,065 calories per day (65 lbs = 29.5 kg times 70 calories per day per kg = 2,065 calories per day).

8. Answer: b
RATIONALE: Because they are role models for their children, parents must first realize the importance of their own behaviors. It is possible that the parents are pressuring the child, but that is not the primary message. Punishment should be appropriate, consistent, and not too severe.

9. Answer: b
RATIONALE: Lymphatic tissue growth is complete by age nine, helping to localize infections and produce antibody–antigen responses. Brain growth will be complete by age ten. Frontal sinuses developed at age seven. Third molars do not erupt until the teen years.

10. Answer: c
RATIONALE: The nurse should tell the parents to investigate the cause of school refusal in the child and help desensitize the child by having him spend part of the day in the counselor's office. Telling the child that he will be punished for absenteeism will further increase the child's fears. The parents should not dismiss the child's fears as baseless, force him to attend school, or ask teachers if they have been harsh with the child without proper investigation.

11. Answer: c
RATIONALE: The nurse should instruct the parent to ensure that her child knows the name, address, and phone number of a trusted neighbor. It is not advisable to allow the child to play outside with friends for unrestricted hours or have friends at home when parents are out. The child should be instructed to tell anyone who comes to the door or who phones that Mom is home but busy.

12. Answer: a
RATIONALE: The nurse could attribute the six-year-old child's lying habit to the fear of being punished. Lying is common in children between six and eight years old. These younger children typically lie to avoid punishment. Children between 8 and 12 years lie because they are unable to meet expectations of family and peers and to impress others. Cheating may be attributed to low self-esteem in the child but is not understood until the child is seven years old. Lying does not suggest low self-esteem.

13. Answer: a
RATIONALE: The nurse should explain to the parent that children between 8 and 12 years of age understand the consequences of their behaviors. They are able to express emotions without using vio-

lence. Children between 6 and 8 years of age begin to see the effects of behaviors on others. Children between 8 and 12 years of age are fully aware of the cause and effect of their behaviors. They also learn discipline techniques with both natural and logical consequences.

14. Answer: b
RATIONALE: The nurse should suggest placing the seven-year-old child in the rear seat with a three-point restraint system. Children under 12 years of age should not be placed in the front seat if the vehicle has an airbag, because it is dangerous. If the child is using a booster seat, the parent should ensure that it is a belt-positioning, forward-facing booster seat with both lap and shoulder belts. The child should not sit in the front seat without a restraint system.

CHAPTER 29

Activity A
1. ossification
2. Exocrine
3. Malocclusion
4. puberty
5. skin
6. function
7. Hispanic
8. identity
9. Peer
10. infancy

Activity B
1. e   **2.** b   **3.** c   **4.** a   **5.** d

Activity C
1.

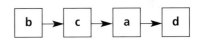

Activity D
1. Completing school prepares the adolescent for college and/or employment. Schools that support peer bonds, promote health and fitness, encourage parental involvement, and strengthen community relationships lead to better student outcomes. Teachers, coaches, and counselors provide guidance and support to the adolescent.
2. To promote appropriate physical growth, the nurse can:
   - Assess parents' and adolescent's knowledge of nutritional needs of adolescents to determine need for further education
   - Educate parents and adolescents about appropriate serving sizes and foods so that they are aware of what to expect for adolescents
   - Determine need for additional caloric intake if necessary

- Plot out height, weight, and body mass index (BMI) to detect a possible pattern
- Assess for risk factors for developing an eating disorder, to refer to if needed, and plan interventions

3. A nurse should suggest the following safety measures:
- Wear a seat belt at all times
- Do not drive with someone who is impaired
- Take a driver education course
- Establish driving rules with parents prior to getting a license
- Have all passengers wear seat belts
- Do not drink and drive
- Do not drive when tired
- Avoid the use of a cell phone while driving
- Maintain car in good condition
- Drive with adult supervision for a period of time after receiving license

4. Practices that prevent and control obesity are
- Proper nutrition and healthy food choices
- Good eating habits
- Decreased fast-food intake
- Exercising for 30 minutes at least four times per week
- Parents/adolescents exercising more at home
- Decreased computer use and television watching

5. Some of the long-term effects and consequences of drug and alcohol use include
- Possibility of overdose and death
- Unintentional injuries
- Irrational behaviors
- Inability to think clearly
- Unsafe driving and legal consequences
- Problems with relationships with family and friends
- Sexual activity and STIs
- Diseases related to the liver and heart

6. The short-term health effects of smoking include damage to the respiratory system, addiction to nicotine, and the associated use of other drug use. Smoking negatively impacts physical fitness and lung growth and increases the potential for addiction in adolescents. Smokeless tobacco may also cause many problems. It can lead to bleeding gums and sores in the mouth that never heal. Smokeless tobacco use leads to discoloration of the teeth and eventually may lead to cancer.

Activity E

1. a. Today, piercings of the tongue, lip, eyebrow, navel, and nipple are common. Generally, body piercing is harmless, but Pamela should be cautioned about undergoing these procedures under nonsterile conditions and about the risk of complications. Qualified personnel using sterile needles should perform the procedure, and proper cleansing of the area at least twice a day is important. Although body piercing is common and considered relatively harmless, complications can occur. Infections usually result from unclean tools. Some of the infections that may occur as a result of unclean tools include hepatitis, tetanus, tuberculosis, and HIV. These complications may not become evident for some time after the piercing has been performed. Also, keloid formation and allergies to metal may occur. The navel is an area prone for infection since it is a moist area that endures friction from clothing. Once a navel infection occurs, it may take up to a year to heal.

b. The nurse should promote effective coping skills by:
- Assessing Pamela's knowledge of normal stress facing teenagers
- Assessing Pamela's present coping skills to determine areas for improvement/support.
- Encouraging Pamela's parents to accept her as a unique individual.
- Discussing with Pamela and her parents normal developmental issues facing teens, to give them knowledge needed to cope.
- Providing different situations Pamela might be faced with and encourage her to develop different solutions.
- Allowing for increasing independence and opportunities to solve her own problems and to improve her coping skills.
- Encouraging Pamela's parents to provide unconditional love to improve her self-esteem.
- Assessing for evidence of any risk-taking behaviors (drugs, smoking, suicide) to identify need for early intervention.

c. Families and parents of adolescents experience changes and conflicts that require adjustments and understanding of the development of the adolescent. The adolescent is striving for self-identity and increased independence. Maintaining open lines of communication is essential but often difficult during this time. Parents sense that they have less influence on the adolescent as the child spends more time with peers, questions family values, and becomes more mobile. To help improve communication, encourage Pamela's mother to set aside an appropriate amount of time to discuss matters without interruptions. Encourage her to talk face-to-face with Pamela and to be aware of both her and Pamela's body language. Suggest that she ask questions about what Pamela is feeling and offer Pamela suggestions and advice. Pamela's mother should choose her words carefully and be aware of her tone of voice and body language. Pamela's mother should listen to what Pamela has to say and should speak to her as an equal. The mother should not pretend to know all the answers and should be able to admit her mistakes. The mother should give praise and approval to Pamela often and to ensure rules and limits are set fairly and discussed.

Activity F

1. Answer: d
RATIONALE: Taking more responsibility for one's behaviors is an Erikson activity for early adolescence. Wondering why things can't change (like wishing her parents were more understanding) and assuming everyone shares her interests are Piaget activities for middle adolescence. Asking broad, unanswerable questions, such as what the meaning of life is, is a Kohlberg activity for early adolescence.

2. Answer: d
RATIONALE: Cheese, yogurt, white beans, milk, and broccoli are good sources of calcium. Strawberries, watermelon, raisins, peanut butter, tomato juice, and whole grain bread are all foods high in iron. Beans, poultry, fish, meats, and dairy products are foods high in protein.

3. Answer: a
RATIONALE: Drowsiness and constricted pupils could be signs of opiate use. Barbiturates typically cause a sense of euphoria followed by depression. Amphetamine use manifests as weight loss, insomnia, tachycardia and hypertension. Marijuana users are typically relaxed and uninhibited.

4. Answer: a
RATIONALE: Checking for signs of depression or lack of friends would be most effective for preventing suicide. All other choices are more effective for preventing violence to others.

5. Answer: b
RATIONALE: The best approach is to describe the proper care (frequent cleansing with antibacterial soap). It is too late for warnings about the dangers of piercing, such as skin- or blood-borne infections, or disease from unclean needles.

6. Answer: d
RATIONALE: If the boy has entered adolescence, he would also have frequent mood changes. A growing interest in attracting girls' attention and understanding that actions have consequences are typical of the middle stage of adolescence. Feeling secure with his body image does not typically occur until late adolescence.

7. Answer: d
RATIONALE: The proper procedure would be to reinsert the tooth into its socket if possible or store it in cold milk or normal saline for transport to the dentist. Asking the child to gargle with cold milk will not help him. Advising him to not play outdoor games in future would not be reasonable. The avulsed tooth should never be discarded as it needs to be reimplanted as soon as possible.

8. Answer: a, b, & d
RATIONALE: Almost all drugs induce euphoria. Weight loss and pressured speech are the manifestations of cocaine. Discoloration of teeth and bleeding gums can be caused by tobacco, not by drugs.

9. Answer: d
RATIONALE: During late puberty, boys will typically experience their first ejaculation, which may occur while they are sleeping (nocturnal emissions). Nurses should provide guidance regarding involuntary nocturnal emissions and assure them that this is a normal occurrence.

10. Answer: d
RATIONALE: It is good if the parents trust their child. However, nurses must remind parents of the importance of peers and the impact they have on the teen's decisions and life choices. Parents must know their teen's friends and continue to be aware of potential problems while allowing the teen the independence to become his or her own person. The other statements do not require any further discussion.

11. Answer: c
RATIONALE: The nurse should discourage the adolescent from squeezing acne lesions to prevent further irritation and permanent scarring. Also, if the adolescent has severe acne, the nurse should encourage him to visit a dermatologist. Washing the face two to three times a day will help him decrease oily skin. The other statements do not call for any further intervention.

12. Answer: a
RATIONALE: The best instruction would be to ask the client to apply and keep reapplying sunscreen or sunblock while being out in the sun. The nurse may warn him about the risk for skin cancer later in life. However, guessing that the boy could have skin cancer can cause unnecessary fear in the adolescent. The other instructions are not helpful.

13. Answer: d
RATIONALE: The best approach for the nurse would be to instruct the boy to cleanse the tattoo with an antibacterial soap and water several times a day. The nurse should also teach him to keep the area moist with an ointment to prevent scab formation. It is too late for warnings that tattoos are wounds or that they could cause an allergic reaction. To ask if it is a mark of a gang membership will not address the immediate health risk caused by the tattoo.

CHAPTER 30

Activity A

1. Developmental
2. medical
3. prevention
4. Screening
5. Inactivated
6. antigens
7. antibodies
8. vision
9. toxins
10. cervical

Activity B

1. The figures show (A) the Weber's test, which screens for hearing by assessing sound conducted via bone, and (B) the Rinne test, which screens for hearing by comparing sound conduction via bone to sound conduction via air.

Activity C

1. d   **2.** c   **3.** a   **4.** b

Activity D

1.

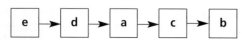

e → d → a → c → b

Activity E

1. There are five types of vaccines.
- Live attenuated vaccines are modified living organisms that are weakened.
- Killed vaccines contain whole dead organisms; they are incapable of reproducing but are capable of producing an immune response.
- Toxoid vaccines contain protein products produced by bacteria called toxins.
- Conjugate vaccines are the result of chemically linking the bacterial cell wall polysaccharide (sugar-based) portions with proteins.
- Recombinant vaccines use genetically engineered organisms.

2. Proper documentation in the child's permanent record includes the following elements:
- Date vaccine was administered
- Name of vaccine (commonly used abbreviation is acceptable)
- Lot number and expiration date of vaccine
- Manufacturer's name
- Site and route by which vaccine was administered
- Edition date of VIS given to the parents
- Name and address of the facility administering the vaccine (where the permanent record will be kept)
- Name of the person administering immunization

3. Rotavirus is the most common cause of severe gastroenteritis among young children. The virus is shed in the stool and easily spreads via the fecal–oral route. Severe, watery, crampy diarrhea quickly leads to dehydration in the infected child. The most severe disease occurs in children ages three to thirty-five months. The rotavirus vaccine is a live vaccine targeting five strains of rotavirus and is administered via the oral route to infants less than thirty-two weeks of age.

4. The psychosocial assessment issues in comprehensive health supervision are as follows:
- Health insurance coverage
- Transportation availability to health care facilities
- Financial stressors
- Family coping effectiveness
- School personnel response to a chronic illness

5. Components of developmental surveillance include:
- Noting and addressing parental concerns
- Obtaining a developmental history
- Making accurate observations
- Consulting with relevant professionals

6. The ability to destroy and remove a specific antigen from the body is called immunity. There are two types of immunity. Passive immunity is produced when the immunoglobulins of one person are transferred to another. This immunity lasts only weeks or months. Passive immunity can be obtained by an injection of exogenous immunoglobulins. It can also be transferred from mothers to infants via colostrum or the placenta. Active immunity is acquired when a person's own immune system generates the immune response. Active immunity lasts for many years or for a lifetime. When an antigen returns, these memory cells very rapidly produce a fresh supply of antibodies to reestablish protection. This immunity can occur after exposure to natural pathogens or after exposure to vaccines.

Activity F

1. a. Other important information would be a nutritional history directly from Jasmine and an activity level history. The nurse should measure her height and weight and plot it on a growth chart to observe a trend.

   b. Screening for iron deficiency is warranted for Jasmine. The increased incidence of iron-deficiency anemia is directly associated with periods of rapid growth and high metabolic demands. The adolescent growth spurt warrants constant iron replacement. The Centers for Disease Control and Prevention recommends universal screening of high-risk children at various age intervals. Jasmine demonstrates risk factors for iron-deficiency anemia, including the rapid growth spurt of adolescence, meal skipping and dieting, and low intake of fish, meat, and poultry. The American Academy of Pediatrics (AAP) recommends universal screening of all adolescent girls during all routine physical examinations, therefore placing Jasmine in this category.

   c. The nurse's focus should be health-centered, not weight-centered. The nurse should emphasize the health benefits of an active lifestyle and nutritious eating pattern. The nurse should educate Jasmine by leveraging her growing autonomy in making self-care decisions. The nurse should encourage healthy eating habits and healthy activity in Jasmine and educate her to limit sedentary activities such as television viewing, computer use, and video games.

Activity G

1. Answer: d

   RATIONALE: The nurse should assess for substandard housing as a contributing factor for asthma in the child. Children from communities experiencing the large-scale breakdown of family relationships and loss of support systems will be at increased risk for depression, violence and abuse, substance abuse, and human immunodeficiency virus (HIV) infection.

2. **Answer: a**

    RATIONALE: Injury prevention and developmental surveillance and screening are additional components of pediatric health supervision visits. Disease prevention and health promotion are also parts of adult health promotion. Immunization is a strategy in disease prevention.

3. **Answer: d**

    RATIONALE: The nurse should use black and white patterns in the infants less than 6 months of age. The nurse can use "tumbling E" and Allen figures for children older than the age of 3 years. These charts allow for a more precise vision assessment and aid the nurse in identifying preschool children with visual acuity problems. By age 5 or 6, most children know the alphabet well enough to use the traditional Snellen chart for vision screening.

4. **Answer: c**

    RATIONALE: Varicella vaccine is administered subcutaneously. Vaccines for influenza, hepatitis A, and pneumococcus are administered intramuscularly.

5. **Answer: a**

    RATIONALE: The client has compromised amino acid metabolism. Phenylketonuria is a disorder of amino acid metabolism and not related to organic-acid metabolism, fatty acid oxidation, and hemoglobin disorders. Multiple carboxylase deficiency is an example of organic acid metabolism disorder. Carnitine uptake defect is an example of fatty acid metabolism disorder. Sickle cell anemia is an example of a disorder of hemoglobin.

6. **Answer: c**

    RATIONALE: Conjugate vaccines drastically increase the immune response when compared with the polysaccharide portion presented alone. Conjugate vaccines are the result of chemically linking the bacterial cell wall polysaccharide (sugar-based) portions with proteins. Live attenuated vaccines are modified living organisms that are weakened. Toxoid vaccines contain protein products produced by bacteria called toxins. Recombinant vaccines use genetically engineered organisms.

7. **Answer: a**

    RATIONALE: Encephalopathy without an identified cause within seven days of the immunization is a contraindication for pertussis vaccination. Immunosuppression, recent blood transfusion, and severe illness with a high fever are reasons for temporary postponement of vaccination.

8. **Answer: c**

    RATIONALE: During hearing screening through Auditory Brainstem Response, the nurse may have to sedate the child if the child is not quiet. When administering pure-tone (conventional) audiom-

etry for children four years and older, the nurse should offer two presentations of stimulus to ensure reliability and administer conditioning trials. When administering Visual Reinforcement Audiometry (VRA) for children between ages six months and two years, the nurse should allow the child to sit in a parent's lap.

9. **Answer: a**

    RATIONALE: Septic arthritis can be prevented by the *Haemophilus influenzae* type B vaccine in children. A combination vaccine of MMR can prevent measles, rubella, and mumps.

10. **Answer: a**

    RATIONALE: The nurse should explain to the mother that poor oral health can have significant negative effects on systemic health. Children who suffer from dental caries have increased incidence of pain, decreased appetite, and sleep pattern disturbances. They are at increased risk for abscesses and systemic infections. Discussing fluoridation and community health are outside the scope of individual dental health discussion. Placing the hands in the mouth exposes the child to pathogens, an issue that is more appropriate to a discussion of personal hygiene promotion. Soft drink consumption is better covered during healthy diet promotion.

11. **Answer: b**

    RATIONALE: Asking about favorite activities would be best for several reasons. It provides assessment of the child's activity preferences, it is health-centered (positive) rather than weight-centered (negative), and it offers variety. If one option does not work, others might. Emphasizing appropriate weight or dietary shortcomings can lead to eating disorders or body hatred. Suggesting softball as the sole activity would limit the success of the healthy weight promotion.

12. **Answer: d**

    RATIONALE: The nurse should use Denver II for developmental screening in the ten-month-old child. Denver II is used to assess personal–social, fine motor–adaptive, language, and gross motor skills. Denver Articulation Screening is used for children two-and-a-half years to seven years of age. Goodenough-Harris Drawing Test is used for screening children who are five to 17 years of age. Battelle Developmental Inventory Screening Test is appropriate for children who are 12 to 96 months of age.

13. **Answer: a, b, & c**

    RATIONALE: The nurse should educate the family members to apply sunscreen lotions, avoid peak sun hours, and wear proper clothing to prevent injury from sunlight. When teaching clients about safe sun exposure, it is very important to remind them that harmful ultraviolet (UV) rays can reflect off water, snow, sand, and concrete. Hand-washing is encouraged when teaching about personal hygiene. Exercise activities would help in maintaining a healthy lifestyle and healthy weight.

14. **Answer: b, c, & e**
    RATIONALE: Hepatitis A is spread through close physical contact and by eating or drinking contaminated food or water. Young children are predisposed to hepatitis A because of their close contact with other children, inadequate hygiene practices, and tendency to place everything in their mouth. Immunosuppression and functional asplenia are indications for pneumococcal vaccines, because these children are at high risk for pneumococcal sepsis.

15. **Answer: c, d, & e**
    RATIONALE: *Streptococcus pneumoniae* (pneumococcus) is the most common cause of pneumonia, sepsis, and meningitis in children under two years of age. Children with long-term health problems such as sickle cell disease, immunosuppression, and diabetes mellitus are immunocompromised;

these conditions place the child at high risk for pneumococcal sepsis. Meningitis and epiglottitis are the infections preventable by the *Haemophilus influenzae* vaccine.

CHAPTER 31

Activity A
1. stadiometer
2. inspection
3. lanugo
4. stridor
5. acrocyanosis
6. vasomotor
7. albinism
8. tympanometer
9. oximetry
10. Cerumen

Activity B
1.

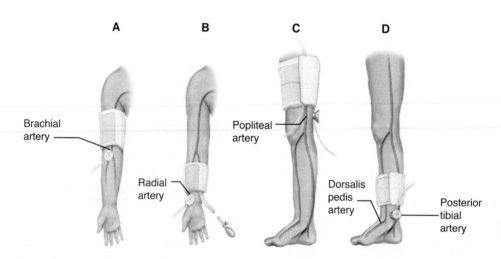

2.

3.

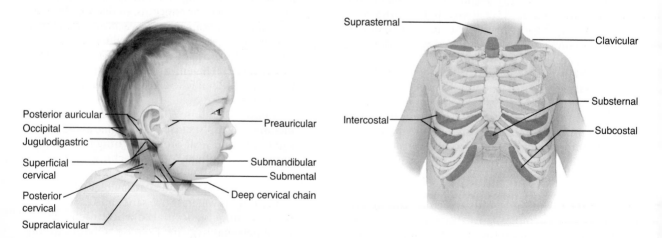

Activity C

1. b   2. a   3. c   4. d

Activity D

1.

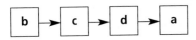

Activity E

1. With the recent increase in obesity in children, BMI is becoming an important measurement. BMI is a measure of body fat and is determined by comparing the child's height and weight. A child whose BMI for age plots at less than the 5th percentile is considered to be underweight. BMI between the 85th and 95th percentiles indicates risk for being overweight. BMI greater than the 95th percentile indicates that the child is overweight. BMI can be calculated by the English formula

$$\frac{\text{Weight in pounds}}{(\text{height in inches}) \times (\text{height in inches})} \times 703$$

and by the metric formula

$$\frac{\text{Weight in kilograms}}{(\text{height in meters}) \times (\text{height in meters})} \times 10{,}000$$

2. The skin is the body's largest organ and reveals information about a child's nutrition, respiratory, cardiac, endocrine, and hydration status, all at a glance. A careful skin examination provides an invaluable understanding of a child's health. Therefore, it is important to inspect the skin.

3. A complete physical examination includes assessment of the general appearance, vital signs, body measurements, and pain, as well as examination of the head, neck, eyes, ears, nose, mouth and throat, skin, thorax and lungs, breasts, heart and peripheral perfusion, abdomen, genitalia and rectum, musculoskeletal system, and neurologic system.

4. The nurse should assess the respiration when the child is resting or sitting quietly, since respiratory rate often changes when infants or young children cry, feed, or become more active. They also tend to breathe faster when they are anxious or scared. The most accurate respiratory rate is obtained before disturbing the infant or child. This can often be done easily when the parent/caregiver is holding the child before any clothing is removed. The nurse should count the respiratory rate for a full minute to ensure accuracy. Infant's respirations are primarily diaphragmatic, so the nurse should count the abdominal movements. After one year of age, the nurse can count the thoracic movements. The nurse should also document the rate, activity of the child, any deviations from normal, and any action taken.

5. Primitive reflexes involve a whole-body response and are subcortical in nature. Most primitive reflexes diminish over the first few months of life.

   Protective reflexes are motor responses related to maintenance of equilibrium. They are necessary for appropriate motor development and remain throughout life once they are established. Selected primitive reflexes present at birth include Moro, root, suck, asymmetric tonic neck, plantar and palmar grasp, step and Babinski. The protective reflexes include the righting and parachute reactions.

6. The PMI is the point on the chest wall where the heartbeat is heard most distinctly. It is just above and outside the left nipple of the infant, at the third or fourth intercostal space. The PMI moves to a more medial and slightly lower area until seven years of age, when it is heard best at the fourth or fifth interspace at the midclavicular line.

Activity F

1. **a.** Blueness of the hands and feet, known as acrocyanosis, results from an immature circulatory system completing the switch from fetal to extrauterine life. It is normal in babies up to several days of age. Therefore, the nurse should assure the client that it is common and does not indicate any lack of care.

   b. The nurse can assess the skin turgor by elevating the skin on the infant's abdomen. The "pinched-up" skin should quickly return to place. If the skin remains tented, it would be a strong indication of moderate to severe dehydration.

   c. Neonatal (erupting by 30 days of age) teeth may pose an aspiration risk, in which case they may have to be extracted. Therefore, the nurse should help them get an appointment with a pediatric dentist.

Activity G

1. **Answer: b**
   RATIONALE: Asking, "What can I help you with today?" is very welcoming and allows for a variety of responses that may include functional problems, developmental concerns, or disease. Asking about the "chief complaint" may not be clear to all parents. Asking if the child feels sick will most likely elicit a yes or no answer and no other helpful details. Asking whether the child has been exposed to infectious agents is unclear and would not open a dialogue.

2. **Answer: b**
   RATIONALE: Preschoolers like to play games. To encourage deep breathing, the nurse could elicit the child's cooperation by engaging the child in a game to blow out the light bulb. Telling the child that he or she may not leave or must breathe deeply would not engage the child. Asking whether the child would allow his or her caregiver to listen would most likely elicit a "no."

3. **Answer: a**
   RATIONALE: The newborn's labia minora are typically swollen from the effects of maternal estrogen. They will decrease in size and be hidden by the labia majora within the first weeks. Lesions on the external genitalia are indicative of sexually transmitted infection. Labial adhesions are not a normal finding for a healthy newborn, nor are swollen labia majora.

4. **Answer: c**
   RATIONALE: The nurse should begin with open-ended questions regarding work, hobbies, activities, and friendships to make the teen feel comfortable. Once a trusting rapport has been established, the nurse should move on to the more emotionally charged questions. Although it is important to ensure confidentiality, the nurse should first establish rapport.

5. **Answer: a**
   RATIONALE: It is best to approach a shy three-year-old by introducing the equipment slowly and demonstrating the process on the girl's doll first. Toddlers are egocentric; referring to how another child performed probably will not be helpful in gaining the child's cooperation. The other questions would most likely elicit a "no" response.

6. **Answer: d**
   RATIONALE: The physical examination of children, just as for adults, always begins with a systematic inspection, followed by palpation or percussion, followed by auscultation.

7. **Answer: b**
   RATIONALE: Touching the thumb to the ball of the infant's foot would elicit the plantar grasp reflex. Palmar grasp reflex is elicited by placing one finger in each of the infant's hands and Babinski by stroking along the lateral aspect of the sole and across the plantar surface. Parachute reflex is elicited when the infant is tilted sideways, forward, or backward.

8. **Answer: d**
   RATIONALE: All infants display some degree of lanugo. Hyperpigmented nevi are a common finding in dark-skinned infants. Cooling or warming the young infant may produce a vasomotor response that causes a mottling of the skin over the trunk and extremities. Rashes are common in children; however, they are often associated with communicable diseases. Therefore, the presence of rashes will need a follow-up.

9. **Answer: b**
   RATIONALE: Visible peristaltic waves are abnormal and should be reported immediately. Because the umbilicus divides the rectus abdominis muscle, an umbilical hernia can protrude through and become larger when the infant or toddler strains or cries. However, it is common and usually disappears as the abdomen becomes stronger. The other observations are normal.

10. **Answer: b**
    RATIONALE: The axillary method works well for children who are neurologically impaired or uncooperative. The thermometer is placed in the axilla and the child's arm is pressed down for 10 seconds to two or three minutes, depending on the model used. The other methods, particularly the oral method of taking temperature, require more cooperation from the client.

11. **Answer: c**
    RATIONALE: This response indicates a positive Romberg test, which warrants further testing for possible cerebellar dysfunction. It is incorrect to interpret that the child has average coordination and balance, as these will be affected by the dysfunction. Leaning when asked to stand still with eyes closed does not indicate an inner ear infection.

12. **Answer: a**
    RATIONALE: The anterior fontanel is usually closed by the age of 9 to 18 months and therefore cannot be felt. Drainage from the ear canal is abnormal. Coarse, dry hair may indicate a thyroid disorder or nutritional deficiency. Dry, brittle nails also indicate a nutritional deficiency. Therefore, the other observations mentioned are not normal and will need further intervention.

13. **Answer: d**
    RATIONALE: Dehydration may be the cause for the sunken fontanels. Most infants have no teeth before the fifth to sixth month. A pink ear canal with tiny hairs and a gray tympanic membrane are normal.

14. **Answer: c**
    RATIONALE: Low-set ears may be associated with genetic abnormalities or syndromes. A newborn may display milia on the forehead, chin, nose, and cheeks, but these recede over time. Similarly, the presence of a greasy, scaly plaque on the scalp is benign and easily treated; therefore, these are not serious health issues. A pink nasal mucosa is normal.

15. **Answer: a**
    RATIONALE: The eyes demonstrate accommodation, or focusing at different distances, if the pupil constricts as the object moves closer. If pupillary reflexive actions are absent, it may indicate blindness. Therefore, unresponsive pupils will not be normal. Blinking of eyes is normal. Strabismus is also not an expected occurrence while checking for accommodation. In fact, persistent strabismus at any age or intermittent strabismus after six months of age should be evaluated by a pediatric ophthalmologist.

CHAPTER 32

Activity A

1. hugging
2. hour
3. bath

4. aversion
5. therapeutic
6. Outpatient
7. protest
8. egocentric
9. motor
10. atraumatic

Activity B

1. The figure shows the cradle method for carrying infants up to three months of age. One hand grasps the infant's thighs; the other arm supports the infant's head and back.
2. The equipment shown in the figure is a wagon with rails and padding used to transport small children.

Activity C

1. e   **2.** a   **3.** b   **4.** d   **5.** c

Activity D

1.

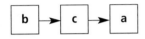

Activity E

1. The nurse caring for the hospitalized child can address and minimize separation anxiety. The nurse should understand the stages of separation anxiety and be able to recognize them in children. Behaviors demonstrated during the first stage do not indicate that the child is "bad." The family should be encouraged to stay with the child. The nurse should help the family deal with various reactions and intervene before the behaviors of detachment occur. The nurse should use guided imagery based on the child's imagination and enjoyment of play to help the child relax.
2. Upon discharge, children and their parents or caregivers receive written instructions about home care, and a copy is retained in the medical record. These instructions are individualized for the child. The nurse needs to assess the family's resources and knowledge level upon admission to determine what education and referrals they may need.
3. Normal fears of childhood include the fear of separation, loss of control, bodily injury, mutilation, or harm. Children's fears are similar to adult fears of the unknown, including fear of unfamiliar environments and losing control. Children may be exposed to equipment, people, situations, and procedures that may be new to them and cause them pain. All these cause fear and increased anxiety for children.
4. The factors affecting a child's response to illness and hospitalization include:
   - Amount of separation from parent/caregiver
   - Age
   - Developmental level
   - Cognitive level
   - Previous experience with illness and hospitalization

- Recent life stresses and changes
- Type and amount of preparation
- Temperament
- Innate and acquired coping skills
- Seriousness of the diagnosis/onset of illness or injury (e.g., acute or chronic)
- Support systems available, including the family and health professionals
- Cultural background
- Parent's reaction to illness and hospitalization

5. The parents of the hospitalized child feel helpless when they play a passive role in their child's care, such as when a medical procedure that hurts or traumatizes the child is required. Then parents attempt to understand by becoming informed and understanding the procedures. Next, they deal with the fear of uncertainty and attempt to promote a sense of comfort by interacting with the hospital staff. Finally, they seek reassurance from the caregivers.
6. The parenting style and the family–child relationship can influence the hospital experience as well as the family members' coping skills. Cultural, ethnic, and religious variations, values, and practices related to illness, general response to stress, and attitudes about the care of a sick child have a significant influence on the family's response and behaviors. Families already in crisis or without support systems have a more difficult time dealing with the added stress of hospitalization.

Activity F

1. **Answer: a**
   INTERVENTION: Assess whether Leslie's irritability is related to the surgery, including pain.
   RATIONALE: The irritability could be related to the surgery, especially pain resulting from the procedure. Once this is ruled out, address the infant's basic needs (trust versus mistrust).
   INTERVENTION: Encourage the family's presence at the bedside and rooming in. Provide consistent nursing staff. Arrange to have a volunteer hold and rock the baby when the family is not present at bedside. Place the baby in a room near the nurses' station.
   RATIONALE: Infants gain a sense of trust in the world through reciprocal patterns of contact. Crying without comfort and lack of stimulation can lead to distress. By 5 to 6 months, infants are acutely aware of the absence of their primary caregiver and may be fearful of unfamiliar persons. Providing caregivers who will address the comfort and care needs of the infant consistently is important for the developing infant. By placing the infant near the nurses' station, response time to crying may be reduced.

Activity G

1. **Answer: b**
   RATIONALE: Children in the first phase of separation anxiety will protest, react aggressively to this separation, and reject others who attempt to comfort

them. In the second phase of separation anxiety, the child displays hopelessness by withdrawing from others, lacking interest in play and food, and exhibiting apathy and depression.

2. **Answer: d**
RATIONALE: It is best to include family members whenever possible so they can help the child cope with any fears. Preschoolers fear mutilation and are afraid of intrusive procedures, and their magical thinking limits their ability to understand things; this requires communication and intervention on their level. Telling the child "we need to put a little hole in your arm" might scare the child. Talking about "taking" or "removing" blood might be interpreted literally.

3. **Answer: a**
RATIONALE: Previous experience with hospitalization can either add to the positive aspects of preparation or distract if the experiences were negative. If the child associates the hospital with the death of a relative, the experience is likely viewed as negative. The other statements would most likely indicate that the child's previous experiences were viewed as positive.

4. **Answer: c**
RATIONALE: Distraction with books or games would be the best way to distract the child from his restricted activity. The other responses would be unlikely to effect a change in the behavior of a six-year-old.

5. **Answer: a**
RATIONALE: Parents who do not tell their child the truth or do not answer his or her questions confuse and frighten the child and may weaken the child's trust in the parents. The other statements are correct and do not indicate a need for further teaching.

6. **Answer: d**
RATIONALE: The initial contact with children and their families forms the foundation for developing a trusting relationship. Asking about a favorite toy would be a good starting point. The nurse should allow the child to participate in the conversation without the pressure of having to comply with a request or undergo any procedures.

7. **Answer: c**
RATIONALE: The nurse needs to describe the procedure and equipment in terms the child can understand. For a four-year-old, a simple explanation along with the chance to touch and feel the tiny tubes would be best. Using the term "tympanostomy tubes" is not age-appropriate and does not teach. Telling the child that she will be asleep the whole time might increase her fears. Showing the child the operating room might increase her fear due to all of the strange and imposing equipment.

8. **Answer: b**
RATIONALE: The nurse understands that a toddler is most likely to develop anxiety and fears due to

separation from the parents. Separation from friends, loss of control, and loss of independence are fears typically experienced by an adolescent.

9. **Answer: c**
RATIONALE: It is important to be honest and encourage the child to ask questions rather than wait for the child to speak up. The other statements are correct and do not indicate a need for further teaching.

10. **Answer: c**
RATIONALE: The best approach would be to write the name of his nurse on a small board and then identify all staff members working with the child (each shift and each day). Reminding the boy he will be going home soon or telling him not to worry does not address his concerns or provide solutions. Encouraging the boy's parents to stay with him at all times may be unrealistic and may place undue stress on the family.

11. **Answer: d**
RATIONALE: The nurse should introduce the child to the health care personnel with whom he or she will come in contact. The nurse should avoid the use of medical terms and instead talk in simple, concrete terms when talking to the child and the parents. The nurse should allow the child to touch and handle some equipment.

12. **Answer: c**
RATIONALE: The nurse should keep one hand on the infant when the crib sides are down, to ensure the infant's safety. The family should be encouraged to maintain home routines while in hospital, planning nursing care around the usual feeding and sleep times. Use of gentle stroking and holding may reduce stress in the infant. A pacifier may be used between feedings to satisfy nonnutritive sucking needs.

13. **Answer: a**
RATIONALE: The nurse should apply an elbow restraint to ensure that the intravenous catheter is not disturbed; it prevents the child from flexing and reaching face, head, IV, and other tubes. A soft limb restraint prevents range of motion of extremities. A mummy restraint secures the whole body of the child or every extremity except for one. A jacket restraint is used to keep children flat in bed, such as after surgery, or safe in a chair.

14. **Answer: d**
RATIONALE: The nurse should ask the parents to offer small cups of fluid and finger foods at frequent intervals, rather than providing large quantities at one time. Children should be offered fluids at different temperatures at different times to promote variety. Children can ingest greater amounts of thin liquids such as gelatin or carbonated drinks than thicker liquids such as cream soups or milkshakes. Ice chips can be included as fluid intake because they supply approximately half the amount of fluid as an equivalent volume of water.

15 Answer: c

RATIONALE: Parents should be allowed to provide all care in the facility; this helps them prepare for discharge from the facility. Parents of children with multiple medical needs benefit from a trial period of caring for the child in the facility. Educational booklets, video-based teaching guides, and a written schedule for medications help the parents when caring for the child at home.

CHAPTER 33

Activity A

1. palliative
2. sensorimotor
3. Technologically
4. screening
5. Home
6. Respite
7. mental
8. family
9. Written
10. Anticipatory

Activity B

1. a   **2.** b   **3.** c   **4.** e   **5.** d

Activity C

1. Vulnerable Child Syndrome is a clinical state in which the parents' reactions to a serious illness or event in the child's past continue to have long-term psychologically harmful effects on the child and parents for many years. Risk factors for the development of Vulnerable Child Syndrome include preterm birth, congenital anomaly, newborn jaundice, handicapping condition, an accident or illness that the child was not expected to recover from, or crying or feeding problems in the first 5 years of life.
2. The inorganic causes of failure to thrive (FTT) include neglect, abuse, behavioral problems, lack of appropriate maternal interaction, poor feeding techniques, lack of parental knowledge, and parental mental illness. Poverty is the single greatest contributing risk factor.
3. Home is the most developmentally appropriate environment for all children, even those who are technology dependent. The child's home provides an emotionally nurturing and socially stimulating environment. Children desire to be cared for at home, and those who are cared for at home display an improved physical, emotional, psychological, and social status.
4. The corrected or adjusted age should be used for evaluating the progression in growth as well as development. For example, if a six-month-old infant was born at 28 weeks' gestation, his growth and development expectations are those for a three-month-old (corrected age). Continue to correct age for growth and development until the child is 3 years old.

5. The Last Acts Palliative Care Task Force has established principles on which palliative care of children should be based. These include
   - Respecting patients' goals, preferences, and choices
   - Comprehensive caring
   - Using the strengths of interdisciplinary resources
   - Acknowledging and addressing caregivers' concerns
   - Building systems and mechanisms of support
6. Hippotherapy is referred to as horseback riding for the handicapped, therapeutic horseback riding, or equine-facilitated psychotherapy. Individuals with almost any cognitive, physical, or emotional disability may benefit from the therapeutic riding or other supervised interaction with horses.

Activity D

1. **a.** The nurse can adopt the following measures to alleviate Georgia's anxiety and fear:
   - Involve the family members in all phases of Georgia's care
   - Explain all aspects of care to Georgia to minimize intervention-related anxiety
   - Answer Georgia's questions honestly
   - Involve Georgia in decision-making whenever possible
   - Limit interventions to those related to palliation
   - Remain with the child when a family member is not around

   b. To support Georgia's family, the nurse should be attuned to their needs and emotions. Families benefit from the presence of the nurse. The nurse should listen to the family and honor the commitment they have made to Georgia. Allowing and encouraging the family customs or rituals in relation to dying and death may help. The nurse may alter the nursing care routine as per the rituals. The nurse should respect the family's need to participate in these rituals and customs.

Activity E

1. **Answer: b**

   RATIONALE: The nurse should teach the parents about cues and behaviors of the baby before the discharge to promote effective home care. Teaching about developmentally appropriate skills, putting emphasis on positive qualities of the baby, and providing consistent caregivers are interventions suitable for promoting growth and development in cases of failure to thrive.
2. **Answer: d**

   RATIONALE: Providing full participation in decision-making gives the adolescent a sense of worth and builds his self-esteem. He also requires direct, honest answers to his questions. However, these actions do not involve self-worth or self-esteem. Helping the child to establish sense of control in daily activities is the best action for a school-going child.

3. **Answer: b**
   RATIONALE: Nurses can help parents build on their strengths and empower them to care for their child by educating them about the course of treatment and the child's expected outcome. Evaluating emotional strength, assessing the home, and preparing a list of supplies would not empower the parents for the task ahead of them.

4. **Answer: c**
   RATIONALE: Young adolescents require time with their peers. Encouraging her to have visitors would best meet this need. Encouraging the child to help make decisions and helping the child to establish a sense of control are interventions suited to school-age children. Explaining her condition in detail meets the needs of an older adolescent.

5. **Answer: a**
   RATIONALE: Serving on his individualized education plan committee will be most beneficial to his education because this plan is designed to meet his educational needs. Collaborating with the school nurse, assessing the health effects of attending school, and discussing future plans would not address his educational needs.

6. **Answer: d**
   RATIONALE: The nurse should educate the child about the illness and course of treatment. Reinforcing that illness is not punishment, beginning developmentally appropriate discipline, and encouraging mastery of self-help skills are the nursing interventions suitable for a preschooler.

7. **Answer: b**
   RATIONALE: Watching the interaction between mother and child to see if the child maintains eye contact may indicate that the child is being neglected, which is an inorganic cause for failure to thrive. Refusing the nipple is a sign of an organic cause for failure to thrive. Prematurity is a risk factor for failure to thrive. Checking the health history may disclose other organic causes for failure to thrive.

8. **Answer: a**
   RATIONALE: The child may be struggling to fit in with his peers by avoiding his treatment regimen in an effort to hide his illness. Monitoring his compliance would disclose this risky behavior. Assessing for depression and encouraging his participation in activities and a support group would not address risky behavior.

9. **Answer: b**
   RATIONALE: Because the child is a toddler, his sense of autonomy would be affected by his medical condition. Sense of trust is affected in infants, sense of initiative is affected in preschoolers, and sense of industry is affected in school-age children.

10. **Answer: c**
    RATIONALE: A former premature baby may develop apnea of prematurity after being discharged from the facility. Attention-deficit disorder, cerebral palsy, and cognitive delay are long-term complica-tions of prematurity. Former premature infants are at higher risk of developing these conditions than the typical infant.

11. **Answer: a**
    RATIONALE: The nurse should provide honest information to the family to help them in end-of-life decision-making. Making judgments on their behalf, asking for clarifications on decisions, and discouraging vacillations in decision-making are inappropriate interventions. The nurse should not make judgments about or question the decisions made by the parents. The nurse should also anticipate that parents may vacillate in the decision-making process.

12. **Answer: d**
    RATIONALE: The nurse should ensure that the transition plan is initiated, because it will help the adolescent in transition to adulthood. Helping to get SSI assistance, informing about online resources, and determining eligibility for insurance would help in strengthening the financial and insurance resources but not in the transition from adolescence to adulthood.

13. **Answer: c**
    RATIONALE: Promoting liaison with community resources is important before the client is discharged from the facility. Encouraging a high level of parental participation, modifying the office routine to promote child comfort, and developing a written health care plan for childcare are nursing interventions suitable for the families of children with special health care needs.

14. **Answer: a**
    RATIONALE: Poor feeding technique is an important inorganic cause of failure to thrive. Inability to swallow correctly, alteration in metabolism, and malabsorption are organic causes of failure of thrive.

15. **Answer: c**
    RATIONALE: The nurse should change the child's position frequently to minimize discomfort. Answering the child's questions honestly, involving the child in decision-making, and explaining all aspects of care to the child would decrease the child's fear and anxiety.

CHAPTER 34

Activity A

1. implanted
2. Pharmacodynamics
3. distraction
4. fifth
5. Hypoglycemia
6. pharmacokinetics
7. Biotransformation
8. residual
9. bolus
10. distal

Activity B

1.

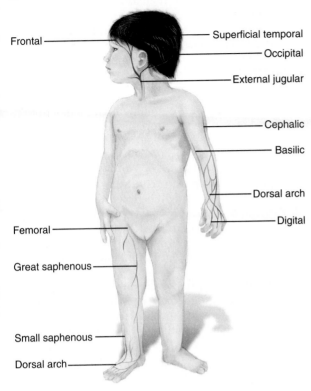

Frontal — Superficial temporal
— Occipital
— External jugular
— Cephalic
— Basilic
— Dorsal arch
— Digital
Femoral —
Great saphenous —
Small saphenous —
Dorsal arch —

2.

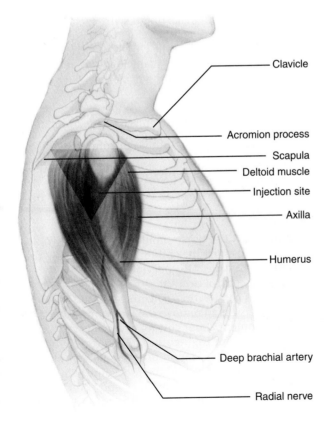

— Clavicle
— Acromion process
— Scapula
— Deltoid muscle
— Injection site
— Axilla
— Humerus
— Deep brachial artery
— Radial nerve

Activity C

1. c   **2.** b   **3.** a   **4.** d

Activity D

1.

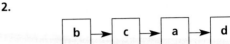

d → b → a → c

2.

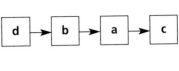

b → c → a → d

Activity E

1. The nurse should check the child's identification. Children may lie about their identity in an attempt to avoid an unpleasant situation, or they may play in another child's bed or remove their ID bracelet. The nurse should confirm the child's identity each time the medication is given and verify the child's name with the caregiver.

2. The physiologic factors affecting distribution of medication in children are:
   - Higher percentage of body water than adults
   - More rapid extracellular fluid exchange
   - Decreased body fat
   - Liver immaturity, altering first-pass elimination
   - Decreased amounts of plasma proteins available for drug binding
   - Immature blood-brain barrier, allowing permeation by certain medications

3. The client should be positioned supine, with the head hyperextended to ensure that the drops will flow back into the nares. The tip of the dropper should be placed just at or inside the nasal opening, and care should be taken not to touch the nares with the dropper. Once the drops are instilled, the child's head should be maintained in hyperextension for at least one minute to ensure that the drops have come in contact with the nasal membranes.

4. - Practice proper hand hygiene
   - Use maximal barrier protection during insertion
   - Check for tube placement before administering any intermittent tube feeding and periodically during continuous tube feeding
   - Assess the site frequently
   - Provide proper site care, using strict sterile technique
   - Ensure that the client's CVC is removed as soon as it is no longer needed

5. A hydroactive dressing method may be used to secure a tube if there is skin breakdown or irritation at the insertion site. The steps are as follows:
   1. Cleanse the skin with soap and water, then rinse; dry well
   2. Cut a 2-by-3-inch piece of hydroactive dressing material, rounding off the corners; cut through to the center and then cut a small hole the size of the tube

3. Remove the paper backing from the hydroactive dressing and apply it to the skin, fitting it snugly around the tube

4. Reapply a new dressing every three to five days or when it becomes wet

6. PPN is used for the short term to supply additional calories and nutrients. TPN provides all the nutrients to meet a child's needs. PPN uses the peripheral vein, whereas TPN involves central venous access. In a case of PPN, the child's nutritional status (prior to PPN) would usually be within acceptable parameters, with decreased or absent oral intake. TPN is administered to a child with a nonfunctioning gastrointestinal (GI) tract, such as with a congenital or acquired GI disorder.

Activity F

1. **a.** When administering a PRN dose of oral acetaminophen, the nurse should
   - Identify the child's condition that warrants PRN medication, based on the order
   - Verify the medication order to ensure that appropriate medication will be administered
   - Calculate the correct dose and the amount to be drawn up from the bottle of acetaminophen
   - Wash hands to prevent infection
   - Verify that the medication is correct and check the expiration date of the medication; verify the time the last dose was given and ensure that it was at least 4 hours ago; verify the ordered route of administration; and draw up the acetaminophen from the bottle with an oral syringe
   - Prepare a bottle of juice, formula, or breast milk
   - Educate Jennifer's parents at the bedside about why the medicine is needed, what the child will experience, the desired effect of the medication, what is expected of the child, and how the parents can participate and support the child
   - Invite the parents to assist and/or give suggestions for techniques
   - Check the child's identification to ensure that medication is given to the right client
   - Administer the medication into the back of the infant's mouth between the teeth and gums; give small amounts and allow the child to swallow before more medicine is placed in the mouth; and have the child upright or at least at a 45-degree angle
   - Offer the infant a sip from the prepared bottle
   - Finally, document the medication administration, and within 30 to 60 minutes document the child's response (recheck temperature)

   b. Dosing for acetaminophen is 10 to 15 mg/kg every 4 to 6 hours. Convert 15 lbs to kg (1 kg = 2.2 lbs). Therefore, 15 lbs equals 6.8 kg; 6.8 kg multiplied by 10 = 68 mg; and 6.8 multiplied by

15 = 102 mg. The range of acetaminophen doses that Jennifer can receive is 68 mg to 102 mg every 4 to 6 hours; therefore, 70 mg q4h is a safe and therapeutic dosage.

   c. 70 mg/× = 80 mg/0.8 mL. Multiply means and extremes and get 56 = 80×. Solve for ×; × = 0.7 mL.

Activity G

1. **Answer: a**
   RATIONALE: The nurse should provide a description of and reason for the procedure in age-appropriate language. The nurse should avoid the use of terms such as *culture* or *strep throat* because they are not age-appropriate for a four-year-old. The nurse should also avoid using confusing terms like *take your blood,* which might be interpreted literally.

2. **Answer: d**
   RATIONALE: Signs of infiltration include cool, puffy, or blanched skin. Warmth, redness, induration, and tender skin are signs of inflammation.

3. **Answer: b**
   RATIONALE: The priority nursing action is to verify the medication ordered. The first step in the eight "rights" of pediatric medication administration is to ensure that the patient is receiving the right medication. After verifying the order, the nurse would then gather the medication and the necessary equipment and supplies; wash hands; and put on gloves.

4. **Answer: c**
   RATIONALE: The parents should never threaten the child in order to make him take his medication. It is more appropriate to develop a cooperative approach that will elicit the child's cooperation, since he needs ongoing, daily medication. The other statements do not indicate a need for further teaching.

5. **Answer: d**
   RATIONALE: The preferred injection site for infants is the vastus lateralis muscle. An alternative site is the rectus femoris muscle. The dorsogluteal site, often used in adults, is not used in children until they have been walking for at least a year. The deltoid muscle is used as an IM injection site in children over 5 years of age because of its small mass.

6. **Answer: b**
   RATIONALE: The nurse should explain what is to occur and enlist the child's help in removing the tape or dressing. This provides the child with a sense of control over the situation and also encourages cooperation. The nurse should avoid using scissors to remove the tape or dressing, and the comment about cutting may be perceived as threatening or frightening. Telling the child to "be a big girl" is inappropriate and does not teach. Telling the child the procedure will not hurt and using the terms "tug" and "pinch" could increase the child's fear and lead to a misunderstanding.

7. Answer: a
RATIONALE: If a dropper is packaged with a certain medication, it should never be used to administer another medication, since the drop size may vary from one dropper to another. The other statements do not require any intervention.

8. Answer: c
RATIONALE: The child's daily requirement is 1,700 mL. Each 24 hours the child will require 100 mL/kg for each of the first 10 kg + 50 mL/kg for each of the next 10 kg + 20 mL/kg for each kg more than 20 kg: $(10 \times 100) + (10 \times 50) + (10 \times 20) = 1,700$.

9. Answer: d
RATIONALE: Yellow, or bile-stained, aspirate indicates intestinal placement. Clear, tan, or green aspirate indicates gastric placement.

10. Answer: a
RATIONALE: Convert the child's weight in pounds into kilograms by dividing it by 2.2 (70 lb/2.2 = 32 kg). Then multiply the child's weight in kilograms by 3 mg (32 kg + 3 mg = 96 mg) for the low end and by 4 mg for the high end (32 kg + 4 mg = 128 mg).

11. Answer: b
RATIONALE: IV therapy may be administered via a peripheral vein or a central vein. Peripheral IV therapy sites commonly include the hands, feet, and forearms. In infants up to about the age of nine months, the scalp veins may be used. Anterior thigh, buttocks, abdomen, and upper arms are the preferred sites for SC administration.

12. Answer: b
RATIONALE: The nurse should always shake the liquid to ensure even drug distribution. The nurse should give the drug in small amounts (0.2 to 0.5 mL). The crushed tablets may taste bitter, so they shouldn't be mixed with essential foods because the child may associate the bitter taste with the food and later refuse to eat it. When a dropper is used, the liquid should be directed toward the posterior side of the mouth.

13. Answer: d
RATIONALE: The nurse should ensure adequate pain relief prior to insertion of the IV device. If possible, the nurse should select a site using hand veins rather than wrist or upper arm veins to reduce the risk of phlebitis. The nurse should encourage parental participation to provide comfort positioning. It is advisable to use a barrier such as gauze, a washcloth, or the sleeve of the child's gown under the tourniquet to avoid pinching or damaging the skin.

14. Answer: b, d, & e
RATIONALE: The nurse should adhere to strict aseptic technique when administering TPN, ensure a closed system at all times, and assess intake and output frequently to reduce the risk of complication. The client will be at risk of hyperglycemia if the TPN infusion is too rapid. No medication, blood, or other solution should be administered through the TPN lumen because it increases the risk for contamination of the system and subsequent infection.

15. Answer: a
RATIONALE: The preferred sites for SC administration include the anterior thigh, buttocks, abdomen, and upper arms. Hands and forearms are among the peripheral IV therapy sites.

CHAPTER 35

Activity A

1. Nociceptors
2. transduction
3. Neuromodulators
4. Oucher
5. tension
6. distraction
7. vasoconstriction
8. brain
9. Epidural
10. depressed

Activity B

1. The figure shows the Oucher pain rating scale.
2. The figure shows a child using the poker chip tool to indicate his degree of "hurt."

Activity C

1. d   2. b   3. a   4. c   5. e

Activity D

1.

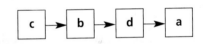

Activity E

1. The point at which the person first feels the lowest intensity of the painful stimulus is termed the pain threshold.
2. Somatic pain refers to pain that develops in the tissues. Superficial somatic pain is also called cutaneous pain. It involves stimulation of nociceptors in the skin, subcutaneous tissue, or mucous membranes. It is typically well localized and is described as a sharp, pricking, or burning sensation. Tenderness is common. Deep somatic pain typically involves the muscles, tendons, joints, fasciae, and bones. It can be localized or diffuse and is usually described as dull, aching, or cramping.
3. Medications bring about effective pain relief. A widely used class of drugs is analgesics. Analgesics typically fall into one of two categories: nonopioid analgesics and opioid analgesics. Anesthetics may also be used for pain relief. Drugs such as sedatives and hypnotics may be used as adjuvant medications to help minimize anxiety or provide or assist with pain relief when typical analgesics are ineffective.

4. Gate control theory explains the process of pain transmission. According to this theory, the dorsal horn of the spinal cord contains interneuronal and interconnecting fibers. These fibers, when stimulated, close the gate or pathway to the brain, thereby inhibiting or blocking the transmission of the pain impulse. Subsequently, the impulse does not reach the brain, where it would be interpreted as pain.

5. The short- and long-term consequences of inadequately treated pain in newborns include hyperalgesia around a wound from occurrences such as repeated heelsticks, an increased risk of developing intraventricular hemorrhage with repeated painful stressors, and a change in the pattern of response to subsequent pain.

6. Imagery involves use of the imagination to create a mental image. This mental image is usually a positive, pleasurable one. It need not be real. When it is used for pain management, the child is encouraged to include details and sensations that are associated with the image, such as specific descriptions of the image's colors, sounds, feelings, and smells. When pain occurs, the child is encouraged to create the mental image or read or listen to the description.

Activity F

1. **a.** Assessment of pain in children consists of both subjective and objective data collection. The acronym QUESTT is an excellent way to remember the key principles of pain assessment.
   - **Q**uestion the child.
   - **U**se a reliable and valid pain scale.
   - **E**valuate the child's behavior and physiological changes to establish a baseline and determine the effectiveness of the intervention. The child's behavior and motor activity may include irritability and protection as well as withdrawal of the affected painful area.
   - **S**ecure the patient's involvement.
   - **T**ake the cause of pain into account when intervening.
   - **T**ake action.

   b. The nurse can use pharmacologic and nonpharmacologic strategies of pain management for the child.
   - The nurse can use topical analgesics as prescribed by the physician.
   - The nurse can use the following nonpharmacologic strategies for pain management in the child:
     - Relaxation techniques, such as instructing the mother to hold closely and stroke the child or telling the child to exhale and inhale slowly
     - Distraction techniques like counting, repetition of specific phrases, listening to music, playing games, blowing bubbles, listening to stories, or watching cartoons
     - Imagery techniques
     - Thought-stopping
     - Positive self-talk

Activity G

1. **Answer: b**
   RATIONALE: The nurse should use the Word–graphic rating scale for pain assessment in the child, because he is 15 years old; this scale is useful for children aged 4 to 17 years. The base age for use of the visual analog and numeric scales is 7 years. The FACES pain-rating scale is suitable for children who are as young as 3 years. The Oucher pain-rating scale is appropriate for children from 3 to 13 years of age. The Poker chip tool is useful for assessing pain in children who are 4 years of age or older.

2. **Answer: a**
   RATIONALE: Clenched fists may indicate pain. Other subtle changes that indicate pain in adolescents include rapid breathing, increased muscle tension, and guarding the affected body part. Physical aggression, intense emotional upset, and a loud cry are responses to pain generally observed in toddlers.

3. **Answer: c**
   RATIONALE: Palmar sweating is a physiologic response to pain. Infants having pain may have palmar or plantar sweating, which can be measured by skin conductivity testing. Infants who have pain will have decreased oxygen saturation, increased heart rate, and decreased vagal tone.

4. **Answer: c**
   RATIONALE: EMLA is contraindicated in children less than 12 months of age who are receiving methemoglobin-inducing agents, such as sulfonamides, phenytoin, phenobarbital, and acetaminophen. Children with dark skin may require longer application times to ensure effectiveness. EMLA is not contraindicated for children less than 6 weeks of age or those undergoing venous cannulation or intramuscular injections.

5. **Answer: d**
   RATIONALE: When caring for a child who has received postoperative epidural analgesia, the priority should be to assess the child for respiratory depression. Respiratory depression, although rare when epidural analgesia is used, is always a possibility. Constipation, easy bruising, and occult blood in the stool are side effects of ibuprofen treatment, and the child should be assessed for these signs.

6. **Answer: a**
   RATIONALE: The nurse should assess for bowel sounds in the child after administering morphine, because it may cause decreased peristalsis and abdominal distension. The nurse should assess for tachycardia and hypertension in clients treated with mixed opioid agents such as pentazocine and butorphanol. Clients who are treated with NSAIDs such as ketarolac and diclofenac should be assessed for signs of bleeding.

7. **Answer: c**
   RATIONALE: Pain-rating scales should be developmentally appropriate for the child to understand

what is being asked. Using the most appropriate tool consistently allows the most accurate assessment of the child's pain. The nurse needs to be consistent in using the same tool so that appropriate comparisons can be made and effective interventions can be planned and implemented. The pain-rating scales should be used 30 minutes to one hour after administering a pain-relief measure.

8. Answer: b
RATIONALE: The score on the Neonatal Infant Pain Scale is 4. Scores for facial expression and state of arousal are 0, and for all the other parameters the score is 1. The scores are then totaled to obtain the final score of 4.

9. Answer: a
RATIONALE: The nurse should use the Riley Infant Pain Scale to assess pain in the infant. It measures these parameters: facial expression, body movement, sleep, verbal or vocal ability, consolability, and response to movements and touch. The Neonatal Infant Pain Scale is used as a behavioral assessment tool for measuring pain in full-term and preterm neonates. The pain observation scale is used for behavioral assessment in children from 1 to 4 years of age. The CRIES scale is the tool used to measure physiologic parameters.

10. Answer: d
RATIONALE: The nurse should instruct the child to create a pleasurable image in his mind as part of imagery for managing pain. When pain occurs, the child is encouraged to create the mental image or read or listen to the description. Repeating positive statements is a part of positive self-talk. Inhaling and exhaling slowly brings about relaxation. Counting numbers is a distraction technique.

11. Answer: c
RATIONALE: The nurse should cover the site with a transparent, occlusive dressing. Applying the cream 30 minutes before the procedure, using two thirds of a five-gram tube for an application, and placing a thin layer of cream on the site of application are inappropriate interventions. The cream should be applied 60 minutes before the procedure. One third to one half of a five-gram tube should be used for an application. The cream should be placed in a thick layer on the site of application.

12. Answer: a, b, & c
RATIONALE: Diaphoresis, tachycardia, and hypertension are due to activation of the sympathetic nervous system occurring during deep somatic pain. Hyperalgia and allodynia are responses to superficial somatic pain caused by thermal, chemical, and mechanical injury or skin disorders.

13. Answer: a, b, & c
RATIONALE: Parameters of facial expressions, increased vital signs, and sleeplessness should be considered when assessing pain in the infant with the CRIES scale. Consolability and vocal

ability are parameters considered when using the Riley Infant Pain Scale.

14. Answer: c, d, & e
RATIONALE: The nurse can use biophysical interventions such as heat application, pressure application, and massage therapy. Biofeedback and thought-stopping are examples of behavioral-cognitive strategies for pain management.

15 Answer: a, c, & e
RATIONALE: When using distraction therapy, the nurse should keep in mind that the type of distraction used depends on the age of the child. For the preschooler client, the nurse may use blowing pinwheels, blowing bubbles, or listening to stories. Computer games and listening to music can be used to distract older children.

CHAPTER 36

Activity A

1. pathogen
2. Antipyretics
3. cryogen
4. Sepsis
5. Pertussis
6. Tetanus
7. exanthems
8. Mumps
9. Parasites
10. Helminthic

Activity B

1. The image shows the rash of scarlet fever. The most striking symptom of scarlet fever is an erythematous rash appearing on the face, trunk, and extremities.
2. The image shows rash associated with Rocky Mountain spotted fever.

Activity C

1. e   2. d   3. c   4. a   5. f   6. b

Activity D

1.

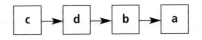

Activity E

1. The risk factors for sepsis related to pregnancy and labor include premature rupture of membranes or prolonged rupture; difficult delivery; maternal infection or fever, including sexually transmitted infections; resuscitation and other invasive procedures; and positive maternal group beta-streptococcal vaginosis.
2. Nursing management of mumps is primarily supportive. Acetaminophen is used for fever manage-

ment. Occasionally narcotic analgesics may be required for pain management. Oral fluids are encouraged to prevent dehydration. If orchitis is present, ice packs to the testicles and gentle testicular support may be helpful. Hospitalized patients are confined to respiratory isolation to prevent the spread of the disease. Infected children are considered not contagious nine days following the onset of parotid swelling.

3. Hyperthermia occurs when normal thermoregulation fails, resulting in an unregulated rise in core temperature. Hyperthermia may occur if disease, drugs, and abnormalities of heat production or thermal stressors impair the central nervous system.

4. Nurses play a key role in educating parents and the community about ways to prevent infectious and communicable diseases. Many infectious diseases can be prevented through frequent handwashing, adequate immunization, proper handling and preparation of food, and judicious antibiotic use.

5. The cellular response to infection involves the arrival of white blood cells to the area. White blood cells are the body's defense against infection or injury. Elevations in certain portions of the white blood cell count reflect different processes occurring in the body, such as infection, allergic reaction, or leukemia.

6. The risk factors that could cause sepsis in a hospitalized child include a stay in the intensive care unit, presence of central line or other invasive lines or tubes, and immunosuppression.

Activity F

1. **a.** When eliciting the history of the present illness, the nurse should inquire about the following:
   - A tick bite
   - Onset of rash
   - Complaints of malaise
   - Mild neck stiffness
   - Headache
   - Fatigue
   - Arthralgia or pain in the joints

   In late disease, the nurse should note recurrent arthritis of the large joints, such as the knees, beginning weeks to months after the tick bite. The child with late disease may or may not have a history of earlier stages of the disease, including erythema migrans.

   b. In most cases Lyme disease can be cured by antibiotics, especially if they are started early in the illness. Doxycycline is the drug of choice for children older than 8 years. Because it can cause permanent discoloration of the teeth, and Nicholas is less than 8, he should be treated with amoxicillin. For patients allergic to penicillin, cefuroxime or erythromycin can be used. Duration of treatment is usually 14 to 21 days.

   c. The nurse can teach the client the following to prevent tick-borne illnesses:

- Wear appropriate protective clothing when entering tick-infested areas. Clothing should fit tightly around wrists, waists, and ankles. Tuck pants into socks, if possible.
- After leaving the area, check for ticks, and remove them promptly.
- Insect repellent may provide temporary relief but may produce toxicity, especially in children, if used frequently, or in large doses.

Activity G

1. **Answer: b**
   RATIONALE: Recurrent arthritis in large joints, such as the knees, is an indication of late-stage Lyme disease. The appearance of erythema migrans would suggest the early-localized stage of the disease. Facial palsy or conjunctivitis would suggest the child is in the early-disseminated stage of the disease.

2. **Answer: c**
   RATIONALE: If the family had been camping or in a wooded area, the girl could have been bitten by a tick, which would not be easy to discover because of her long hair. Ticks like dark, hair-covered areas, and the signs and symptoms presented are neurologic, with a rapid onset, which can be characteristic of a tick bite. The other questions are important but do not focus on the causative agent.

3. **Answer: c**
   RATIONALE: It is very important to ensure that the correct dose is given at the proper interval because an overdose can be toxic to the child. Concerns about allergies and taking the entire prescribed dose are appropriate precautions when administering antibiotics and all medications. Drowsiness is not a side effect of antipyretics.

4. **Answer: d**
   RATIONALE: The nurse should obtain the urine specimen before antibiotics are administered to ensure that the sensitivity result is accurate. The entire volume of urine is not required for culture; the specimen is obtained by midstream clean-catch or catheterization. Stool specimen for culture is obtained on three different days. Placing bags on the perineum is not acceptable because of the high chance of contamination.

5. **Answer: a**
   RATIONALE: The usual sites for obtaining blood specimens are the veins on the dorsal side of the hand or the antecubital fossa. A young infant will benefit from the use of oral sucrose via pacifier before and during the capillary puncture. Accessing an indwelling venous access device may be appropriate if the child is in an acute care setting. An automatic lancet device is used for capillary puncture of an infant's heel.

6. **Answer: a**
   RATIONALE: Infants and young children are more susceptible to infection due to the immature responses of their immune systems. Cellular immu-

nity is generally functional at birth. Humoral immunity develops after the child is born. Newborns have a decreased inflammatory response. Young infants lose the passive immunity from their mothers, but disease protection from immunizations is not complete.

7. Answer: a
RATIONALE: The presence of petechiae can indicate serious infection in an infant. Grunting is abnormal, indicating respiratory difficulty. Fever and irritability in the two-month-old is normal after immunizations. The four-month-old needs to be watched but is adequately hydrated. The eight-month-old also needs to be watched, but restlessness and irritability is common in infants who are teething and is not indicative of illness.

8. Answer: d
RATIONALE: Penicillin V and erythromycin are the preferred antibiotics for treatment of scarlet fever. Scarlet fever transmission is airborne, not via droplet. Lymphadenopathy occurs with cat-scratch disease and diphtheria. Close monitoring of airway status is critical with diphtheria because the upper airway becomes swollen.

9. Answer: c
RATIONALE: The nurse should avoid squeezing the foot during specimen collection, because it may contribute to hemolysis of the specimen. The nurse should clean the site of the heel puncture with an antiseptic prep pad and allow it to dry. The first drop of blood should be wiped with dry gauze or a cotton ball. After obtaining the sample, the nurse should hold a dry gauze over the site until bleeding stops and then apply a bandage.

10. Answer: c
RATIONALE: The nurse should provide the child with mitts, gloves, or socks to cover the hand or keep the child's fingernails short to prevent injury to the skin, leading to increased pain. The child is offered warm fluids to ease the discomfort of a sore throat. Cool compresses or a cool bath provides comfort to the child with pruritus. The child should be dressed in light clothing, not warm clothing, because diaphoresis can lead to increased pruritus.

11. Answer: d
RATIONALE: The nurse should encourage parents to give an antipyretic to the child before sponging. Parents need to call the physician if the child's temperature is greater than 40.6° C. The child should be dressed lightly; warm, binding clothes or blankets should be avoided. Parents should use tepid water, not cold water or alcohol, for sponging; they should also ensure that sponging does not produce shivering.

12. Answer: a, b, & e
RATIONALE: Ticks should be removed with the help of fine-tipped tweezers. Fingers should be protected with tissue, a paper towel, or latex gloves.

After removal of the tick, the site should be cleaned with soap and water and the hands washed thoroughly. Grasp the tick as close to the skin as possible and pull upward with steady, even pressure, without twisting or jerking.

13. Answer: c
RATIONALE: The nurse should inform the parents that all wounds should be cleaned thoroughly and a proper antiseptic used. Booster immunizations are given every ten years, not five years. Tetanus is not manifested as rash; initial signs include headache, spasms, crankiness, and cramping of the jaw (lockjaw), which are followed by difficulty swallowing and a stiff neck. Booster immunization may be needed if the wound is contaminated and it has been more than five years since the last tetanus dose.

14. Answer: b, c, & e
RATIONALE: Parents should be asked to ensure that cats do not lick open wounds on the child. Any bites or scratches should be washed thoroughly with soap and running water. Parents should ensure control of fleas in pet cats. There is no immunization available for cat scratch disease. Transmission-based isolation is not required, because the disease is not transmitted from person to person.

15 Answer: b, c, & e
RATIONALE: The nurse should ask the caregiver to soak combs in pediculicide, shampoo, or hot water. Headgear, towels, and pillowcases should be washed in hot water and dried in the hot cycle. Household and other close contacts should be examined and treated if infested; bedmates should be treated prophylactically. Parents need not isolate the child or avoid sending the child to school. In cases of scabies, bedding and clothing worn four days prior to treatment are washed in hot water.

CHAPTER 37

Activity A

1. Myelinization
2. microcephaly
3. Sunset
4. febrile
5. Kernig's
6. Aseptic
7. Hypoxia
8. Migraines
9. plagiocephaly
10. contusion

Activity B

1. (A) Decorticate: the child is curled up, similar to a fetal position. (B) Decerebrate: the child's limbs are extended.
2. (A1) Kernig's sign is tested by flexing legs at the hip and knee. (B1) Brudzinski's sign is tested by having the child lay supine with the neck flexed.

3. A newborn is positioned for a lumbar puncture. The newborn is positioned upright with head flexed forward.

Activity C

1. a   **2.** e   **3.** c   **4.** b   **5.** d

Activity D

1.

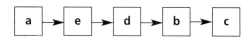

Activity E

1. An infant displaying the opisthotonic posture will hyperextend its head and neck to relieve discomfort due to bacterial meningitis.
2. The Pediatric Glasgow Coma Scale is a popular scale used to standardize degrees of consciousness. It consists of three parts: eye opening, verbal response, and motor response.
3. The following precautions should be taken for a child with seizures:
   - Padding the side rails and other hard objects
   - Keeping side rails raised at all times when child is in bed
   - Keeping oxygen and suction at bedside
   - Supervising, especially during bathing, ambulation, or other potentially hazardous activities
   - Having child use a protective helmet during activity may be appropriate
   - Having child wear a medical alert bracelet
4. Neonatal seizures occur within the first 4 weeks of life and are most commonly seen within the first 10 days. They are different from those in the child or adult because generalized tonic-clonic seizures tend not to occur during the first month of life. Seizures in newborns are associated with underlying conditions such as hypoxic-ischemic encephalopathy, metabolic disorders (hypoglycemia and hypocalcemia), neonatal infection (meningitis and encephalitis), and intracranial hemorrhage.
5. Breath-holding is usually triggered by the child becoming angry or stressed after not getting his or her way. It can also occur as a reflexive response to fear, pain, or being startled.
6. A cerebral vascular disorder is a sudden disruption of the blood supply to the brain. It affects neurologic functioning, such as movement and speech. Two major types of cerebral vascular disorders are seen in children just as in adults: ischemic stroke and hemorrhagic stroke.

Activity F

1. **a.** Has Jessica been taking the medication as directed? When was the phenobarbital level last determined? What is the dosing of Jessica's phenobarbital? Has Jessica been sick or had a fever lately? Does Jessica have a history of a head injury? Did Jessica hit her head during the seizure? What was Jessica doing before the seizure? Could Jessica have accidentally ingested a medication or chemical? Physical assessment should include vital signs, oxygen saturation, neurological assessment, and overall assessment for any signs of injury.

   b. The nurse should anticipate the following tests:
   - CBC
   - Electrolytes
   - Culture (if febrile)
   - Phenobarbital level
   - Toxicology, if ingestion of medicine or chemicals is suspected
   - Lumbar puncture, if signs of central nervous system infection are present
   - Imaging studies, such as CT or MRI, if head injury is suspected

   c. If the child is standing or sitting, ease her to the ground if possible, cradle her head, and place her on a soft area. Do not attempt to restrain her. Place her on one side and open her airway if possible. Place blow-by oxygen by the child and have suction ready if needed. Remove any sharp or potentially dangerous objects. Tight clothing and jewelry around the neck should be loosened if possible. Observe length of seizure and activity such as movements, as well as cyanosis or loss of bladder or bowel control, and any other characteristics about the child's condition during the seizure. If the child's condition deteriorates or seizures persist, call for help. Report seizures to the health care provider promptly. Administer anticonvulsants as ordered. Remain with the child until she is fully conscious. Allow postictal behavior without interfering while providing environmental protection. When possible, reorient the child. Accurately document information in the chart, including preseizure activity. Provide emotional support and education to the family. Obtain anticonvulsant levels as ordered.

   d. Discuss seizure warning signs. Teach the family to recognize warning signs and how to care for the patient during and after a seizure. Discuss the disease process and prognosis of the condition and the need for lifelong treatment if indicated. Teach parents the need for routine medical care and the importance of having the child wear a medical bracelet. Review the medication regimen and the importance of maintaining a therapeutic medication level and administering all prescribed doses. Encourage the parents to discuss with the child why she does not want to take the medicine. Explain to the child in simple terms why the medicine is needed and how it will help her. Encourage participation from the health care provider and parents. Discuss alternative ways to administer phenobarbital, such as crushed tablets or elixir, with the health care provider and family. Urge the family to use an understanding and gentle—yet firm—approach with medication administration. Encourage the family to give medicine at the same time and place, which helps create a routine. Help the family to identify creative strategies to gain the child's cooperation, such as using a sticker chart and allowing the child to do more, such as administering the medication. Offer choices when possible, such as, "Do you want your medicine before or after your bath, and would you like to have apple or grape juice after your medicine?" Praise the child's improvements.

Activity G

1. **Answer: a**
RATIONALE: The nurse should place the infant on the abdomen when awake and supervise the infant. The use of a car seat outside of the automobile should be discouraged. A rolled washcloth should be placed along the right side to discourage turning the head in that direction. Placing the infant in a left-lateral or supine position will cause flattening of the skull on the left side or in the back, respectively. It is important to keep changing the infant's position.

2. **Answer: c**
RATIONALE: Horizontal nystagmus is a symptom of lesions on the brain stem. Vertical nystagmus indicates brainstem dysfunction. Sunset eyes indicate increased intracranial pressure. One dilated but reactive pupil indicates intracranial mass.

3. **Answer: b, c, & e**
RATIONALE: The nurse should assess for poor feeding, weak cry, constipation, listlessness, and generalized weakness in an infant with botulism. Continual vomiting and hyperreflexia are seen in children with Reye's syndrome.

4. **Answer: a**
RATIONALE: Signs and symptoms for contusions include disturbances in vision, strength, and sensation. A child with a concussion will be distracted and unable to concentrate. Vomiting is a sign of a subdural and epidural hematoma. Bleeding from the ear is a sign of a basilar skull fracture.

5. **Answer: b**
RATIONALE: The child's level of consciousness is obtunded if the child has limited responses to the environment and falls asleep unless stimulated. Confusion is defined as a state in which disorientation exists; the child may be alert but responds inappropriately to questions. Stupor exists when the child responds only to vigorous stimulation. Coma defines a state in which the child cannot be aroused, even with painful stimuli.

6. **Answer: c**
RATIONALE: Video electroencephalograms determine the precise localization of the seizure area in the brain. Cerebral angiography is used to diagnose vessel defects or space-occupying lesions. Lumbar puncture diagnoses hemorrhage, infection, or obstruction. Computed tomography is used to diag-

nose congenital abnormalities such as neural tube defects.

7. **Answer: b**
RATIONALE: A "cracked pot" sound on percussing the infant's head indicates separation of the sutures. This finding is known as Macewen's sign. It does not indicate smallness of the skull, swelling in the brain, or intracranial hemorrhage.

8. **Answer: a, c, & e**
RATIONALE: The nurse should know that a normal EEG, absence of tachycardia and elevated blood pressure, and suppression of nonepileptic movement by gently restraining the limb are characteristics of a nonepileptic seizure. A nonepileptic seizure is accompanied by tremors and jitteriness. Ocular deviation may be seen with seizure activity but will not be present with nonepileptic seizure.

9. **Answer: c**
RATIONALE: A febrile seizure lasts a few seconds to ten minutes. The nurse should also know that the seizure may stop before the child receives medication. The child's core temperature is likely to increase to 39°C or higher. A febrile seizure usually presents as a generalized tonic-clonic seizure.

10. **Answer: b**
RATIONALE: The nurse should recognize projectile vomiting as an early sign of intracranial pressure. Lowered level of consciousness, bradycardia, and fixed and dilated pupils are late signs of intracranial pressure.

11. **Answer: c**
RATIONALE: The nurse should instruct the parents not to restrain the child during a seizure. The child should be placed on his or her side and the airway opened if possible. The child's jaws should not be opened with a tongue blade or fingers. If the child has a seizure while sitting, he or she should be eased to the ground if possible.

12. **Answer: b**
RATIONALE: The nurse should look for signs of spasticity and upper extremity weakness in an adolescent client with type II Arnold-Chiari malformation. Choking and gagging, weight loss, and coarse upper airway sounds are signs seen in infants with type II Arnold-Chiari malformation; symptoms in older clients are subtler and less frequently life-threatening.

CHAPTER 38

Activity A

1. conjunctivitis
2. adenoids
3. tympanic
4. Blepharitis
5. myopia
6. diplopia
7. Infantile

8. sensorineural
9. Tympanometry
10. antibiotics

Activity B

1. The figure explains the variation in the length and positioning of eustachian tubes between children and adults. The child's eustachian tube is relatively shorter and wider and is positioned horizontally.
2. (A) Bacterial conjunctivitis: redness of conjunctiva and eyelid swelling are seen in bacterial conjunctivitis.
   (B) Allergic conjunctivitis: clear, watery discharge is identified, along with redness of the conjunctiva.

Activity C

1. d   **2.** c   **3.** a   **4.** e   **5.** b

Activity D

1.

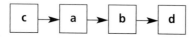

Activity F

1. Children with astigmatism have blurry vision and difficulty seeing letters as a whole. Their ability to read is affected and they may have headaches or dizziness. Older children may complain of eye fatigue or strain. Children with astigmatism often learn to tilt their head slightly so that they can focus more effectively.
2. Strabismus refers to misalignment of the eyes. It is common and occurs in about 4% of children. The most common types of strabismus are exotropia and esotropia. In exotropia the eyes turn outward and in esotropia they turn inward. The complications of strabismus include amblyopia and visual deficits.
3. Legal blindness is a term used to refer to vision less than 20/200 or peripheral vision less than 20 degrees. In most cases, vision may be augmented with corrective lenses. Some blind children can differentiate light versus dark, while others live in total darkness.
4. Conductive hearing loss results when transmission of sound through the middle ear is disrupted. When the fluid fills the middle ear, the tympanic membrane is unable to move properly, and partial or complete hearing loss occurs.
5. Risk factors for otitis media with effusion (OME) include passive smoking, absence of breast-feeding, frequent viral upper respiratory infections, allergy, young age, male sex, adenoid hypertrophy, Eustachian tube dysfunction, and certain congenital disorders.
6. Nystagmus refers to a very rapid, irregular eye movement. It is described by some as bouncing of the eyes. It may occur in children with congenital cataracts, but the most common cause is a neurologic problem. It is difficult for the brain and eyes

to communicate when the eyes are in continuous motion; thus, visual development may be affected.

Activity F

1. **a.** The nurse can adopt the following interventions to relieve pain in the child:
   - Administer analgesics as prescribed.
   - Apply a warm compress or heating pad to the affected ear.

   The nurse can adopt the following interventions to treat the infection in the child's ear:
   - Administer antibiotic or antifungal eardrops as prescribed.
   - Place a wick in the ear to keep the antibiotic drops in contact with the skin of the ear canal and promote healing.
   - Restrain the child for his safety, during wick insertion, because it can be extremely painful.

   b. The nurse should suggest the following measures to the mother to prevent otitis externa:
   - Avoid the use of cotton swabs, headphones, and earphones.
   - Wear earplugs when swimming.
   - Promote ear canal dryness and alternate pH. Use one or more of the following methods:
     - Dry the ear canals with a hair dryer set on a low setting.
     - Administer solutions that have a drying effect on the auditory canal skin and change the pH of the canal to discourage organism growth in susceptible children. The following solutions can be used:
       - A few drops of Domeboro solution can be placed in the canal and then allowed to run out.
       - A mixture of half rubbing alcohol and half vinegar (squirted into the canal and then allowed to run out). The alcohol solution should be used only when the ear canals are healthy. Using it while the canals are inflamed will cause stinging and increased pain.

Activity G

1. **Answer: a**
   RATIONALE: A mixture of half rubbing alcohol and half vinegar squirted into the canal and then allowed to run out is a good preventive measure, but not when inflammation is present. Cotton swabs should not be used to dry the ears. The boy can wash his hair as needed. Antibiotics should be used only for otitis media with bacterial infection.
2. **Answer: d**
   RATIONALE: Proper hand-washing by the care provider is the single most important factor to reduce the spread of acute infectious conjunctivitis. Not sharing face cloths or towels with the child, keeping the child home from school until she is no longer infectious, and encouraging the child to keep her hands away from her eyes are sound pre-

ventive measures but not as important as frequent hand-washing.

3. **Answer: a**
RATIONALE: Teaching the parents the importance of patching the child's eye as prescribed is most important for the treatment of strabismus. Ultraviolet-protective glasses are needed after surgery for cataracts. Multiple operations may be needed for infantile glaucoma. Teaching the importance of completing the full course of oral antibiotics is appropriate for periorbital cellulitis.

4. **Answer: a**
RATIONALE: Therapeutic management of amblyopia may be achieved by using atropine drops in the better eye, so educating parents on how to use atropine drops would be the most helpful intervention. While follow-up visits to the ophthalmologist are important, compliance with treatment is the first priority. Protecting the operative site with eye patching is the nursing intervention for strabismus. The child who has a refractive error should be encouraged to wear glasses regularly.

5. **Answer: a**
RATIONALE: Assessing for asymmetric corneal light reflex would be the priority intervention, because strabismus may develop in the child with regressed retinopathy of prematurity. Observing for signs of visual impairment would not be critical for this child, nor would teaching the parents to check whether his glasses fit. Referral to an early intervention program would be appropriate if the child were visually impaired.

6. **Answer: d**
RATIONALE: The nurse should assess for the presence of photophobia. Erythema will be present in scleral hemorrhage; bruising and edema of the lid would be present in black eye.

7. **Answer: b**
RATIONALE: Recurrent viral URTI contributes to the development of otitis media with effusion. Frequent swimming would put the child at risk for otitis externa. Although otitis media is a risk factor for infective conjunctivitis, infective conjunctivitis is not a risk factor for otitis media with effusion. Having moisture in the ear canal will cause otitis externa.

8. **Answer: c**
RATIONALE: Deep suturing may result in ptosis at a later date, so the child should be referred to an ophthalmologist. Scleral hemorrhage resolves gradually without intervention. Black eye needs ice, observation, and analgesics. Corneal abrasions may self-heal.

9. **Answer: d**
RATIONALE: The nurse should be aware of tympanosclerosis as a complication of acute otitis media. Chlamydial pneumonia is a complication of chlamydial conjunctivitis in neonates. Orbital cellulitis is a complication of periorbital cellulitis. Amblyopia is a complication of strabismus.

10. **Answer: a**
RATIONALE: Glaucoma is a complication that occurs after cataract surgery. Blindness and myopia are complications of retinopathy of prematurity. Strabismus is also a complication of retinopathy of prematurity but occurs in regressed retinopathy of prematurity (ROP).

11. **Answer: a**
RATIONALE: Reassessing for language acquisition would be most important to the health of the child. There is a risk that otitis media with effusion may cause hearing loss as well as speech, language, and learning problems. Parents should not use over-the-counter drugs to alleviate the child's symptoms, nor should they smoke around her. Also, children who were bottle-fed have a higher occurrence of this disorder. However, these concerns are not as important as language acquisition.

12. **Answer: d**
RATIONALE: The corneal light reflex is extremely helpful in the assessment of strabismus. It consists of shining a flashlight into the eyes to see if the light reflects at the same angle in both eyes. Strabismus is present if the reflections are not symmetrical. The visual acuity test measures how well the child sees at various distances. Refractive and ophthalmologic examinations are comprehensive and are performed by optometrists and ophthalmologists.

13. **Answer: c**
RATIONALE: By age two to three years, the visual acuity of most children is 20/50. At birth, acuity ranges from 20/100 to 20/400; 20/20 visual acuity is achieved between 6 and 7 years of age.

14. **Answer: c**
RATIONALE: In the postoperative period, the nurse should restrain the child's elbow to prevent the child from rubbing the eyes. Encouraging the parents to comply with ongoing visual assessment and teaching the parents how to administer postoperative medications are important interventions after surgery for infantile glaucoma but not immediately after surgery. Encouraging muscle exercise of the eye is an important intervention in children with amblyopia.

15. **Answer: a**
RATIONALE: Low birth weight increases the risk for developing retinopathy of prematurity. Developmental delay and genetic syndrome are risk factors for developing visual impairment. Astigmatism is a risk factor for strabismus.

CHAPTER 39

Activity A
1. Clubbing
2. Stridor

3. expiration
4. Reye
5. pharyngitis
6. atelectasis
7. tracheostomy
8. tachypnea
9. pancreatic
10. Pallor

Activity B

1. The figure explains the variation in diameter of a child's airway under normal circumstances and in the presence of edema.
2. It is a chest x-ray that shows the presence of a foreign body in the bronchus.

Activity C

1. a   2. b   3. c   4. e   5. d

Activity D

1.

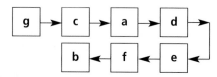

Activity E

1. Nasopharyngitis is normally known as common cold. It is also referred to as a viral upper respiratory infection (URI). Colds can be caused by a number of different viruses, including rhinoviruses, parainfluenza, RSV, enteroviruses, and adenoviruses. Recently, human meta-pneumovirus has been identified as an important cause of the common cold.
2. Cystic fibrosis is an autosomal recessive disorder. A deletion occurring on the long arm of chromosome 7 at the cystic fibrosis transmembrane regulator (CFTR) is the responsible gene mutation. DNA testing can be used prenatally and in newborns to identify the presence of the mutation.
3. A collection of air in the pleural space is called a pneumothorax. It can occur spontaneously in an otherwise healthy child, or as a result of chronic lung disease, cardiopulmonary resuscitation, surgery, or trauma. Trapped air consumes space within the pleural cavity, and the affected lung suffers at least partial collapse. Needle aspiration and/or placement of a chest tube is used to evacuate the air from the chest.
4. Common laboratory and diagnostic studies ordered for the assessment of pneumonia include pulse oximetry, chest x-ray, sputum culture, and white blood cell count.
5. The complications of respiratory distress syndrome include tachypnea, retractions, nasal flaring, grunting, and varying degrees of cyanosis. Auscultation reveals fine rales and diminished breath sounds. If untreated, RDS progresses to seesaw respirations, respiratory failure, and shock.

6. Epistaxis occurs most frequently in children younger than adolescent age. The nursing assessments include exploring the child's history for initiating factors such as local inflammation, mucosal drying, or local trauma (usually nose picking). Inspect the nasal cavity for blood.

Activity F

1. The nurse should teach parents to:
   - Avoid letting the child play with toys with small parts and keep coins and other small objects out of the reach of children.
   - Avoid feeding peanuts and popcorn to the child until he or she is at least three years old.
   - When children progress to table food, chop all foods so that they are small enough to pass down the trachea if the child does not chew them up thoroughly.
   - Carrots, grapes, and hot dogs should be cut into small pieces.
   - Harmful liquids should be kept out of the reach of children.

Activity G

1. **Answer: d**
   RATIONALE: The nurse should provide continuous ventilatory and oxygen support for the newborn. Anti-inflammatory inhaled medications are used for maintenance, and short-acting bronchodilators are used as needed for wheezing episodes. Chest physiotherapy with postural drainage may be required in infants with cystic fibrosis but is not recommended in infants with bronchopulmonary dysplasia. The nurse may have to restrict fluids rather than keep the infant well hydrated. The nurse should provide a high caloric intake to promote growth and to compensate for the calories expended by the increased work of breathing. Therefore, providing a light, low-calorie intake is not recommended.

2. **Answer: d**
   RATIONALE: Oxygen administration is indicated for the treatment of hypoxemia. Suctioning removes excess secretions from the airway caused by colds or flu. Saline lavage loosens mucus that may be blocking the airway so that it may be suctioned out. Saline gargles are indicated for relieving throat pain, as with pharyngitis or tonsillitis.

3. **Answer: a**
   RATIONALE: Secretions in the lower trachea cause wheezing that clears with coughing. Wheezing, a high-pitched sound that usually occurs on expiration, results from obstruction in the lower trachea or bronchioles. Wheezing caused by obstruction in the bronchioles does not clear with coughing. Fluid-filled alveoli do not cause wheezing; they cause rales. Intrathoracic foreign body causes prolonged expiration.

4. Answer: a
RATIONALE: Rales, or crackling sounds, are heard on auscultation in the child with pneumonia due to fluid-filled alveoli. Wheezing results from obstruction of the bronchioles, as in bronchiolitis, asthma, and chronic lung disease.

5. Answer: a
RATIONALE: Clubbing might occur in children with a chronic respiratory illness. It is an enlargement of the terminal phalanx of the finger, resulting in a change in the angle of the nail to the fingertip. Clubbing is the result of increased capillary growth as the body attempts to supply more oxygen to distal body cells. Epistaxis, pneumonia, and influenza are acute conditions and do not cause clubbing.

6. Answer: d
RATIONALE: Eyelid edema is a characteristic of involvement of the ethmoid sinus. Irritability, halitosis, and facial pain are generally observed in children with sinusitis; they are not indicative of involvement of the ethmoid sinus.

7. Answer: a
RATIONALE: Atelectasis in the client manifests as absent fremitus. Increased tactile fremitus might occur in a case of pneumonia or pleural effusion. Fremitus might be decreased in the case of barrel chest, as with cystic fibrosis.

8. Answer: a
RATIONALE: If the airway becomes completely occluded due to epiglottitis, respiratory arrest and death may occur. Additional complications include pneumothorax and pulmonary edema. Otitis media may be a complication of influenza; aseptic meningitis is a complication of infectious mononucleosis; and children with pneumonia would present with retraction of the chest wall.

9. Answer: d
RATIONALE: Performing nasal washes with normal saline may keep the nasal mucus from becoming thickened, preventing secondary bacterial infection. The nasal wash also decongests the nose, allowing for improved nasal airflow. Oral antihistamines are used to treat allergic conditions. Anti-inflammatory (corticosteroid) nasal sprays can help to decrease the inflammatory response to allergens. Teaching parents how to avoid allergens such as tobacco smoke, dust mites, and molds helps prevent recurrence.

10. Answer: a
RATIONALE: Infants consume twice as much oxygen (6 to 8 liters) as adults (3 to 4 liters). This is due to their higher metabolic and resting respiratory rates. Term infants are born with about 50 million alveoli, which is only 17% of the adult number of around 300 million. The tongue of the infant, relative to the oropharynx, is larger than

in adults. Infants and children will develop hypoxemia more rapidly than adults when in respiratory distress.

11. Answer: c
RATIONALE: The child is at risk for developing pneumonia if she has aspirated a foreign body. If the child is allergic to dust, then the child may be at risk for allergic rhinitis. The child may be at increased risk for tuberculosis if there is concurrent HIV infection. If the child was born prematurely, the child may be at risk for chronic lung disorder.

12. Answer: c
RATIONALE: A flutter valve device is used to help mobilize secretions for older children and adolescents with cystic fibrosis. The family would not need to learn about metered-dose inhalers, nebulizers, and peak flow meters because these are used for asthma therapy.

13. Answer: c
RATIONALE: Complications of chronic tracheostomy include the formation of granulation tissue around the insertion site. Other complications include infection and cellulitis. Hemorrhage, air entry, pulmonary edema, anatomic damage, and respiratory arrest are the immediate postoperative complications.

14. Answer: a
RATIONALE: Until the family adjusts to the demands of the disease, they can become overwhelmed and exhausted, which can lead to noncompliance. However, over time, they will gain understanding of the illness and the required treatments and will become experts on the child's care. Typical challenges for the family are that they become overly vigilant, the child feels fearful and isolated, and the siblings are jealous or worried.

CHAPTER 40

Activity A

1. electrophysiologic
2. Coarctation
3. Cardiomyopathy
4. Kawasaki
5. Hypothermia
6. Hypercyanosis
7. Congenital
8. Aortic
9. Prehypertension
10. apex

Activity B

1. The figure shows fetal and newborn circulation with oxygen-rich, poor, and mixed blood.

2. The figure shows an opening between the two atria, revealing atrial septal defect.

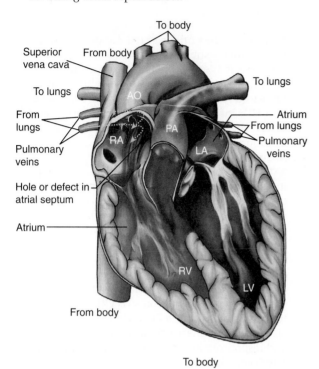

Superior vena cava

To body

From body

To lungs

AO

From lungs

To lungs

Atrium

From lungs

PA

Pulmonary veins

RA

LA

Pulmonary veins

Hole or defect in atrial septum

Atrium

RV

LV

From body

To body

Activity C

1. c   **2.** a   **3.** b   **4.** d

Activity D

1. The three types of ASDs are identified according to the location of the opening. In ostium primum (ASD1), the opening is located at the lower portion of the septum. In ostium secundum (ASD2), the opening is located near the center of the septum. In sinus venosus defect, the opening is located near the junction of the superior vena cava and the right atrium.

2. The fetal heart is developed within the first 21 days of gestation, with development of the heart rate and fetal blood circulation. The four chambers of the heart and arteries are formed during gestational months 2 through 8. During fetal development, oxygenation of the fetus occurs via the placenta. The lungs, though perfused, do not perform oxygenation and ventilation. The foramen ovale, an opening between the atria, allows blood flow from the right to the left atrium. The ductus arteriosus allows blood flow between the pulmonary artery and the aorta.

3. Tetralogy of Fallot is a congenital heart defect that actually comprises four heart defects: pulmonary stenosis, VSD, overriding aorta, and right ventricular hypertrophy. Surgical intervention is usually required during the first year of life. The rate for survival into adulthood with a good functional long-term result is greater than 90%.

4. TAPVC is a rare congenital heart defect in which the pulmonary veins do not connect normally to the left atrium; instead, they connect to the right atrium, often by way of the superior vena cava. Males exhibit this disorder more often than females.

5. The common manifestations of heart failure in a child with CHD are:
- Failure to gain weight or rapid weight gain
- Failure to thrive
- Difficulty feeding
- Fatigue
- Dizziness, irritability
- Exercise intolerance
- Shortness of breath
- Sucking and then tiring quickly
- Syncope
- Decreased number of wet diapers

6. Orthotopic transplantation is a process of transplantation in which the recipient's heart is removed and the donor heart is implanted in its place in the normal anatomic position. Cardiopulmonary bypass and hypothermia are used to maintain circulation, protect the brain, and oxygenate the recipient during the procedure. Postoperatively the child may have near-normal heart function and capacity for exercise.

Activity E

1. a. The nurse should carry out the following preprocedural assessments:
- Obtain vital signs
- Note fever or other symptoms of infection
- Obtain the child's weight to aid in medication dosage calculation
- Check the results of laboratory tests of blood and urine
- Perform a complete physical examination
- Assess peripheral pulses, with particular attention to pedal pulses
- Mark the pedal pulses with indelible marker

b. The postprocedural nursing interventions are as follows:
- Closely monitor the baby for complications of bleeding, arrhythmia, hematoma, thrombus formation, and infection.
- Evaluate vital signs, neurovascular status of lower extremities, and pressure dressing over catheterization area.
- Monitor cardiac rhythm and oxygen saturation via pulse oximetry.
- Assess the baby's pedal pulses.
- Assess the color and temperature of the extremity.
- Check capillary refill and sensation in the extremities.
- Monitor intake and output regularly.
- Provide the parents with education prior to discharge.

Activity F

1. **Answer: a**
   RATIONALE: The normal infant heart rate averages 120 to 130 bpm; the toddler's or preschooler's is 80 to 105; the school-age child's is 70 to 80 bpm; and the adolescent's is 60 to 68 bpm.

2. **Answer: d**
   RATIONALE: Clubbing of fingers and toes indicates congenital heart disease due to severe hypoxia. Narrow or thready pulse may occur in children with heart failure or severe aortic stenosis. Prominence of precordial chest wall is seen in children with cardiomegaly. Edema in lower extremities indicates left ventricular failure.

3. **Answer: a**
   RATIONALE: The nurse should monitor serum potassium in the child receiving Aldactone. Platelet count, serum glucose, and liver enzymes should be monitored in the client who is receiving indomethacin.

4. **Answer: b**
   RATIONALE: The normal adolescent's blood pressure is 100–120/50–70 mm Hg. The normal infant's blood pressure is about 80/40 mm Hg. The toddler or preschooler's blood pressure averages 80–100/64 mm Hg. The normal school-age child's blood pressure averages 94–112/56–60 mm Hg.

5. **Answer: a**
   RATIONALE: The nurse should expect to hear a soft or moderately loud systolic murmur at the base of the heart when auscultating the child with coarctation of the aorta. Systolic murmur at the left sternal border is heard in aortic stenosis. Systolic ejection murmur is heard at the upper left sternal border in pulmonary stenosis. Fixed splitting of the second heart sound is heard in total anomalous pulmonary venous connection.

6. **Answer: d**
   RATIONALE: Early surgical correction is required for a ventricular septal defect to prevent pulmonary hypertension. Ventricular dysrhythmia and AV block are the postoperative complications of a ventricular septal defect. Infective endocarditis develops as a complication of an untreated ventricular septal defect.

7. **Answer: b**
   RATIONALE: The nurse should monitor for complete heart block when caring postoperatively for an infant who underwent pulmonary artery banding surgery. Monitoring for ventricular dysrhythmias is the postoperative intervention for ventricular septal defect. Monitoring for atrial arrhythmias and left ventricular dysfunction is important when monitoring a child after surgery for tricuspid atresia.

8. **Answer: d**
   RATIONALE: The nurse should withhold the administration of digoxin if the apical pulse is <90 in the infant. A serum digoxin level between 0.8 ng/ml and 2 ng/ml is therapeutic and does not require discontinuation. Signs of hypotension and a BP

range falling more than 15 mm Hg are considered when administering antihypertensive agents.

9. **Answer: d**
   RATIONALE: Pulsed-dose corticosteroids are used to prevent coronary dilatation in Kawasaki disease. In the acute phase of management, a high dose of aspirin in four divided doses and a single intravenous immunoglobulin dose are used. If fever persists longer than 48 hours after the initiation of aspirin therapy, the child may receive a second dose of intravenous immunoglobulin.

10. **Answer: d**
    RATIONALE: During the acute phase of Kawasaki disease a CBC would reveal an elevation of the white blood cell count. Platelet count is elevated in the later phase of the disease. Hematocrit and RBC count are elevated in children with congenital heart diseases such as tetralogy of Fallot.

11. **Answer: a**
    RATIONALE: Some medications taken by pregnant women, such as lithium, may be linked with the development of congenital heart defects (CHDs). Febrile illness during the first trimester, not the third, may be linked to an increased risk of congenital heart defects. Repeated exposure to x-rays and strong cleaning products after pregnancy is not linked with CHD.

12. **Answer: b**
    RATIONALE: A bounding pulse is a characteristic of patent ductus arteriosus. Clients with coarctation of the aorta demonstrate weak pulses in the lower extremities. Presence of chest pain similar to angina is usually found in the client with aortic stenosis. Dyspnea and cyanosis are common findings in the client with pulmonary stenosis.

13. **Answer: c**
    RATIONALE: Edema of the lower extremities is characteristic of right ventricular heart failure in older children. In infants, peripheral edema occurs first in the face and then the presacral region and the extremities.

14. **Answer: c**
    RATIONALE: A mild to late ejection click at the apex is typical of a mitral valve prolapse. Abnormal splitting or intensifying of S2 sounds occurs in children with major heart problems, not mitral valve prolapse. Clicks on the upper left sternal border are related to the pulmonary area.

15. **Answer: a**
    RATIONALE: Malar rashes should be inspected for in the hypertensive client. Polymorphus rash, desquamation, and erythema should be inspected for in the client with Kawasaki disease.

CHAPTER 41

Activity A

1. regurgitation
2. Dysphagia

3. retching
4. fungal
5. Cholelithiasis
6. Hepatobiliary
7. omphalomesenteric
8. hypovolemic

9. Diarrhea
10. pylorus

Activity B

1. A colostomy is a stoma from the colon; an ileostomy is a stoma from the ileum.

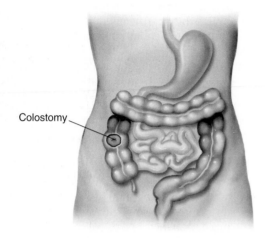

Colostomy

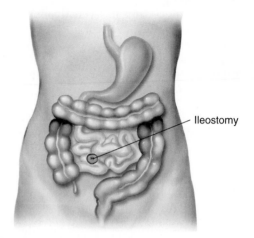

Ileostomy

Activity C

1. d   2. c   3. a   4. b

Activity D

1. The basal metabolic rate in infants and children is higher than that of adults in order to support growth. This higher metabolic rate, even in states of wellness, accounts for increased insensible fluid losses and increased need for water for excretory functions. The young infant's renal immaturity does not allow the kidneys to concentrate urine as well as in older children and adults. This puts infants at particular risk for dehydration or overhydration, depending upon the circumstances.

2. The child's hydration status often indicates how severe the current GI illness is. The oral mucosa should be checked to see if it is pink and moist. Skin turgor should be checked for its elasticity. Decreased turgor and tenting indicate dehydration. Assessing the amount of urine output the patient has had in the past 24 hours is another way to check hydration status.

3. Appendicitis is an acute inflammation of the appendix. It is the most common cause of emergent abdominal surgery in children. It occurs in all age groups; the median range in the pediatric population is four to 15 years. Appendicitis is considered a surgical emergency because, if left uncorrected, the appendix may perforate. Surgical removal of the appendix is necessary and is often accomplished via minimally invasive laparoscopic technique. In cases of perforation, an open surgical procedure is usually required, and lavage of the abdominal cavity may

be performed to cleanse it of the infected fluid released from the appendix.

4. A nurse can make the following interventions to help maintain appropriate nutrition in children with GI disorders:
   - Encourage favorite foods (within prescribed diet restrictions if present) to maximize oral intake.
   - Administer enteral tube feedings as ordered to maximize caloric intake.
   - Add butter, gravy, or cheese as appropriate to foods (if allowed within diet restrictions) to increase caloric intake.
   - Encourage high-quality, high-calorie snacks between meals, so as not to interfere with meal intake.
   - Document response to feeding to determine feeding tolerance.
   - Limit intake of calorie-free beverages; beverages should contain nutrients and calories.
   - Consult nutritionist for appropriate diet supplementation recommendations.

5. Intussusception is a process that occurs when a proximal segment of bowel "telescopes" into a more distal segment, causing edema, vascular compromise, and ultimately partial or total bowel obstruction. Intussusception usually occurs in otherwise healthy infants under age two. A barium enema is successful at reducing a large percentage of intussusception cases; other cases are reduced surgically. If surgical reduction is unsuccessful or bowel necrosis has occurred, a portion of the bowel must be resected.

6. Gastroesophageal reflux is passage of gastric contents into the esophagus. It is considered a normal

physiologic process that occurs in healthy infants and children. However, when complications develop from the reflux of gastric contents back into the esophagus or oropharynx, it becomes more of a pathologic process known as gastroesophageal reflux disease (GERD).

Activity E

1. **a.** The nurse should encourage parents to hold the medically stable infant immediately after delivery to encourage bonding. The nurse should acknowledge normal feelings of guilt, anger, and sadness, and support the parents in providing care for the infant, particularly in feeding, which is viewed as a significant nurturing function. The nurse must also provide education about the surgical procedures and eventual normal appearance of the child's lip.

   b. To prevent injury to the facial suture line and to the palatal operative sites, the nurse should ask the parents to:
   - Not allow the infant to rub the facial suture line or the palatal operative sites. To prevent this, position the infant in a supine or side-lying position.
   - Use arm restraints, if necessary, to stop the hands from touching the face or entering the mouth.
   - Clean the suture as ordered by the surgeon.
   - Use possible care options of petroleum jelly on the facial suture line or a lip-protective device such as a Logan bow or a butterfly adhesive.
   - Avoid putting items in the infant's mouth that might disrupt the sutures (e.g., suction catheter, spoon, straw, pacifier, or plastic syringe).
   - Prevent vigorous or sustained crying in the infant, because this may cause tension on either suture line. Ways to prevent crying include administering medications as needed for pain and providing other comfort or distraction measures, such as cuddling, rocking, and anticipation of needs.

Activity F

1. **Answer: b**
   RATIONALE: Palpable kidneys, except in neonates, may indicate a tumor or hydronephrosis. The liver should be palpated during inspiration below the right costal margin. The sigmoid colon can be palpated in the left lower quadrant. The cecum may be felt in the right lower quadrant as a soft mass.

2. **Answer: a**
   RATIONALE: The ostomy pouch should fit closely around the stoma to avoid acidic stool contact with skin and thereby prevent its irritation. Liquid stool output can be acidic, causing irritation and severe burn-like areas on the surrounding skin, so special attention to skin care around the ostomy site is essential. Products such as powders and pastes can be used to help protect the skin. The ostomy pouch should also be emptied and measured for stool output several times a day.

3. **Answer: a**
   RATIONALE: A nurse should help the toddler maintain a clear liquid diet, though not longer than 24 hours, because a prolonged diet of clear liquids will result in continued liquid stools. Milk products should be avoided until diarrhea improves. The nurse should encourage complex carbohydrate foods to bulk up the stools. Fats can be added to carbohydrates to increase intestinal transit time to encourage water absorption.

4. **Answer: c**
   RATIONALE: Tap water, milk, undiluted fruit juice, soup, and broth are not appropriate for oral rehydration. The other statements do not indicate any need for further intervention.

5. **Answer: d**
   RATIONALE: Anorexia is one of the few intestinal symptoms of Crohn's disease. The other features mentioned are of symptoms of ulcerative colitis.

6. **Answer: d**
   RATIONALE: Positioning after feedings is important. For infants, the head of the crib should be elevated 30 degrees. The other statements do not require any further intervention.

7. **Answer: c**
   RATIONALE: The only current treatment for celiac disease is a strict gluten-free diet. Eliminating gluten will cause the villi of the intestines to heal and function normally, with subsequent improvement of symptoms. Even very small amounts of gluten introduced back into the diet can cause damage to the villi, so the patient must adhere to a gluten-free diet throughout life. Because of this, it would be inappropriate to say that gluten intake should be restricted only until he is an adolescent.

8. **Answer: a, c, & d**
   RATIONALE: Children at risk for thrush include those with immune disorders and those receiving therapy that suppresses the immune system (e.g., chemotherapy for cancer). Children who use corticosteroid inhalers are also at increased risk for the development of thrush. Antibiotic use may also contribute to thrush. Excessive intake of formula can cause chronic diarrhea. Excessive vomiting is a risk factor for dehydration.

9. **Answer: a, c, & e**
   RATIONALE: The common signs and symptoms of intussusception include:
   - sudden onset of intermittent and crampy abdominal pain
   - severe pain
   - vomiting
   - diarrhea
   - lethargy
   - currant-jelly stools, gross blood, or Hemoccult-positive stools

Abdominal distention and tachycardia are symptoms of malrotation. Abdominal distention can also indicate enterocolitis.

10. **Answer: a, c, & d**
    RATIONALE: Heartburn or chest pains, halitosis (mostly in older children), and poor dentition (caused by acid erosion) are a few of the signs and symptoms of GERD. Explosive stools and rectal bleeding are signs of enterocolitis.

11. **Answer: c, d, & e**
    RATIONALE: The most common causes of short bowel syndrome are necrotizing enterocolitis, small intestinal atresia, gastroschisis, malrotation with volvulus, and trauma to the small intestine. Stretched rectal vault is associated with encopresis. Lack of ganglion cells in the bowel can cause Hirschsprung's disease.

12. **Answer: a, c, & d**
    RATIONALE: The clinical presentation of a child with autoimmune hepatitis includes hepatosplenomegaly, jaundice, fever, fatigue, and right upper quadrant pain. Abdominal distention and steatorrhea are symptoms of celiac disease.

13. **Answer: c**
    RATIONALE: Hemoccult checks for occult blood in the stool, which helps determine bleeding in the GI tract. In ERCP, a fiberoptic endoscope is used to view the hepatobiliary system. Esophageal manometry tests the esophagus. A small bowel series is done in conjunction with an upper GI series to visualize the small intestine contour, position, and motility.

14. **Answer: b**
    RATIONALE: When symptoms have lessened or resolved, the nurse should reintroduce a regular diet to reduce the number of stools, provide adequate nutrition, and shorten the duration of the effects of illness. The nurse should offer small amounts of oral rehydration solution frequently to maintain balance. High-carbohydrate fluids should be avoided, because they are low in electrolytes, and increased simple carbohydrate consumption can decrease stool transit time. The nurse should discourage ingestion of fluids and milk products that contain high levels of sugar during the acute phase of illness, because these products may worsen diarrhea.

15 **Answer: b**
    RATIONALE: The nurse should assess whether the hernia can be reduced. If it is possible, the nurse should teach the patient and family how to reduce the hernia. Most umbilical hernias are not corrected surgically. Surgical correction is necessary only for the largest umbilical hernias that have failed to close by age five years. The use of home remedies to reduce an umbilical hernia should be discouraged because of the risk of bowel strangulation. This includes taping a quarter over a reduced umbilical hernia and the use of "belly bands."

CHAPTER 42

Activity A
1. suppression
2. Vesicostomy
3. urethral
4. cystourethrogram
5. Renal
6. hypoalbuminemia
7. glomerulonephritis
8. Dipstick
9. Peritoneal
10. Circumcision

Activity B
1. The figure shows bladder exstrophy. The bladder has a bright-red color.
2. The figure shows hydronephrosis and the variation of the pelvis in a normal and a distended kidney.

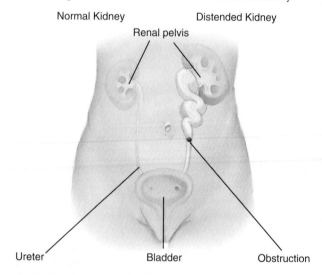

Normal Kidney   Distended Kidney
Renal pelvis

Ureter   Bladder   Obstruction

3. A: Arteriovenous fistula; B: Arteriovenous graft

Activity C
1. e   2. a   3. b   4. d   5. c

Activity D
1.

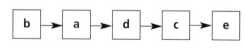

b → a → d → c → e

Activity E
1. Following cystoscopy, the nurse should encourage ingestion of fluids and monitor vital signs. The nurse must also be aware that the child may feel burning with voiding after the procedure and the urine may have a pink tinge.
2. Vesicoureteral reflux is a condition in which urine from the bladder flows back up the ureters. This reflux of urine occurs during bladder contamination with voiding. Reflux may occur in one or both ureters. If the reflux occurs when the urine is in-

fected, the kidney is exposed to bacteria and pyelonephritis may result.

3. Hydronephrosis is a condition in which the pelvis and calyces of the kidney are dilated. It occurs as a congenital defect, as a result of obstructive uropathy, or secondary to vesicoureteral reflux. It may be revealed on prenatal ultrasound. Complications include renal insufficiency, hypertension, and eventually renal failure.

4. There are four types of enuresis: primary, secondary, nocturnal, and diurnal.
   - Primary enuresis: enuresis in the child who has never achieved voluntary bladder control.
   - Secondary enuresis: urinary incontinence in the child who previously demonstrated bladder control over a period of at least 3 to 6 consecutive months.
   - Diurnal enuresis: daytime loss of urinary control.
   - Nocturnal enuresis: nighttime bedwetting.

5. Vitamin D and calcium are used to correct hypocalcemia and hyperphosphatemia; ferrous sulfate for anemia; Bicitra or sodium bicarbonate tablets to correct acidosis; multivitamins to augment nutritional status; erythropoietin injections to stimulate red blood cell growth; and growth hormone injections to stimulate growth in stature.

6. Hydrocele (fluid in the scrotal sac) is usually a benign and self-limiting disorder. It is usually noted early in infancy and often resolves spontaneously by 1 year of age. Varicocele (a venous varicosity along the spermatic cord) is often noted as a swelling of the scrotal sac. Complications of varicocele include low sperm count or reduced sperm motility, which can result in infertility.

Activity F

1. a. Kevin presented with fatigue and abdominal pain, which are common signs of acute glomerulonephritis. His age, which is above two years, and sex (male) are risk factors, too. However, the following signs and symptoms may also help confirm acute glomerulonephritis:
   - Fever
   - Lethargy
   - Headache
   - Decreased urine output
   - Vomiting
   - Anorexia

   The nurse should also assess the child's current and past medical history for risk factors such as a recent episode of pharyngitis or other streptococcal infection.
   b. Though there is no specific medical treatment for APSGN, the nurse can perform the following interventions when caring for Kevin:
   - Administer antihypertensives such as labetalol or nifedipine and diuretics as ordered
   - Monitor blood pressure frequently
   - Maintain sodium and fluid restrictions as prescribed during the initial edematous phase

- Weigh the child daily on the same scale and wearing the same amount of clothing
- Monitor increasing urine output and note improvement in the urine color
- Document resolution of edema
- Provide careful neurological evaluation, because hypertension may cause encephalopathy and seizures
- Ensure bed rest during the acute phase, when children with APSGN are generally fatigued
- Provide the child with age-appropriate activities and cluster care to allow rest periods
- Enable management at home if edema is mild and if the child is not hypertensive. The nurse should teach the family to monitor urine output and color, take blood measurements, and restrict the diet as prescribed. The child cared for at home should not participate in strenuous activity until proteinuria and hematuria are resolved.
- If renal involvement progresses, dialysis may become necessary

Activity G

1. **Answer: c**
   RATIONALE: Urinalysis is ordered to reveal preliminary information about the urinary tract. The test evaluates the color, pH, specific gravity, and odor of urine. Urinalysis also assesses for presence of protein, glucose, ketones, blood, leukocytes, esterase, RBCs, WBCs, bacteria, crystals, and casts. Total protein, globulin, albumin, and creatinine clearance would be ordered for suspected renal failure or renal disease. Urine culture and sensitivity are used to determine the presence of bacteria and determine the best choice of antibiotic.

2. **Answer: c**
   RATIONALE: The nurse should administer the drug in the morning and encourage fluids and voiding during and after administration to decrease the risk of hemorrhagic cystitis. Drug allergy is checked before antibiotic administration. When the client is on human chorionic gonadotropin for a long term, the nurse should monitor the client for precocious puberty. Cyclophosphamide is administered in the morning.

3. **Answer: b**
   RATIONALE: The nurse should note the condition as secondary enuresis because the child has become incontinent after demonstrating bladder control over a period of three to six consecutive months. Primary enuresis occurs in the child who has never achieved voluntary bladder control. Diurnal enuresis is the daytime loss of urinary control. Nocturnal enuresis refers to nighttime bedwetting.

4. **Answer: c**
   RATIONALE: Hemolytic uremic syndrome is defined by these three features: hemolytic anemia, thrombocytopenia, and acute renal failure. Dirty green-colored urine, elevated erythrocyte sedimentation

rate, and depressed serum complement level are indicative of acute glomerulonephritis. Hypertension, not hypotension, would be seen, and the child would have decreased urinary output, which would not cause nocturia.

5. **Answer: a**
RATIONALE: The nurse should immediately notify the physician if there is absence of a bruit. The nurse should always auscultate the site for the presence of a bruit and palpate for the presence of a thrill. Dialysate without fibrin or cloudiness indicates infection in the client who is undergoing peritoneal dialysis. Alteration in blood pressure is an important parameter in both peritoneal dialysis and hemodialysis that should be reported to the physician but may not necessitate immediate notification, as would an absence of bruit.

6. **Answer: c**
RATIONALE: The nurse should withhold routine medications on the morning that hemodialysis is scheduled because they would be filtered out through the dialysis process. His medications should be administered after he returns from the dialysis unit. Liberal diet and fluid intake should be allowed in peritoneal dialysis. A Tenckhoff catheter is used for peritoneal dialysis, not Hemodialysis. The nurse should avoid measuring blood pressure in the extremity with the AV fistula as it may cause occlusion.

7. **Answer: a**
RATIONALE: The nurse should monitor renal function and electrolytes when administering Lasix to the client. Monitoring for hyperkalemia is important when administering angiotensin converting enzymes (ACEs). Monitoring for the development of pulmonary edema is important when administering Muromonab–CD3. Monitoring for the signs of infection is necessary when administering cytotoxic drugs.

8. **Answer: b**
RATIONALE: The nurse should avoid prolonged use of the tourniquet while drawing the blood for serum calcium because it may cause a false increase in calcium levels. Allowing the child to be NPO after midnight is considered when sending the blood for phosphorus levels. Obtaining a specimen prior to the testing is done when sending urine for culture and sensitivity. The child must have a full bladder when undergoing urodynamic studies.

9. **Answer: d**
RATIONALE: Epispadias is characterized by the presence of the urethral opening on the dorsal surface of the penis. In hypospadias, the urethral opening is on the ventral surface of the penis. Bladder exstrophy is a structural disorder where a midline closure defect occurs during the embryonic period of gestation, leaving the bladder open and exposed outside of the abdomen. Hydronephrosis is a con-

dition in which the pelvis and calyces of the kidney are dilated.

10. **Answer: d**
RATIONALE: History of intrauterine growth retardation is a risk factor for the child with nephrotic syndrome. Prune belly syndrome and chromosome abnormalities are risk factors for obstructive uropathy. Neurogenic bladder is the risk factor for UTI.

11. **Answer: b**
RATIONALE: Wearing cotton underwear will reduce the incidence of perineal irritation. Bubble bath increases the risk of developing urinary tract infection, so it should be avoided. The nurse should instruct the client not to wipe from back to front after voiding. Wiping from front to back after each voiding will prevent contamination of the urethra with rectal material. The client should be discouraged from holding urine to prevent stasis and infection.

12. **Answer: a**
RATIONALE: The nurse should consider testicular torsion a surgical emergency because necrosis of the testis may occur, causing gangrene and subsequently infertility. Management of hydrocele, phimosis, and varicocele is not an emergency and surgery is done only after the child has reached one year of age.

13. **Answer: c**
RATIONALE: The nurse should monitor for signs of muscle twitching in the child to assess hypocalcemia. Muscle weakness, abdominal cramps, and irregular pulse are signs of hyperkalemia.

14. **Answer: c**
RATIONALE: Presence of a yellowish-gray discharge in the client with vulvovaginitis indicates infection with *Trichomonas vaginalis*. White cottage-cheese-like discharge can be seen when *Candida albicans* is the causative organism. Thin gray discharge indicates presence of *Bordetella* or *Gardnerella* species organisms. Brownish-green discharge indicates unhygienic practices.

15. **Answer: a**
RATIONALE: Vesicoureteral reflux is an indication for undergoing voiding cystourethrogram. Urinary outlet obstruction and kidney tumor are indications for intravenous pyelogram. Hydronephrosis is an indication for renal ultrasound.

CHAPTER 43

Activity A

1. autoimmune
2. atrophy
3. dystrophy
4. contractures
5. neurogenic
6. lumbosacral
7. Meningocele

8. corticosteroids
9. scoliosis
10. Kernicterus

Activity B

1. **A:** Meningocele; **B:** Myelomeningocele
2. The neuromuscular disorder is known as spinal muscular atrophy (SMA). It is a genetic motor neuron disease that affects the spinal nerves' ability to communicate with the muscles.

Activity C

1. b   2. a   3. c   4. e   5. d

Activity D

1.

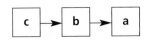

Activity E

1. The four classifications of cerebral palsy are spastic, athetoid (dyskinetic), ataxic, and mixed. Spastic is the most common form and ataxic is the rarest.
2. Nursing management of a child with myelomeningocele focuses on preventing infection, promoting bowel and urinary elimination, promoting adequate nutrition, preventing latex allergic reaction, maintaining skin integrity, providing education and support to the family, and recognizing complications such as hydrocephalus or increased intracranial pressure (ICP) associated with the disorder.
3. Fairly symmetrical flaccid weakness or paralysis, ataxia, and sensory disturbances are commonly seen during the illness. Serial measurement of tidal volumes may reveal respiratory deterioration in the child with GBS.
4. The following laboratory and diagnostic tests are used to diagnose muscular dystrophy:
   - Electromyography (EMG) to demonstrate that the problem lies in the muscles, not in the nerves
   - Serum creatine kinase levels, which are elevated early in the disorder
   - Muscle biopsy, providing a definitive diagnosis
   - DNA testing, revealing the presence of the gene
5. The risk factors for myelomeningocele are:
   - Lack of prenatal care
   - Lack of preconception and/or prenatal folic acid supplementation
   - Previous child born with neural tube defect or family history of neural tube defects
   - Maternal consumption of certain drugs that antagonize folic acid, such as anticonvulsants (carbamazepine and phenobarbital)
6. The perinatal causes of cerebral palsy are:
   - Prematurity (<32 weeks)
   - Asphyxia
   - Hypoxia
   - Breech presentation
   - Sepsis or central nervous system infection

- Placental complications
- Electrolyte disturbance
- Cerebral hemorrhage
- Kernicterus
- Chorioamnionitis

Activity F

1. **a.** Cerebral palsy (CP) is a term used to describe a range of nonspecific clinical symptoms characterized by abnormal motor pattern and postures caused by nonprogressive, abnormal brain function. The majority of causes of CP occur before or during delivery, and it is often associated with brain anoxia. Many times, no specific cause can be identified. A prolonged, complicated, difficult delivery and prematurity are risk factors for CP. CP is the most common movement disorder of childhood and is a lifelong, nonprogressive condition. It is one of the most common causes of physical disability in children. There is a large variation in symptoms and disability among those with CP. For some it may be as mild as a slight limp; for others it may result in severe motor and neurologic impairments. Its primary signs include motor impairments such as spasticity, muscle weakness, and ataxia. Complications of CP include mental impairments, seizures, growth problems, impaired vision or hearing, abnormal sensation or perception, and hydrocephalus. It is impossible to predict intelligence, but many children with cerebral palsy also have some degree of mental retardation. Most children can survive into adulthood, but the disorder may have substantial effects on function and quality of life.

   b. Earliest signs of cerebral palsy include abnormal muscle tone and developmental delay. Primary signs include spasticity, muscle weakness, and ataxia. Children with CP may demonstrate abnormal use of muscle groups, such as scooting on their back instead of crawling or walking. Hypertonicity and increased resistance to dorsiflexion and passive hip abduction are common early signs. Sustained clonus may be present after forced dorsiflexion. Children with CP often demonstrate prolonged standing on their toes when supported in an upright standing position.

   c. Nursing management focuses on promoting growth and development through the promotion of mobility and maintenance of optimal nutritional intake. Treatment modalities to promote mobility include physiotherapy, pharmacologic management, and surgery. Physical or occupational therapy as well as medications may be used to address musculoskeletal abnormalities, to facilitate range of motion, to delay or prevent deformities such as contractures, to provide joint stability, to maximize activity, and to encourage the use of adaptive devices. The nurse's role in relation to the various therapies is to provide ongoing follow-through with prescribed exercises, positioning, or bracing. Children with CP may experience difficulty eating and swallowing due to poor motor control of the throat, mouth, and tongue. This may lead to poor nutrition and problems with growth. The child with CP may require a longer time to feed because of the poor motor control. Special diets, such as soft or puréed, may make swallowing easier. Proper positioning during feeding is essential to facilitate swallowing and reduce the risk of aspiration. Speech or occupational therapists can assist in strengthening swallowing muscles as well as developing accommodations to facilitate nutritional intake. Consult a dietitian to ensure adequate nutrition for children with CP. In children with severe swallowing problems or malnutrition, a feeding tube such as a gastrostomy tube may be placed. Providing support and education to the child and family is also an important nursing function. From the time of diagnosis, the family should be involved in the child's care. Refer caregivers to local resources, including education services and support groups.

Activity G

1. **Answer: d**
   RATIONALE: The persistence of a primitive reflex in a nine-month-old would warrant further evaluation. Symmetrical spontaneous movement, absence of the Moro and tonic neck reflexes, and a flexed resting posture would be expected in a normally developing nine-month-old child.

2. **Answer: b**
   RATIONALE: Dimpling and skin discoloration in the child's lumbosacral area can be an indication of spina bifida occulta. It would be best to respond that the dimpling and discoloration is a normal variation with no adverse effects and indicate that the doctor will want to take a closer look. Spina bifida is a term that is often used to generalize all neural tube disorders that affect the spinal cord. This can be confusing and a cause of concern for parents. It is probably best to avoid the use of the term initially until a diagnosis is confirmed. Nursing care would then focus on educating the family.

3. **Answer: c**
   RATIONALE: Symptoms of constipation and bladder dysfunction may result from a growing lesion. Increasing intracranial pressure (ICP) and head circumference would point to hydrocephalus. Leaking cerebrospinal fluid would indicate the sac is leaking.

4. **Answer: b**
   RATIONALE: Parents must always wash their hands very well with soap and water before catheterization. The other statements are correct.

5. **Answer: a**
   RATIONALE: A hallmark finding of DMD is the presence of Gower's sign: the child cannot rise from the floor in standard fashion because of increasing weakness. Signs of hydrocephalus are not typically associated with DMD. Kyphosis and scoliosis occur more frequently than lordosis. The calf muscles of a child with DMD appear enlarged because of pseudohypertrophy of the calves.

6. **Answer: a**
   RATIONALE: Tickling is often a successful technique for assessing the level of paralysis in the child either initially or in the recovery phase. Symmetrical flaccid weakness, ataxia, and sensory disturbances are other symptoms seen during the illness.

7. **Answer: b**
   RATIONALE: The central nursing priority is to prevent rupture or leaking of cerebrospinal fluid. Keeping the infant in the prone position will help prevent pressure on the lesion. Keeping the lesion free from fecal matter or urine is important as well, but the priority is to prevent rupture or leakage. The nurse should consider the lesion first when maintaining the infant's body temperature.

8. **Answer: c, d, & e**
   RATIONALE: The nurse should suggest using a wheelchair for mobility, participating in computer activities, and avoiding overexertion to maximize the quality of life of the child with Duchenne muscular dystrophy. The nurse should discourage long periods of bed rest, as it may contribute to further weakness. Avoiding sports altogether is not necessary; the child could participate in the Special Olympics appropriate to his age.

9. **Answer: c**
   RATIONALE: The nurse should assess for uncontrolled, slow, wormlike writhing or twisting movements in the child with athetoid cerebral palsy. Hypertonicity of affected extremities, continuation of primitive reflexes, and exaggeration of deep tendon reflexes are characteristics noted in the spastic type of cerebral palsy.

10. **Answer: b**
    RATIONALE: Splinting may be used to maintain muscle strength in a child with cerebral palsy. Braces are used in young children to combat scoliosis that develops from spasticity. Serial casting may be used to increase the muscle and tendon length. Walkers are assistive devices for gross motor movements used by children with cerebral palsy.

11. **Answer: d**
    RATIONALE: The nurse should assess for scissor-crossing of the legs with plantarflexion in the infant with cerebral palsy. Lack of response to touch and pain stimuli, absence of deep tendon reflexes, and a relaxed anal sphincter may be seen in infants with myelomeningocele.

12. **Answer: b**
    RATIONALE: The nurse should know that a high cervical injury will result in damage to the phrenic nerve, which innervates the diaphragm. Damage to this nerve may leave the child unable to breathe

without assistance. A neurogenic bladder is not the direct result of a spinal cord injury but is seen in children with congenital neuromuscular disorders such as myelomeningocele. Paradoxical breathing, or use of the diaphragm without intercostal muscle support, is not possible in a child with damage to the phrenic nerve; it is noted in children with spinal muscular atrophy (SMA) type 1 and 2.

13. **Answer: c**
    RATIONALE: Although all four answers are appropriate, for this child the *most* important nursing action is to promote pulmonary function.

14. **Answer: b**
    RATIONALE: It is important to maintain the medication regimen in order to prevent calcinosis (calcium deposits) and joint deformity in the future. Children with dermatomyositis should be excused from physical education classes while the disease is active. Anticholinergics and IV IgG, as well as appropriate stress management and the avoidance of extreme temperatures, are important for a child with myasthenia gravis.

15 **Answer: d**
    RATIONALE: The nurse should instruct the parents on complications of pump placement, including infection, rupture, dislodgement, or blockage of catheter. The pump needs to be refilled with medication approximately every three months. The pump should be replaced every 5–7 years. There is no need to limit the child's activity and encourage bed rest if proper care is taken during activity.

CHAPTER 44

Activity A
1. Ossification
2. Casts
3. Narcotic
4. Arthrography
5. Polydactyly
6. Dysplasia
7. Torticollis
8. Gastrointestinal
9. Scoliosis
10. Sprains

Activity B
1. The figure demonstrates the Cotrel-Dubousset method, in which the rods are fused to the vertebrae and connected to a distracting rod to rotate the vertebral column.

Activity C
1. c   2. b   3. a   4. d

Activity D
1.

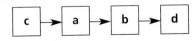

Activity E
1. Pectus excavatum and pectus carinatum are anterior chest wall deformities. Pectus excavatum, a funnel-shaped chest, accounts for 87% of anterior chest wall deformities. A depression that sinks inward is apparent at the xiphoid process. Pectus carinatum, a protuberance of the chest wall, accounts for only 5% of anterior chest wall deformities. The remainder are mixed deformities.

2. Clubfoot may be classified into four categories: postural, neurogenic, syndromic, and idiopathic. Postural clubfoot often resolves with a short series of manipulative casting. Neurogenic clubfoot occurs in infants with myelomeningocele. Clubfoot in association with other syndromes (syndromic) is often resistant to treatment. Idiopathic clubfoot occurs in otherwise normal healthy infants. The approach to treatment is similar, regardless of the classification.

3. Treatment of rickets is aimed at correcting the calcium imbalance so that the skeleton may develop properly and without deformity. Calcium and phosphorus supplements are given, and some children also require vitamin D supplements.

4. Osteomyelitis is acquired hematogeneously. Bacteria from the bloodstream mainly invade the most rapidly growing portion of the bone. The invading bacteria trigger an inflammatory response, formation of pus, and edema and vascular congestion. Small blood vessels thrombose and the infection extends into the metaphyseal marrow cavity. As the infection progresses, the inflammation extends throughout the bone, and blood supply is disrupted, resulting in death of the bone tissues.

5. Transient synovitis of the hip (also called toxic synovitis) is the most common cause of hip pain in children. It occurs in children as young as nine months of age through adolescence, most commonly affecting children three to eight years old. Boys are affected twice as often as girls.

6. The laboratory findings of septic arthritis include
   • White blood cell count normal or elevated, with elevated neutrophil counts
   • Elevated erythrocyte sedimentation rate and C-reactive protein levels
   • Fluid from joint aspiration demonstrates elevated white blood cell count; culture determines responsible organism
   • Joint x-ray may show subtle soft-tissue changes or an increase in the joint space
   • Positive blood culture for the causative organism

Activity F
1. a. The nurse should perform the following assessments for a person diagnosed with osteogenesis imperfecta:
   • Elicit a health history, which may reveal a family history of osteogenesis imperfecta, a pattern of frequent fractures, or screaming as-

sociated with routine care and handling of the newborn
- Inspect the eyes for sclerae that have a blue, purple, or gray tint
- Note abnormalities of the primary teeth
- Inspect skin for bruising and note joint hypermobility with active range of motion

b. The nurse can teach the following to Oliver's parents to prevent injuries:
- Never push or pull on an arm or leg
- Do not bend an arm or leg into an awkward position
- Lift the baby by placing one hand under the legs and buttocks and one hand under the shoulders, head, and neck
- Do not lift the baby's legs by the ankles to change the diaper
- Do not lift the baby or small child from under the armpits
- Provide supported positioning
- If fracture is suspected, handle the limb minimally

Activity G

1. **Answer: c**
   RATIONALE: In type II metatarsus adductus, the forefoot is flexible passively past neutral, but only to midline actively. The forefoot is flexible past neutral actively and passively in type I. The forefoot is rigid and does not correct to midline even with passive stretching in type III. An inverted forefoot turned slightly upward is indicative of clubfoot.

2. **Answer: a**
   RATIONALE: The child with rickets would have an elevated alkaline phosphatase level. Elevated white blood cell count, erythrocyte sedimentation rate, and C-reactive protein level are found in children with osteomyelitis.

3. **Answer: a**
   RATIONALE: Asymmetry of the thigh or gluteal folds indicates developmental dysplasia of the hip. The lower extremities of the infant typically have some normal developmental variations due to in utero positioning. Internal tibial torsion (genu varum) and in-toeing are common findings that typically resolve as the musculoskeletal system matures.

4. **Answer: b**
   RATIONALE: It is very important to teach parents to identify the signs of neurovascular compromise (pale, cool, or blue skin) and tell them to notify the physician immediately. The nurse should teach the mother to avoid causing depression on the cast. The mother should be told to encourage the child to keep the casted arm still. The mother should also be aware of odor or drainage from the cast.

5. **Answer: c**
   RATIONALE: The nurse should emphasize that the child should not be allowed to lie on his side for four weeks following the surgery, to ensure the

band does not shift. The parents should be aware of signs of infection, but the position must be emphasized to protect the band. The nurse would be expected to monitor the child's vital capacity, not the parents. Log-rolling the child is not permitted.

6. **Answer: b**
   RATIONALE: Because the baby is less than six months of age, she would be treated with a Pavlik harness. Children from six months to two years of age often require closed reduction. Closed reduction with skin or skeletal traction would be followed by spica cast. Children over two years of age would require an open surgical reduction.

7. **Answer: d**
   RATIONALE: Blue sclera is a common finding of OI. Inversion of the heel is a common finding in congenital clubfoot. Medial deviation of the forefoot is found in metatarsus adductus. Extra digits in the hand are a characteristic finding in polydactyly.

8. **Answer: b**
   RATIONALE: The nurse should monitor the client for constipation after administering Ketorolac in tablet form. Heartburn, abdominal discomfort, and regurgitation are side effects of oral alendronate.

9. **Answer: a**
   RATIONALE: Brown, flaky skin is a normal sign after removal of a cast. Skin coolness, prolonged capillary refill, and pale or blue skin are the signs of neurovascular compromise in the client with a cast.

10. **Answer: c**
    RATIONALE: The nurse should ensure the head halter does not place pressure on the ear while caring for a client with skin traction applied with a skin strap. Ensuring that the ankle and heel are free from pressure is an important intervention for children with Bryant's traction. A Buck's traction should be removed every eight hours and the underlying skin should be assessed. In a child with side arm 90-90 traction, maintaining elbow flexion at 90 degrees is important.

11. **Answer: a**
    RATIONALE: When caring for the child with balanced suspension traction, the nurse should avoid pressure to the popliteal area. Ensuring that the leg is slightly abducted is an intervention for a child with Buck's traction. Assessing the fingers and hands for coolness is an important intervention for a child with side arm 90-90 traction. Ensuring proper replacement of sling is an intervention for a client with Russell's traction.

12. **Answer: a**
    RATIONALE: C-Reactive proteins and erythrocyte sedimentation rate will be elevated in the client with septic arthritis. White blood cell count will be normal or elevated with elevated neutrophil counts.

13. **Answer: c**
    RATIONALE: The client with Osgood–Schlatter disease will exhibit painful swelling in the anterior

portion of the tibial tubercle. Tenderness in the proximal humerus is found in children with epiphysiolysis of the proximal humerus. Children with calcaneal apophysitis usually present with pain over the posterior aspect of the calcaneus. Pain in the anterior aspect of the middle part of the lower leg is a common finding in shin splints.

14. Answer: a
RATIONALE: The nurse should change the baby's diaper while the baby is in the harness to ensure that the harness is worn at all times. The harness should be manually washed with a mild detergent. Clothes should not be kept under the harness, and the child should be allowed to sleep on his or her back.

15 Answer: a
RATIONALE: Chronic renal disease is a risk factor for rickets. Renal osteodystrophy and orthogenesis imperfecta are risk factors for fracture. Infected varicella lesions are a risk factor for osteomyelitis.

CHAPTER 45

Activity A

1. increases
2. IgE
3. Seborrhea
4. androgens
5. Cellulitis
6. versicolor
7. Psoriasis
8. toes
9. Superficial
10. Sunburn

Activity B

1. The figure shows keloid formation, which is more common in dark-skinned than light-skinned children.
2. The figure shows tinea corporis, characterized by a raised scaly border with clearing in the center.
3. The figure shows severe cradle cap, characterized by yellow, greasy-appearing plaques.

Activity C

1. c   2. b   3. a   4. d

Activity D

1.

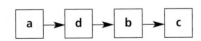

Activity E

1. Dark-skinned children tend to have more pronounced cutaneous reactions compared to children with lighter skin. Hypopigmentation or hyperpigmentation in the affected area following the healing of a dermatologic condition is common. Dark-skinned children tend to have hypertrophic

scarring, keloid formation, and more prominent papules, follicular response lichenification, and vesicular or bullous reaction than lighter-skinned children with the same disorder.

2. Impetigo is a readily recognizable skin rash. Nonbullous impetigo generally follows some type of skin trauma or may arise as a secondary bacterial infection of another skin disorder, such as atopic dermatitis. Bullous impetigo demonstrates a sporadic occurrence pattern and develops on intact skin, resulting from toxin production of *Staphylococcus aureus*.

3. Therapeutic management of atopic dermatitis includes good skin hydration, application of topical corticosteroids or immune modulators, oral histamines for sedative effects, and antibiotics if secondary infection occurs.

4. The risk factors for development of pressure ulcers in children include immobility or decreased activity, decreased sensory perception, increased moisture, impaired nutritional status, inadequate tissue perfusion, and the forces of friction and shear.

5. Burns are classified according to the extent of injury, as follows:
   - Superficial burns
   - Partial-thickness burns
   - Deep partial-thickness burns
   - Full-thickness burns

6. The following precautions should be taken to prevent frostbite:
   - Dressing warmly in layers, and keeping warm and dry
   - Avoiding exertion
   - Not playing outside when wind chill advisories are in effect, and locking doors with high locks to prevent toddlers from going outside

Activity F

1. a. A nurse conducting a primary survey should do the following:
   - Assess the child's airway, noting whether it is patent, maintainable, or unmaintainable
   - Suspect airway injury from burn or smoke inhalation if any of the following are present: burns around the mouth, nose, or eyes; carbonaceous (black-colored) sputum; hoarseness or stridor
   - Evaluate the child's skin color, respiratory effort, symmetry of breathing, and breath sounds
   - Determine the pulse strength, perfusion status, and heart rate; note extent and location of edema

   b. A nurse conducting a secondary survey should do the following:
   - Determine burn depth
   - Estimate burn extent by determining the percentage of body surface area affected; use a chart for estimation or rapidly estimate by using the child's palm size, which is equivalent to about one percent of the child's body surface area
   - Inspect the child for other traumatic injuries

c. A nurse can take the following measures to promote fluid balance:
- Assess fluid volume status at least every shift—more frequently if disrupted—to obtain baseline for comparison
- Strictly monitor intake and output to detect imbalance or need for additional fluid intake
- Weigh the child daily on the same scale, at the same time, in the same amount of clothing, because changes in weight are an accurate indicator of fluid volume status in children
- Provide intravenous fluid resuscitation in the initial period, followed by encouragement of oral fluid intake by the burned patient, to compensate for fluid loss through burned areas

Activity G

1. **Answer: c**
   RATIONALE: Presence of stridor indicates airway injury from burn or smoke inhalation. Cervical spine injury is a traumatic injury and does not indicate airway injury. Internal traumatic injury may be present if the child had jumped from a house but does not indicate airway injury from burns. Red, dry lesions on the abdomen do not indicate airway injury.

2. **Answer: c**
   RATIONALE: The child may have staphylococcal scalded skin syndrome, which results from infection with *Staphylococcus aureus;* it produces a toxin that then causes exfoliation. It is abrupt in onset and results in diffuse erythema and skin tenderness. It is most common in infancy and rare beyond 5 years of age. Bullous impetigo presents with red macules and bullous eruptions on an erythematous base. Cellulitis presents with localized erythema, pain, and edema. Folliculitis presents with red raised hair follicles.

3. **Answer: d**
   RATIONALE: The nurse should emphasize that the parents should avoid hot water. The child should be bathed twice a day in warm water, not hot water. The parents should avoid skin products containing perfumes, or fragrances, and should use a mild soap like unscented Dove for sensitive skin. The soap should be used only to clean dirty areas of the body.

4. **Answer: a**
   RATIONALE: Tinea pedis presents with a red scaling rash on the soles and between the toes. Tinea capitis presents with patches of scaling on the scalp with central hair loss and the risk of development of an inflamed boggy mass filled with pustules. Tinea cruris presents with erythema, scaling, and maceration in the inguinal creases and inner thighs.

5. **Answer: d**
   RATIONALE: Erythema multiforme typically manifests in the form of lesions over the hands and feet and extensor surfaces of the extremities with spread to the trunk. Thick or flaky greasy yellow scales on the neck and trunk are the signs of seborrhea. Silvery or yellow-white scale plaques and sharply demarcated borders define psoriasis. Hypopigmented oval scaly lesions, especially on the upper back and chest and proximal arms, are indicative of tinea versicolor.

6. **Answer: c**
   RATIONALE: The nurse should administer diphenhydramine as soon as possible after the sting in an attempt to minimize a reaction. The other actions are important for an insect sting, but the priority intervention is to administer diphenhydramine.

7. **Answer: b**
   RATIONALE: Second-degree frostbite demonstrates blistering with erythema and edema. First-degree frostbite results in superficial white plaques with surrounding erythema. In third-degree frostbite, hemorrhagic blisters occur; these progress to tissue necrosis and sloughing in the fourth degree.

8. **Answer: b**
   RATIONALE: When administering the systemic antifungal medication Griseofulvin to the child, the nurse should give the medication along with fatty food to increase absorption. The nurse should monitor for Cushing syndrome and taper the doses before stopping when the child is on systemic corticosteroids. The child should be monitored for suicidal risk if the child is treated with isotretinoin.

9. **Answer: a**
   RATIONALE: The nurse should turn the child frequently to avoid development of pressure ulcers. Assessing the entire surface of the child's skin at least every shift, using pressure-alleviating beds and mattresses, and maintaining the child's nutritional status are other preventive measures against pressure ulcers. Applying topical antibiotics, applying a cold compress, and dressing the client in layers are inappropriate interventions. Applying topical antibiotics may help the child who has a bacterial infection. The child who has sunburns may benefit from applying a cold compress. A client should be dressed in layers to prevent frostbite.

10. **Answer: c**
    RATIONALE: The nurse should teach the parents to let the child go diaperless for a period of time each day to allow the rash to heal. The diaper area should be wiped with a soft cloth. Harsh soaps, rubber pants, and baby wipes with preservatives or fragrance should not be used for the child.

11. **Answer: b**
    RATIONALE: Acne is a skin condition that involves the pilosebaceous unit; it is characterized by inflammatory papules and pustules. Hair follicles are involved in folliculitis. Skin and subcutaneous tissue are involved in cellulitis, and the epidermis is involved in psoriasis.

12. **Answer: d**
    RATIONALE: The nurse should suggest the adolescent use noncomedogenic cosmetic products to prevent development of comedones. The adolescent should avoid oil-based cosmetics and hair products because their use may block pores, contributing to noninflammatory lesions. Headbands, helmets, and hats may exacerbate the lesions by causing friction. The adolescent should avoid alcohol-based cleaners on the acne.

13. **Answer: a**
    RATIONALE: The most important nursing implication for the adolescent girl on Isotretinolin treatment is to be on a pregnancy prevention program because the drug causes defects in fetal development. Monitoring of lipid profile, complete blood cell count, and beta-human chorionic gonadotropin and monitoring for suicidal risk are general implications for all clients treated with Isotretinolin.

14. **Answer: d**
    RATIONALE: The nurse should document this as a full-thickness burn because the area is painless with an edematous, leathery, waxy appearance. Superficial burns are painful, red, dry, and possibly edematous. Partial-thickness and deep partial-thickness burns are very painful and edematous and have a wet appearance or blisters.

15. **Answer: a**
    RATIONALE: Presence of spatter-type burns rule out child abuse–induced burns because they usually result from the child pulling a container of hot fluid onto himself. Intentional scald injuries usually yield a uniform sock or glove distribution when the child's extremity is held under hot water as punishment. Flexor-sparing burns that involve the dorsum of the hand indicate abuse-induced burns. Porcelain-contact sparing pattern is seen when the portion of the child's skin that was in contact with the tub or sink is not burned.

CHAPTER 46

Activity A

1. hemogram
2. placenta
3. aplastic
4. lead
5. hemoglobinopathies
6. Hemosiderosis
7. chelation
8. minor
9. Hemophilia
10. protoporphyrin

Activity B

1. **a.** The findings are related to a disorder known as thalassemia.

    b. Iron overload related to thalassemia leads to bony changes such as frontal bossing and maxillary prominence.

Activity C

1. a 2. c 3. b 4. f 5. d 6. e

Activity D

1. Folic acid deficiency is caused by a low dietary intake of green leafy vegetables, liver, and citrus. It can also be caused by malabsorption from medication such as Dilantin or parasitic infections. Pernicious anemia is a deficiency in vitamin B12. Management of folic acid deficiency involves ensuring compliance with dietary changes. Pernicious anemia is managed with monthly injections of vitamin B12.

2. The recommended action is to confirm the result with a repeat lab study within one week and to educate the family on how to decrease lead exposure. Refer the family to the local health department for investigation of the home for lead reduction, with referrals for support services.

3. Color changes to the skin such as pallor, bruising, and flushing can indicate hematologic problems. Changes in mental status such as lethargy can also indicate a decrease in hemoglobin and a decrease in oxygen getting to the brain.

4. Physical examination of the child with iron deficiency anemia includes the following:
   - Observing the child for fatigue and lethargy
   - Inspecting the skin, conjunctivae, oral mucosa, palms, and soles for pallor
   - Noting spooning of the nails (concave shape)
   - Obtaining a pulse oximeter reading
   - Evaluating the heart rate for tachycardia
   - Auscultating the heart for the presence of a flow murmur
   - Palpating the abdomen for splenomegaly

5. Complications of sickle cell anemia include the following:
   - Recurrent vaso-occlusive pain crises, stroke, sepsis, acute chest syndrome, splenic sequestration, reduced visual acuity related to decreased retinal blood flow, chronic leg ulcers, cholestasis and gallstones, delayed growth and development, delayed puberty, and priapism
   - In children, an increased incidence of enuresis due to the kidneys not concentrating urine effectively; as they reach adulthood, multiple organ dysfunction is common

6. The fetus receives iron through the placenta from the mother. The preterm infant misses out on the final weeks or months of transplacental iron transfer, putting him or her at increased risk for anemia.

Activity E

1. **a.** How much milk does Jayda drink per day? Excessive cow's milk consumption (greater than 24 ounces a day) is a risk factor for iron deficiency

anemia. When did Jayda start drinking cow's milk? Cow's milk consumption before 12 months of age is another risk factor for iron deficiency anemia. Was Jayda formula-fed, and if so, with what type? Low-iron formula can lead to iron deficiency anemia. Was Jayda breastfed, and if so, did she receive iron supplementation (including eating iron-fortified cereal) after 6 months of age? What are Jayda's food preferences and usual eating patterns? Is she on any restricted diet? Is she taking any medications? Certain medications, such as antacids, can interfere with iron absorption.

b. Teach Jayda's parents to precisely measure the amount of iron to be administered. Teach them to place the liquid behind the teeth, because iron in liquid form can stain the teeth; use of a straw and brushing teeth after administration may help. Constipation can result from iron administration; in some cases, reducing the amount of iron can resolve this problem, but stool softeners may be necessary to relieve painful or difficult-to-pass stools. Encourage the parents to increase their child's fluid intake and maintain adequate consumption of fiber to avoid the development of constipation. Instruct the parents that stools may appear dark because of the iron. Instruct the parents to keep iron supplements and all medications in a safe place to avoid accidental overdose. Providing juice enriched with vitamin C can help aid absorption of iron. Limit cow's milk intake to 24 ounces per day. Limit fast food consumption and encourage iron-rich foods such as red meats, tuna, salmon, eggs, tofu, enriched grains, dried beans and peas, dried fruits, leafy green vegetables, and iron-fortified breakfast cereals (iron from red meat is the easiest for the body to absorb). Encourage parents to provide nutritious snacks and finger foods that are developmentally appropriate for Jayda. Toddlers are often picky eaters. This often becomes a means of control for the child, and parents should guard against getting involved in a power struggle with their child. Referring the parents to a developmental specialist who can assist them in their approach to diet with their child may prove beneficial. Encourage appropriate follow-up and review the signs and symptoms of anemia.

c. Low socioeconomic status, which can lead to a lack of adequate food supply; recent immigration from a developing country; culturally based food influences that lead to dietary imbalances; and child abuse or neglect, leading to improper nutrition

Activity F

1. **Answer: b**
RATIONALE: If neurologic deficits are assessed, immediate reporting of the findings is necessary so that treatment can begin to prevent permanent damage. The nurse would continue to monitor the neurologic signs, evaluate the respiratory status of the child, and inspect for signs of bleeding

2. **Answer: d**
RATIONALE: A concave shape of the fingernails, termed spooning, can occur with iron deficiency anemia. Capillary refill in less than two seconds, pink palms and nail beds, and absence of bruising are normal findings.

3. **Answer: a**
RATIONALE: Although iron from red meat is the easiest for the body to absorb, the nurse should discourage fast food consumption, because this type of food is also high in fat, fillers, and sodium. The other statements are correct.

4. **Answer: b**
RATIONALE: The best response for a seven-year-old is to use distraction and involve him in the infusion process in a developmentally appropriate manner. A seven-year-old is old enough to assist with the dilution and mixing of the factor. Asking for help with the Band-Aid would be best for a younger child. Teens should be taught to administer their own factor infusions. Telling him to be brave is not helpful and does not teach.

5. **Answer: a**
RATIONALE: The priority is to emphasize that the parents must precisely measure the amount of iron to be administered to avoid overdosing. The other instructions are important, but the priority is to emphasize precise measurement.

6. **Answer: c**
RATIONALE: Symmetrical swelling of the hands and feet in the infant or toddler is termed dactylitis; aseptic infarction occurs in the metacarpals and metatarsals and is often the first vaso-occlusive event seen with sickle cell disease.

7. **Answer: a**
RATIONALE: Laboratory evaluation for iron deficiency anemia will reveal decreased hemoglobin (Hgb) and hematocrit (Hct), decreased reticulocyte count, microcytosis, hypochromia, decreased serum iron and ferritin levels, and an increased FEP level.

8. **Answer: b, c, & d**
RATIONALE: The nurse should assess for behavioral problems, skin pallor, and irritability and hyperactivity in the child. Blurred vision and dehydration are not related to lead poisoning.

9. **Answer: b, c, & e**
RATIONALE: When caring for a child with aplastic anemia, the nurse would assess for oral ulcerations, increased bleeding with menstruation, and tachycardia or tachypnea. Evaluation of oxygen-carrying capacity is an assessment related to a decrease in hemoglobin production. An elevation in WBCs would require an evaluation for infection.

10. **Answer: d**
RATIONALE: The presence of fetal hemoglobin (Hgb F) in infants with sickle cell anemia usually causes them to remain asymptomatic until 3 to 4 months

of age because Hgb F protects against sickling. Hgb A is present in the blood at any given time; it does not protect against sickling. Hgb A (adult hemoglobin) develops only over the first several months of life and replaces Hgb F in the older infant. The healthy older infant then displays the presence of Hgb AA. Hgb AS is passed on from parents who have the sickle cell gene or trait, which may cause sickle cell anemia in the infant.

11. **Answer: a, c, & d**
    RATIONALE: When auscultating the child with sickle cell anemia, the nurse should assess for adventitious breath sounds, heart murmur, and an elevated heart rate. Crackles and wheezing are not heard in a child with sickle cell anemia.

12. **Answer: b, c, & e**
    RATIONALE: The nurse should assess the child with thalassemia major for pathologic fractures, growth retardation, and skeletal deformities. Cardiac complications are observed in clients with clotting disorders such as Henoch-Schonlein purpura. Bleeding episodes are seen in clients with clotting disorders such as hemophilia, von Willebrand disease, and disseminated intravascular coagulation.

13. **Answer: a, b, & e**
    RATIONALE: The nurse should instruct the parents to avoid aspirin, as well as nonsteroidal anti-inflammatory drugs (NSAIDs) and antihistamines, because these medications may precipitate the development of anemia in children with idiopathic thrombocytopenia purpura (ITP). The use of acetaminophen is more appropriate when necessary for pain control. The nurse should discourage participating in contact sports because direct contact can lead to injury or trauma; activities such as swimming provide physical activity with less risk of trauma and may be encouraged.

CHAPTER 47

Activity A

1. autoantibodies
2. positive
3. passive
4. Vertical
5. Hypogammaglobulinemia
6. butterfly
7. Allergy
8. absent
9. Vasodilation
10. food

Activity B

1. c   2. d   3. b   4. a

Activity C

1.

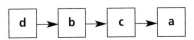

Activity D

1. The four different types of hypogammaglobulinemia are:
   - Selective IgA deficiency
   - X-linked agammaglobulinemia
   - X-linked hyper-IgM syndrome
   - IgG subclass deficiency
2. Polymerase chain reaction (PCR) is preferable for the detection of HIV infection in infants. Virologic testing for HIV-exposed infants with PCR is done at birth, 4 to 7 weeks of age, and 8 to 16 weeks of age. This test is positive in infected infants over 1 month of age. Serologic testing at 12 months of age or older is done with PCR to document disappearance of HIV-1 antibody.
3. Juvenile idiopathic arthritis is an autoimmune disorder in which the autoantibodies mainly target the joints. Inflammatory changes in the joints cause pain, redness, warmth, stiffness, and swelling.
4. Delayed hypersensitivity reactions are mediated by T cells rather than antibodies. An infant's skin test response is diminished most likely because of a decreased ability to mount an inflammatory response.
5. Anaphylaxis is an acute IgE-mediated response to an allergen that involves many organ systems and may be life-threatening. As much as 1% to 2% of the population is at risk for anaphylaxis due to food allergies or insect stings. The reaction is severe and usually starts within 5 to 10 minutes of exposure, though delayed reactions are possible.
6. Wiskott-Aldrich syndrome is an X-linked genetic disorder that results in immunodeficiency, eczema, and thrombocytopenia. The defective gene responsible for this disorder was recently identified as Wiskott-Aldrich syndrome protein. The complications include autoimmune hemolytic anemia, neutropenia, skin or cerebral vasculitis, arthritis, inflammatory bowel disease, and renal disease.

Activity E

1. a. To assess the presence of infections in the child, the nurse collects the history of severe infections. The nurse should inspect the mouth for persistent thrush and auscultate the lungs, noting adventitious sounds related to pneumonia. The nurse should also look at the child's body, head to toe, for any signs of integumentary infection.
   b. The prevention of infection in the child with SCID is critical. The nursing interventions are as follows:
      - Teach the family to practice good handwashing.
      - Do not expose the child to persons outside the family.
      - Encourage adequate nutrition; supplemental enteral feedings may be necessary.
      - Instruct families to administer prophylactic antibiotics if prescribed.
      - Administer IVIG infusions as prescribed and monitor for adverse reactions.

Activity F

1. Answer: a
RATIONALE: Premedication with diphenhydramine or acetaminophen may be indicated in children who are IVIG-naïve, have not had an infusion in over 8 weeks, have had a recent bacterial infection, or have a history of serious infusion-related adverse reactions. Assessing baseline blood urea nitrogen and creatinine is a common laboratory test that is performed in all clients before administration of IVIG. Observing for the signs of anaphylaxis reaction should be done during the infusion. Epinephrine and corticosteroids should be administered in cases of anaphylaxis reaction.

2. Answer: d
RATIONALE: The ELISA will be positive in infants of HIV-infected mothers because of transplacentally received antibodies. These antibodies may persist and remain detectable up to 24 months of age, making the ELISA test less accurate in detecting true HIV infection in infants and toddlers than the PCR. The PCR is positive in infected infants over the age of 1 month. Rheumatoid factor and antinuclear antibody are not indicated for HIV infection. Rheumatoid factor is tested in cases of juvenile idiopathic arthritis and systemic lupus erythematosus. An antinuclear antibodies test is done in cases of systemic lupus erythematosus.

3. Answer: d
RATIONALE: Alopecia is a common clinical manifestation of SLE. A history of persistent diarrhea and oral thrush indicates severe combined immune deficiency; history of bruising and skin color change indicates Wiskott-Aldrich syndrome.

4. Answer: b
RATIONALE: Lip edema, urticaria, stridor, and tachycardia are common clinical manifestations of anaphylaxis. Severe polyarticular juvenile idiopathic arthritis, systemic lupus erythematosus, and severe combined immune deficiency are not appropriate candidates because they are not manifested by lip edema, urticaria, stridor, and tachycardia.

5. Answer: c
RATIONALE: The nurse should instruct children and their families to avoid foods with a known cross-reactivity to latex, such as bananas. Blueberries, pumpkin, and pomegranate do not have cross-reactivity to latex.

6. Answer: a
RATIONALE: Polyarticular JIA is defined by the involvement of five or more joints. These are frequently the small joints, and they are affected symmetrically. Pauciarticular JIA is defined by the involvement of four or fewer joints. Systemic JIA presents with fever and rash in addition to joint involvement at the time of diagnosis. The child with JIA is not at greater risk for anaphylaxis.

7. Answer: d
RATIONALE: The nurse would find a low platelet count in the child with SLE. The child will also exhibit a low WBC count. Elevated IgA concentration and low IgM concentrations are found in children with Wiskott-Aldrich syndrome.

8. Answer: c
RATIONALE: The nurse should monitor salicylate levels when administering aspirin to the client with juvenile idiopathic arthritis. Potassium and CBC should be monitored when administering immunosuppressant drugs. Monitoring for liver enzymes is important when administering NSAIDs.

9. Answer: d
RATIONALE: The nurse should assess for respiratory infections in the client with agammaglobulinemia. A client with X-linked hyper-IgM syndrome should be assessed for malabsorption, autoimmune disorders, and neutropenia.

10. Answer: d
RATIONALE: The nurse should observe the skin for butterfly rashes in the client with SLE. Auscultating the lungs for pneumonia and palpating for the presence of lymphadenopathy are nursing assessments for HIV infection. Inspecting the skin for nonpruritic macular rashes is done in cases of juvenile idiopathic arthritis.

11. Answer: c
RATIONALE: The EpiPen® Jr. should be jabbed into the outer thigh at a 90-degree angle, not the upper arm. The other statements are correct.

12. Answer: d
RATIONALE: The nurse should instruct the parent to avoid durum for the client who is allergic to wheat. Whey, casein, and yogurt should be avoided in clients who are allergic to milk.

13. Answer: d
RATIONALE: Nasal congestion is the common clinical manifestation that the nurse should assess in the client with a latex allergy. Photosensitivity, skin rashes, and stomatitis are the clinical manifestations of systemic lupus erythematosus.

14. Answer: a
RATIONALE: The client with polyarticular juvenile idiopathic arthritis will have lymphadenopathy as a non-joint manifestation. Severe anemia, hepatomegaly, and splenomegaly are the non-joint manifestations of systemic juvenile idiopathic arthritis.

15 Answer: a, b, & c
RATIONALE: To help promote a normal life for the client with juvenile idiopathic arthritis after hospital discharge, the nurse should teach the client and his parents to provide adequate pain relief through medications so that the child can perform activities. Applying warm compresses to affected joints would decrease the pain and promote sleep. The

parents should encourage the child to attend school to prevent social isolation. Protecting against cold weather with layered clothing and applying sunscreen daily to prevent rashes are nursing interventions suitable for a child with systemic lupus erythematosus.

CHAPTER 48

Activity A

1. homeostasis
2. pancreas
3. polyuria
4. hypopituitarism
5. Acromegaly
6. cretinism
7. Radioimmunoassay
8. glucocorticoids
9. hypoglycemic
10. Endocrine

Activity B

1. **a.** The newborn has congenital hypothyroidism.
   b. Congenital hypothyroidism usually results from the failure of the thyroid gland to migrate during fetal development. This results in malformation or malfunction of the thyroid gland, which leads to insufficient production of the thyroid hormones that are required to meet the body's metabolic and growth and development needs.

Activity C

1. c   2. b   3. d   4. a

Activity D

1.

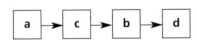

Activity E

1. The process of hormone production and secretion involves the principle of feedback control. One gland produces a hormone that affects another endocrine gland. Once the physiologic effect is achieved, the target organ inhibits the further release of the original hormone. If the original gland does not release enough of the hormone, the inhibition process stops so that the gland increases the production of the hormone.
2. The hypothalamus affects the pituitary by releasing and inhibiting hormones and may be the cause of pituitary disorders. Pituitary disorders are classified as anterior pituitary hormones and posterior pituitary hormones. Anterior pituitary disorders in children include growth hormone deficiency, hyperpituitarism, and precocious puberty. Posterior pituitary disorders include diabetes insipidus and syndrome of inappropriate antidiuretic hormone secretion.

3. A bone age radiograph is the study of the wrist or hand to determine bone maturation compared to national standards. This diagnostic test is performed to determine if bone age is consistent with chronologic age to rule out GH deficiency or excess or hypothyroidism.
4. Psychosocial dwarfism results from emotional deprivation that causes suppression of production of the pituitary hormones, resulting in decreased growth hormone. The child is withdrawn, has bizarre eating and drinking habits, and has primitive speech. With normalized eating and behavioral habits, pituitary secretion is restored and the child dramatically catches up in growth parameters.
5. An insulin pump is a device that administers a continuous infusion of rapid-acting insulin. It comprises a computer, a reservoir of rapid-acting insulin, thin tubing through which the insulin is delivered, and a small needle inserted into the abdomen. A continuous basal rate of insulin is maintained, and a bolus of insulin can be delivered if glucose testing results show that it is needed.
6. The child with hypoglycemia may display behavioral changes, confusion, slurred speech, belligerence, diaphoresis, tremors, palpitations, and tachycardia. The child with hyperglycemia may display mental status changes, fatigue, weakness, dry, flushed skin, blurred vision, abdominal cramping, nausea, vomiting, and fruity breath odor.

Activity F

1. **a.** Historically, DM type 2 occurred in adults, with only a few cases seen in childhood. However, since the early 1990s, the incidence has increased significantly in children. Many of these children have a relative with type 2 diabetes or they are overweight; African-American, Hispanic-American, Asian-American, or Native American heritage also seems to be a risk factor.

   Type 2 diabetes begins when the pancreas produces insulin as usual, but the body develops a resistance to insulin or no longer uses the insulin properly. As the need for insulin rises, the pancreas gradually loses its ability to produce sufficient amounts of insulin to regulate blood sugar. Eventually, insulin production decreases, with a result similar to type 1 diabetes mellitus.
   b. Nursing management should focus on regulating glucose control, monitoring for complications, and educating and supporting the child and family. Other important interventions involve nutritional guidelines and exercise protocols.

   In DM type 2, oral hypoglycemic medications are used to regulate glucose levels. If these oral hypoglycemics fail to maintain a normal glucose level, then insulin will be required. Nutritional guidelines will be established with the help of a dietitian to ensure that the diet reflects the needs of the growing child. The dietitian will develop detailed meal planning and dietary guidelines.

Review basic nutritional information with the child and family and provide sample meal plans. Incorporate family culture and food preferences into meal planning. Encourage the child and family to keep a food diary to assist with any problem areas. Offer low-carbohydrate snacks if the child needs to lose weight. Encourage appropriate daily physical activity. The child with DM type 2 is often overweight, so an exercise plan is very important to help him lose weight, as well as assisting with the hypoglycemic effects of the medications.

Education is the priority intervention to empower the child and family toward self-management of DM. Education will continue over a period of time and is often done in an outpatient setting. This gives the family an opportunity to adjust to the diagnosis of a chronic illness that will require self-management. DM is a life-long condition that requires regular follow-up visits three or four times a year to a diabetes specialty clinic. With appropriate therapeutic management, involvement of the community, and confidence and compliance by the family, the child can maintain a happy, productive life.

The initial goal of education is for the family to start developing basic management and decision-making skills. Assess the family's ability to learn the concepts, and offer psychological support to the family. Develop a teaching plan that will include specific topics in sessions of 15 to 20 minutes for the children and 45 to 60 minutes for the caregivers. Teaching must be geared toward the child's level of development and understanding.

Topics to include in the teaching plan are fingerstick method and blood glucose measurement; urine ketone testing; medication use (oral hypoglycemic agents, glucagon); signs and symptoms of hypoglycemia and hyperglycemia; complications associated with DM; sick day instructions; and requirements related to laboratory testing and follow-up care.

Children with diabetes and their families may have difficulty with coping, related to lack of confidence in their self-management skills. Assess the ability of the child and family to handle past situations. Role-play specific situations to help them see different ways to solve problems depending on the situation that arises related to symptoms or complications associated with diabetes. Work with children and families to enhance conflict resolution skills. Provide opportunities for children and families to express their feelings. Observe for signs of depression, especially in adolescents. Refer families to local support groups, parent-to-parent networks, camps for children with diabetes, or one of many national support resources and foundations.

c. Children lack the maturity to understand the long-term consequences of this serious chronic illness. Children do not want to be different from their peers, and having to make lifestyles changes may result in anger or depression. Families may demonstrate unhealthy behaviors, making it difficult for the child to initiate change because of the lack of supervision or role modeling. Family dynamics are affected because management of diabetes must occur all day, every day.

Activity G

1. **Answer: d**
   RATIONALE: Administering intravenous calcium gluconate as ordered will restore normal calcium and phosphate levels, as well as relieve severe tetany. Providing calcium and vitamin D is an intervention for nonacute symptoms. Ensuring patency of the IV site to prevent tissue damage due to extravasation or cardiac arrhythmias, and monitoring fluid intake and urinary calcium output, are secondary interventions.

2. **Answer: b**
   RATIONALE: Observing pubic hair and hirsutism in a preschooler indicates congenital adrenal hyperplasia. Auscultation revealing an irregular heartbeat and palpation eliciting pain due to constipation may be signs of hyperparathyroidism. Hyperpigmentation of the skin would suggest Addison's disease.

3. **Answer: c**
   RATIONALE: Monitoring blood glucose levels during a growth hormone stimulation test is the priority task, along with observing for signs of hypoglycemia, diaphoresis, and somnolence. Providing ice chips to suck on would be more appropriate for a child who is on therapeutic fluid restriction, such as with syndrome of inappropriate antidiuretic hormone. Monitoring intake and output would not be necessary for this test but would be appropriate for a child with diabetes insipidus. Although it is important to educate the family about this test, it is not the priority task.

4. **Answer: a**
   RATIONALE: This child may have syndrome of inappropriate antidiuretic hormone (SIADH). The priority intervention for this child is to notify the physician of the neurologic findings. Remaining interventions will be to restore fluid balance with IV sodium chloride to correct hyponatremia, set up safety precautions to prevent injury due to altered level of consciousness, and monitor fluid intake, urine volume, and specific gravity.

5. **Answer: b**
   RATIONALE: Observation of an enlarged tongue, along with an enlarged posterior fontanel, and feeding difficulties are key findings for congenital hypothyroidism. The mother would report constipation rather than diarrhea. Auscultation would

reveal bradycardia rather than tachycardia, and palpation would reveal cool, dry, scaly skin.

6. **Answer: d**
   RATIONALE: Acanthosis nigricans, in addition to the obesity and amenorrhea, is a further indication of polycystic ovary syndrome. Blurred vision and headaches may be due to diabetes mellitus. Auscultation revealing an increased respiratory rate points to diabetes insipidus. Palpation revealing hypertrophy and weakness is typical of hypothyroidism.

7. **Answer: a**
   RATIONALE: A history of rapid weight gain and long-term corticosteroid therapy suggests this child may have Cushing's disease, which could be confirmed with an adrenal suppression test. A round, child-like face is common to both Cushing's and growth hormone deficiency. A high weight-to-height ratio and delayed dentition are findings in a child with growth hormone deficiency.

8. **Answer: c**
   RATIONALE: The primary nursing diagnosis would be deficient fluid volume due to electrolyte imbalance. It is important to increase the child's hydration to minimize renal calculi formation. Disturbed body image due to hormone dysfunction is a diagnosis for growth hormone deficiency. Imbalanced nutrition: more than body requirements would be important for a child with diabetes mellitus. Deficient knowledge related to treatment of the disease is appropriate for hyperparathyroidism, but it is not a priority diagnosis.

9. **Answer: b**
   RATIONALE: Obtaining glucose levels before bedtime snacks focuses on blood glucose monitoring. Ensuring consistency of food intake, maintaining proper injection schedules, and identifying carbohydrate, protein, and fat foods are teachings relating to diet and exercise.

10. **Answer: d**
    RATIONALE: The nurse should instruct both child and family to report side effects of hypothyroidism, such as restlessness, inability to sleep, and irritability. The nurse educates the family of the child with hypoparathyroidism on how to recognize vitamin D toxicity. Teaching the parents how to maintain fluid intake regimens is important for a child with diabetes insipidus. Children with hyperthyroidism are administered methimazole with meals.

11. **Answer: a, b, & e**
    RATIONALE: The nursing implications for a child undergoing a water deprivation study include monitoring the child for orthostatic hypotension, weighing the child before, during, and after the test, and rehydrating the child after the test. Serial blood samples are obtained at specific times and blood glucose levels are monitored for the child un-

dergoing the procedure for growth hormone stimulation.

12. **Answer: b, d, & e**
    RATIONALE: Palpitations, diaphoresis, and tremors are signs of hypoglycemia due to a fall in the blood glucose levels. An increase in the blood glucose levels or hyperglycemia causes blurred vision and fruity breath odor.

13. **Answer: c**
    RATIONALE: A child with acquired hypothyroidism has vague complaints of cold intolerance, fatigue, weakness, weight gain, dry skin, and constipation. Weight loss, oily skin, and diarrhea are not observed in the child with acquired hypothyroidism.

14. **Answer: a, b, & e.**
    RATIONALE: A cervical fat pad (buffalo hump) developing over time, tendency to bruise due to thin fragile skin, and reddish-purple striae on the abdomen indicate Cushing's syndrome. Rapid weight gain and water retention are also observed in Cushing's syndrome. Gradual onset of weight loss and dehydration may be seen in Addison's disease, not Cushing's syndrome.

15. **Answer: b**
    RATIONALE: The nurse should inform the parents to check the pulse before administering medication. An adverse effect of the medication is increased pulse rate, which may indicate an overdose of thyroid hormone. The nurse should inform the family that the medication will be needed throughout the child's life, not just for six months. Medication should not be administered with soy-based formulas and iron preparations, because they affect medication absorption. Medication may be mixed with a small amount of formula and placed in the nipple, but it should not be placed in a full bottle of formula because the infant will not ingest all the medication if he or she does not finish the bottle.

CHAPTER 49

Activity A

1. Neuroblastoma
2. Leukemia
3. Rhabdomyosarcoma
4. retinal
5. Chicken pox
6. Maintenance
7. Lymphohematopoietic
8. Nadir
9. nomogram
10. autologous

Activity B

1. The figure shows phases of the cell cycle: S, G1, G2, G0, and M.
2. The figure shows a maculopapular rash on the skin as the first sign of graft-versus-host disease (GVHD).

Activity C

1. e   **2.** a   **3.** b   **4.** c   **5.** f   **6.** d

Activity D

1.

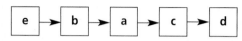

Activity E

1. The signs and symptoms related to location of rhabdomyosarcoma are as follows:
- Orbit – Proptosis
- Middle ear – Drainage, pain, facial nerve palsy
- Sinuses – Discharge, pain, sinusitis, facial swelling
- Nasopharynx – Pain, epistaxis, dysphagia, nasal quality to speech, airway obstruction
- Neck – Dysphagia, hoarseness
- Thorax, testicle, extremities – Enlarging mass, painless
- Retroperitoneum – Gastrointestinal and urinary tract obstruction, pain, weakness, paresthesia
- Bladder, prostate – Hematuria, urinary obstruction
- Vagina – Mass, vaginal disease, bleeding or chronic discharge

2. Allopurinol, antibiotics, antiemetics, antifungals, mesna, leucovorin, analgesics, and topical antibiotics.

3. The nursing interventions promoting skin integrity are as follows:
- Assess skin frequently for erythema, erosions, or blisters to provide baseline data, and intervene early if skin is impaired.
- Use mild soap for cleansing and pat dry rather than rubbing to avoid skin irritation.
- Use aloe vera lotion to moisturize the skin.
- Avoid perfumed lotions or soaps, and heat, cold, or sun, because these will further irritate the skin in the irradiated area.
- Do not scrub ink from marked radiation field and avoid adhesive tape in that area to avoid further skin irritation.
- Administer diphenhydramine or apply hydrocortisone 1% cream to reduce itching and the urge to scratch.

4. General guidelines related to the preparation and administration of chemotherapy include:
- Chemotherapy should be prepared and administered only by specifically trained personnel.
- Personal protective equipment in the form of double gloves and nonpermeable gowns should be worn when preparing or administering chemotherapy. If splashing is possible or a spill occurs, then a face shield and/or mask may also be necessary.
- Dispose all equipment used in chemotherapy preparation and administration in a puncture-resistant container.

5. To calculate the absolute neutrophil count (ANC):
- Add together the percentage of banded and segmented neutrophils reported on the complete blood cell count with differential (CBC with diff).
- Multiply the total number of WBCs reported on the CBC by the sum above. This yields the ANC (total number of neutrophils present).

    Example: Bands 5%, Segs 15%, WBCs 2,500
        5% + 15% = 20% (0.20)
        2,500 × 0.20 = 500
        ANC = 500

6. Massive hepatomegaly is managed in the following ways:
- Tumor resection or debulking
- Mechanical ventilation, inotropic support
- Nasogastric decompression
- Blood transfusions
- Comfort measures

Activity F

1. a. Nursing assessment for this toddler includes:
- Obtain a health history
- Determine whether other symptoms such as strabismus, orbital inflammation, vomiting, or headache have occurred
- Inquire about risk factors such as family history of retinoblastoma, other cancer, or presence of chromosomal anomalies
- Assess pupils for size and reactivity to light
- Note presence of leukocoria in the affected eye
- Assess the eyes for erythema, orbital inflammation, or hyphema

b. When caring for the child who is to undergo magnetic resonance imaging, the nurse must ensure that
- There are no metal objects on the child
- The child is motionless for the entire scan
- The younger child is sedated if necessary

c. The nurse should provide routine postoperative care to the toddler. If the eye is enucleated, the nurse should observe the larger pressure dressing on the eye socket for bleeding. Dressing changes to the socket may include sterile saline rinses or application of an antibiotic ointment or both. If chemotherapy is necessary, monitor for the side effects of chemotherapy. Follow-up will include eye examinations every three to six months until age six and then annually to check for further tumor development.

Activity G

1. Answer: b

RATIONALE: Along with the symptoms reported by the mother, the fact that the child has Beckwith-Wiedemann syndrome suggests that the child could have a Wilms' tumor. Down syndrome would point to leukemia or brain tumor. Schwachman syndrome is a risk factor for leukemia. A family history of neurofibromatosis is a risk factor for brain tumor, rhabdomyosarcoma, or acute myelogenous leukemia.

2. **Answer: a**
   RATIONALE: Coupled with the mother's complaints, observation of nystagmus and head tilt would suggest the child may have a brain tumor. Elevated blood pressure of 120/80 might be indicative of Wilms' tumor. Fever and headaches are common symptoms of acute lymphoblastic leukemia. A cough and labored breathing point to rhabdomyosarcoma near the child's airway.

3. **Answer: d**
   RATIONALE: Increased heart rate, murmur, and respiratory distress are symptoms of hyperleukocytosis, which is associated with leukemia with a high white blood cell count. Increased heart rate and blood pressure are indicative of tumor lysis syndrome, which may occur with ALL, lymphoma, and neuroblastoma. Wheezing and diminished breath sounds are signs of superior vena cava syndrome related to non-Hodgkin's lymphoma or neuroblastoma. Respiratory distress and poor perfusion are symptoms of massive hepatomegaly, which is caused by a neuroblastoma filling a large portion of the abdominal cavity.

4. **Answer: a**
   RATIONALE: It would be more accurate and appropriate for the nurse to stress that self-examination is an excellent way to screen for testicular cancer. Testicular cancer is one of the most curable cancers, if diagnosed early. The girls should know that they can take responsibility for their own sexual health by getting a Papanicolaou smear, which does not require parental consent in most states. Cervical cancer has a high response rate to therapy.

5. **Answer: b**
   RATIONALE: Ewing's sarcoma may result in swelling and erythema at the tumor site. Common sites are the chest wall, pelvis, vertebrae, and long bone diaphyses. Dull bone pain in the proximal tibia is indicative of osteosarcoma. Persistent pain after an ankle injury is equivocal. Many times bone tumors are attributed to trauma. An asymptomatic mass on the upper back suggests rhabdomyosarcoma.

6. **Answer: a**
   RATIONALE: The priority intervention is to monitor for increases in intracranial pressure because brain tumors may block cerebral fluid flow or cause edema in the brain. Lower-priority interventions include providing a tour of the ICU to prepare the child and parents for after the surgery, and educating the child and parents about shunts.

7. **Answer: c**
   RATIONALE: According to the formula BSA (m^2) = the square root of height in cm × weight in kgs divided by 3600:
   Body weight = 35 kgs, height = 150 cms
   35 × 150 = 5250 / 3600 = 1.458 and the square root of 1.458 is 1.20
   So the BSA is 1.20.

8. **Answer: c**
   RATIONALE: The parents should seek medical care immediately if the child has a temperature of 101°F or greater. This is because many chemotherapeutic drugs cause bone marrow suppression; the parents must take action at the first sign of infection to prevent overwhelming sepsis. The appearance of earache, stiff neck, sore throat, blisters, ulcers, or rashes and difficulty or pain when swallowing are reasons to seek medical care but are not as grave as the risk of infection.

9. **Answer: b**
   RATIONALE: The nurse should inform the oncologist about the decreased serum calcium level, which is a characteristic feature in tumor lysis syndrome. Decreased bicarbonate levels and pH levels are found in clients with hyperleukocytosis. Decreased platelet count levels are found in clients with sepsis.

10. **Answer: a**
    RATIONALE: The nurse should assess for dyspnea in the client with superior vena cava syndrome associated with neuroblastoma. Anorexia would be found in the client with typhlitis. Back pain is the characteristic feature of spinal cord compression, and hypotension should be assessed in a client with massive hepatomegaly.

11. **Answer: a**
    RATIONALE: The nurse should use corticosteroid eye drops to prevent conjunctivitis due to high doses of cytarabine. Maintaining adequate hydration is a general nursing implication for all chemotherapies. Monitoring urine for change of color is important when administering doxorubicin because the color of the urine may turn to red-orange. The nurse should monitor for Cushing syndrome while administering dexamethasone.

12. **Answer: a**
    RATIONALE: Ondansetron, when administered intravenously, causes dry mouth. Wheezing occurs due to administration of methotrexate antidote. Mucositis is a side effect of antimetabolite administration. Drowsiness is a side effect of antimicrotubulars.

13. **Answer: a**
    RATIONALE: The nurse should administer gammaglobulin during the pretransplantation phase of stem cell transplantation. Mycophenolate, cyclosporine, and tacrolimus are immunosuppressant drugs administered if a graft–versus-host disease (GVHD) occurs.

14. **Answer: d**
    RATIONALE: The nurse should expect to find erythema and swelling on inspection in the client with osteosarcoma. Bluish-gray papular lesions and salmon-colored lesions can be seen in the client with acute myelogenous leukemia. Petechiae and purpura can be found in the client with acute lymphoblastic leukemia.

15 Answer: a
RATIONALE: Neurofibromatosis is a risk factor for brain tumor. Down syndrome, ataxiatelangiectasia, and Schwachman syndrome are risk factors for acute lymphoblastic leukemia.

CHAPTER 50

Activity A

1. hepatosplenomegaly
2. maternal
3. mutant
4. Down
5. Hypoxemia
6. masculinization
7. Brushfield
8. Neurocutaneous
9. fibrillin
10. methionine

Activity B

1. The disorder is known as Trisomy 18, also known as Edwards' syndrome. This genetic disorder is characterized by the presence of three number 18 chromosomes.
2. **a.** The disorder is known as Fragile X syndrome, which is the outcome of a mutation of a gene (FMR1 [fragile X mental retardation]) on the X chromosome. This mutation essentially "turns off" the gene, triggering fragile X syndrome.
   b. Typical behavior problems include attention deficits, hand flapping and biting, hyperactivity, shyness, social isolation, low self-esteem, and gaze aversion.
3. This is a neurocutaneous genetic disorder known as neurofibromatosis. The hallmark of this disorder is the light-brown macules known as café-au-lait spots. These are usually present at birth but can appear during the first year of life and usually increase in size, number, and pigmentation.

Activity C

1. b   2. a   3. d   4. c

Activity D

1. A few major complications in a child with Down syndrome are cardiac defects, hearing or vision impairment, developmental delays, mental retardation, gastrointestinal disorders, recurrent infections, sleep apnea, etc.
2. When eliciting the health history of a child with a genetic disorder, the nurse should include questions related to the following:
   - Age when the disorder was diagnosed
   - Developmental delay
   - Complications of the disorder
   - Medications the child takes for complications associated with the disorder
   - Dietary restrictions
   - Compliance with management regimen

3. When three or more minor anomalies are present, the risk for a major anomaly or mental retardation is approximately 20%. When one major anomaly is present, the possibility of a genetic cause must be investigated.
4. Management of Down syndrome will involve multiple disciplines, including a primary physician, specialty physicians such as a cardiologist, ophthalmologist, and gastroenterologist, nurses, physical therapists, occupational therapists, speech therapists, dietician, psychologist, counselors, teachers, and parents.
5. Turner syndrome can be suspected prenatally by ultrasound findings such as fetal edema or redundant nuchal skin or by abnormal results of the triple screen. It can be diagnosed by chromosomal analysis, either prenatally or after birth. Most children are diagnosed at birth or in early childhood when slow growth or growth failure are noted.
6. Inborn errors of metabolism are a group of hereditary disorders. They are collectively common but individually rare. Most follow an autosomal recessive inheritance pattern. They are caused by gene mutations that result in abnormalities in the synthesis or catabolism of proteins, carbohydrates, or fats.

Activity E

1. **a.** Newborn screening is used to detect disorders before symptoms develop. Recent developments in screening techniques (tandem mass spectrometry) allow dozens of metabolic disorders or inborn errors of metabolism to be detected from a single drop of blood. Chloe's test results tell us that additional testing is needed to rule out a false-positive or confirm the diagnosis. Most inborn errors of metabolism presenting in the neonatal period are lethal or can result in serious complications such as mental retardation if specific treatment is not initiated immediately. This is why additional testing is so important.

   Inborn errors of metabolism are a group of hereditary disorders. Most follow an autosomal recessive inheritance pattern, meaning that two abnormal genes are needed for the child to demonstrate signs and symptoms of the disorder. For each child born to two carriers, there is a 25% chance that the child will be born with the defective gene, a 50% chance the child will be a carrier of the defective gene, and a 25% chance that the child will not be a carrier or have the disease. Inborn errors of metabolism are caused by gene mutations that result in abnormalities in the making or breakdown of proteins, carbohydrates, or fats. Therefore, the body is not able to turn food into energy as it normally would. This results in either an accumulation of a byproduct that can be harmful to the child or a deficiency or absence of a necessary product. Presentation can occur at any time, even in adulthood, but many show signs in the newborn period or shortly after.

b. In fatty acid oxidation disorders (such as medium-chain acyl-CoA dehydrogenase deficiency), the goal is to prevent or avoid prolonged fasts and to provide frequent feeds. Special consideration during illness is very important. If Chloe is unable to tolerate food, then she needs to be seen by a physician immediately; intravenous dextrose may be required. Again, the goal is to avoid prolonged fasting. Supplementation with specific vitamins may also be important in the treatment, and a dietitian and the physician will work with the caregivers. Strict adherence to frequent meals is necessary to prevent complications.

Nursing management will focus on education and support for the family and caregivers. Ensure that they have thorough knowledge about medium chain acyl-CoA dehydrogenase deficiency and its management. Refer the family to a dietitian and other appropriate resources, including support groups. Monitor the developmental progress of Chloe and initiate therapies if concern arises.

Activity F

1. **Answer: c**
   RATIONALE: Numerous café-au-lait spots on the trunk of the child are the hallmark of this disorder. These will increase in size, number, and pigmentation within the first year of life. A grandparent having had neurofibromatosis; a slightly larger head size; and freckles in the child's axilla are symptoms of the disorder but are not as definitive unless they appear in groups of two or more symptoms.

2. **Answer: c**
   RATIONALE: Children with phenylketonuria will have a mousy odor to their urine, as well as an eczema-like rash, irritability, and vomiting. Increased reflex action and seizures are typical of maple sugar urine disease. Signs of jaundice, diarrhea, and vomiting are typical of galactosemia. Seizures are a sign of biotinidase deficiency or maple sugar urine disease.

3. **Answer: a**
   RATIONALE: A major anomaly is an anomaly or malformation that creates significant medical problems and requires surgical or medical management. Café-au-lait macules are a major anomaly. Polydactyly (extra digits), syndactyly (webbed digits), and protruding ears are minor anomalies. Minor anomalies are features that do not cause an increase in morbidity in and of themselves.

4. **Answer: b**
   RATIONALE: Galactosemia is a deficiency in the liver enzyme needed to convert galactose into glucose. This means that the child will have to eliminate milk and dairy products from her diet for life. Ad-

hering to a low-phenylalanine diet is an intervention in phenylketonuria. Eating frequent meals and never fasting is an intervention in medium-chain acyl-CoA dehydrogenase deficiency. Maple sugar urine disease requires a low-protein diet and supplementation with thiamine.

5. **Answer: b**
   RATIONALE: A delay in attaining developmental milestones will most likely be the first clue found in assessment of a child with fragile X syndrome. Low self-esteem, problems with abstract reasoning, and gaze aversion may be present but may not be noted as the first sign of fragile X syndrome.

6. **Answer: a, b, & d**
   RATIONALE: Children with Sturge-Weber syndrome will have a facial nevus, or port wine stain, most often seen on the forehead and one eye, intracranial calcification, and hemiparesis. Vision and hearing loss and scoliosis are seen in children with neurofibromatosis.

7. **Answer: c**
   RATIONALE: The nurse should tell the parents that surgical interventions can help remove bone malformations in a child with neurofibromatosis. The inheritance pattern is autosomal dominant; therefore, offspring of affected individuals have a 50% chance of inheriting the altered gene and presenting with symptoms. There is no cure for neurofibromatosis; therapeutic management is aimed at controlling symptoms. Neurofibromatosis does not subside in adulthood; it is a progressive disease and tends to worsen over time.

8. **Answer: b**
   RATIONALE: The nurse should note underdeveloped labia in the girl with CHARGE syndrome. Tall stature with long limbs, minimal subcutaneous fat, and a long, narrow face are signs of Marfan syndrome. AQ7

9. **Answer: d**
   RATIONALE: The nurse should look for hypoplastic vertebrae in the child with VATER association. Craniocystosis, bilateral symmetrical syndactyly, and a prominent forehead may be noted in children with Apert syndrome.

10. **Answer: d**
    RATIONALE: Angelman syndrome is characterized by jerky ataxic movements, similar to a puppet's gait. Short stature is seen in Prader-Willi syndrome. A moonlike face may be noted in cri-du-chat syndrome. Cleft palate is a symptom of velocardiofacial/DiGeorge syndrome.

11. **Answer: b, d, & e.**
    RATIONALE: The nurse should look for epicanthal folds, arched palate, and a flattened occiput in the child with Down syndrome. Wide-spaced nipples and a low posterior hairline are characteristics of Turner syndrome.

12. **Answer: c**
    RATIONALE: A client with Klinefelter syndrome will have increased breast size caused by testosterone

deficiency. The client will also have long rather than short, stubby limbs and decreased pubic hair. Mental retardation is not present, but cognitive impairments may be present in varying degrees.

13. Answer: a, d, & e
RATIONALE: Homocystinuria is a deficiency in the enzyme needed to digest a component of food called methionine. The child with homocystinuria will need to adhere to a methionine-restricted diet and include cystine supplements and vitamin B6 and B12 supplements. Adhering to a low-protein diet may be needed for a child with maple sugar urine disease. Ensuring frequent meals is a necessary intervention for medium-chain acyl-CoA dehydrogenase deficiency.

14. Answer: a, d, & e
RATIONALE: The nurse should tell the parents that their child may have a learning disability and may be prone to skeletal deformities, and that there is no cure for Turner syndrome. Children with Turner syndrome have slow growth, no development of secondary sex characteristics, and may not be fertile. The risk of recurrence in future pregnancies does not increase, because Turner syndrome appears to be a sporadic event.

15 Answer: b
RATIONALE: Diagnosis of Klinefelter syndrome is usually not made until adolescence or adulthood because of nonspecific findings during childhood, not failure to report signs or social stigma. Prenatal diagnosis takes place only if amniocentesis is performed for genetic testing; it is possible but rare. Klinefelter syndrome presents with physical signs such as more than average height, lack of secondary sex characteristics, decreased facial hair, and gynecomastia.

CHAPTER 51

Activity A

1. dyslexia
2. inflicted
3. Neglect
4. psychostimulant
5. Hypnosis
6. Dyspraxia
7. comorbidity
8. psychopharmacology
9. Bulimia
10. Milieu

Activity B

1. c   **2.** a   **3.** b   **4.** d   **5.** e

Activity C

1. Set limits with the child, holding him responsible for his behavior. Do not argue, bargain, or negotiate about the limits, once established. Provide consistent caregivers (unlicensed assistive person-

nel and nurses for the hospitalized child) and establish the child's daily routine. Use a low-pitched voice and remain calm. Redirect the child's attention when needed. Ignore inappropriate behaviors. Praise the child's self-control efforts and other accomplishments. Use restraints only when necessary.

2. Radiographic skeletal survey or bone scan (for current or past fractures); CT scan of the head (intracranial hemorrhage); and rectal, oral, vaginal, or urethral specimens for sexually transmitted infections such as gonorrhea or chlamydia.

3. Generalized anxiety disorder is characterized by unrealistic concerns over past behavior, future events, and personal competency. Social phobia may result, in which the child or teen demonstrates a persistent fear of formal speaking, eating in front of others, using public restrooms, or speaking to authorities.

4. Mental retardation refers to a functional state in which significant limitations in intellectual status and adaptive behavior (functioning in daily life) develop before the age of 18 years. As defined by the American Association on Intellectual and Developmental Disabilities (AAIDD, 2007), mental retardation includes:
- Deviations in IQ of two or more standard deviations (IQ of less than 70 to 75)
- Coexisting deficits in at least two adaptive skills; communication, community use, functional academics, health and safety, home living, leisure, self-care, self-direction, social skills, and work
- Occurrence before the age of 18 years

5. Warning signs of Münchausen syndrome by proxy include:
   a. Child with one or more illnesses that do not respond to treatment or that follow a puzzling course; a similar history in siblings
   b. Symptoms that do not make sense or that disappear when the perpetrator is removed or not present; the symptoms are witnessed only by the caregiver
   c. Physical and laboratory findings that do not fit with the reported history
   d. Repeated hospitalizations failing to produce a medical diagnosis, transfers to other hospitals, and discharge against medical advice
   e. Parent who refuses to accept that the diagnosis is not medical

6. The following indications shown by the child will require a nurse to refer him or her for evaluation for a learning disability:
- Cannot speak in sentences by 30 months of age
- Does not have understandable speech 50% of the time by age 3 years
- Cannot sit still for a short story by three to five years of age
- Cannot tie shoes, cut, button, or hop by five to six years of age

Activity D

1. Obtain a health history from Greg and his father separately. Assess for a history of recent changes in behavior, changes in peer relationships, alterations in school performance, withdrawal from previously enjoyed activities, sleep disturbances, changes in eating behaviors, and increases in accidents or sexual promiscuity. Ask about potential stressors, conflicts with parents or peers, school concerns, dating issues, and abusive events. If possible, use a standardized depression-screening questionnaire.
   - Assess for history of weight loss
   - Observe for apparent apathy
   - Inspect the entire body surface for the presence of self-inflicted injuries
   - Assess for risk factors of suicide, including a change in school performance, changes in sleep or appetite, loss of interest in formerly preferred activities, feelings of hopelessness, depression, thoughts of suicide, and any previous attempts at suicide

2. Autism spectrum disorder (ASD) is a developmental disorder that has its onset in infancy or early childhood. Autistic behaviors may be first noted in infancy as developmental delays or between 12 and 36 months when the child loses previously acquired skills. Children with ASD demonstrate impairments in social interactions and communication. Most children with autism are mentally retarded, though in some cases they are gifted. The child with autism may be mute or may utter only sounds or repeat words or phrases over and over. The infant or toddler may spend hours in repetitive activity and demonstrate bizarre motor and stereotypic behaviors. The child may resist cuddling, lack eye contact, be indifferent to touch or affection and show little change in facial expressions. A hypersensitivity to touch or hyposensitivity to pain may be noted. The child may not look at objects when pointed to, may not point to himself, and may not let his needs be known.

3. The nurse or Rob's parents can take the following steps to improve his nutritional intake:
   - Mutually establish a contract related to treatment to promote the child's sense of control
   - Provide mealtime structure, because clear limits let the child know what the expectations are
   - Encourage the child to choose foods and timing of meals to develop independence in eating habits
   - Ensure that the eating environment is pleasant and relaxed, with minimal distractions, to minimize the child's anxiety and guilt about not eating
   - Withdraw attention if child refuses to eat (secondary gain is minimized if refusal to eat is ignored)
   - Provide continuous supervision during the meal and for 30 minutes following it so that the child cannot conceal or dispose of food or induce vomiting

Activity E

1. **Answer: b**
   RATIONALE: The nurse should pay particular attention to reports of a child spending hours in a repetitive activity, such as lining up cars rather than playing with them. Most three-year-olds are very busy and would rather play than sit on a parent's lap. The other statements are not outside the normal range and do not warrant further investigation.

2. **Answer: d**
   RATIONALE: The nurse should encourage the family to explore with their physician the option of one of the newer extended-release or once-daily medications for ADHD. The other statements are not helpful and do not address the mother's or boy's concerns.

3. **Answer: b**
   RATIONALE: Sudden, rapid, stereotypical sounds are a hallmark finding with Tourette syndrome. Toe walking and unusual behaviors such as hand-flapping and spinning are indicative of autism spectrum disorder. Lack of eye contact is associated with autism spectrum disorder but is also noted in children without a mental health disorder.

4. **Answer: a**
   RATIONALE: The nurse should emphasize the importance of adhering to a rigid, unchanging routine, because children with autism spectrum disorder often act out when their routine changes. The other statements would not warrant additional referral or follow-up.

5. **Answer: b**
   RATIONALE: An IQ of 35 to 50 is classified as moderate. An IQ of 50 to 70 is classified as mild. An IQ of 20 to 35 is classified as severe, and an IQ less than 20 is considered profound.

6. **Answer: b**
   RATIONALE: It is important to continue the usual routine when a child is hospitalized, particularly a child with mental retardation. By asking about a typical day, the nurse can identify routines that may be able to be duplicated in the hospital. Telling the girl she will be going home soon or asking if she wants art supplies does not address her concerns. Asking whether she has talked to her parents is unhelpful. (Also, for some families the caretaking burden is extensive and lifelong. The child's hospitalization may be providing some respite to the parents.)

7. **Answer: c**
   RATIONALE: Adolescents with anorexia may have a history of constipation, syncope, secondary amenorrhea, abdominal pain, and periodic episodes of cold hands and feet.

8. **Answer: a**
   RATIONALE: The nurse should carefully assess the mouth and oropharynx for eroded dental enamel, red gums, and an inflamed throat from self-in-

duced vomiting. The other findings are typically noted with anorexia nervosa.

9. **Answer: a**
RATIONALE: If burns occur only on the soles or palms, they would be highly suspicious for inflicted burns. However, for injury, the abdomen would be a highly suspicious site for physical abuse.

10. **Answer: c**
RATIONALE: It is important to remind the parents that medications for the management of ADHD are not a cure but help to increase the child's ability to pay attention and decrease the level of impulsive behavior. The other statements are correct.

11. **Answer: a**
RATIONALE: It is incorrect that medication can completely cure autism spectrum disorder. The other approaches mentioned such as complementary and alternative medical therapies, restrictive diets, and nutritional supplements have not been scientifically proven to improve autism.

12. **Answer: d**
RATIONALE: Complications of bulimia include fluid and electrolyte balance, decreased blood volume, cardiac arrhythmias, esophagitis, rupture of the esophagus or stomach, tooth loss, and menstrual problems. Paralysis, hernia, and severe acne are not associated with bulimia.

13. **Answer: c**
RATIONALE: Therapeutic management of anxiety disorders generally involves the use of pharmacologic agents such as anxiolytics and antidepressants. It can also involve psychological approaches such as cognitive-behavioral therapy and individual, family, or group psychotherapy. Psychostimulants are used in case of attention-deficit/hyperactivity disorder (ADHD). Antipsychotic medications are sometimes helpful for children with repetitive and aggressive behaviors. It may not best suit the condition of post-traumatic stress. Sensory integration technique is attempted for autism, and it is not scientifically proved.

14. **Answer: c**
RATIONALE: A bipolar disorder can be suspected if the history reveals rapid, pressured speech, increased energy, decreased sleep, flamboyant behavior, or irritability during the manic episodes. Social phobia is a possible consequence of an anxiety disorder. There can be various reasons for poor performance in school. Vocal tics are associated with Tourette syndrome.

15. **Answer: b, c, & e**
RATIONALE: The nurse should encourage discussion of the client's thoughts and feelings rather than having her suppress them. The nurse should also set clear limits on behavior as needed, instead of removing them, so that the client has a structure to adhere to. The other steps mentioned are good ways to promote coping skills.

CHAPTER 52

Activity A

1. Intubation
2. defibrillation
3. hyperventilation
4. Asystole
5. hypocapnia
6. Ventricular
7. Bradycardia
8. hypovolemic
9. barotrauma
10. circumoral

Activity B

1. The figure illustrates a head-tilt/chin-lift maneuver. This maneuver is applied to open the airway in an unconscious child.
2. The figure depicts nursing management of pediatric trauma. (A) The infant and young child's prominent occiput encourages flexion of the neck and may result in airway occlusion. (B) Putting a towel roll under the shoulders helps to open the infant's or young child's airway by placing it in the neutral, or "sniff," position.

Activity C

1. b   2. a   3. e   4. d   5. c

Activity D

1.
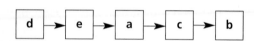

Activity E

1. The ABCs of the rapid cardiopulmonary assessment are A: airway; B: breathing; and C: circulation. Because pediatric arrests are usually related primarily to airway and breathing, and usually only secondary to the heart, the assessment and interventions using the ABCs of resuscitation are necessary. The assessment and interventions are always performed in that order. If the pediatric airway is properly managed and breathing is assisted, the child may not experience a full arrest requiring chest compressions.
2. Cricoid pressure, also known as the Sellick's maneuver, is the use of gentle pressure to occlude the esophagus, preventing air from entering the stomach. Cricoid pressure may help to prevent vomiting secondary to gastric distention. Vomiting during resuscitative efforts can complicate the situation because the child is at risk of aspirating abdominal contents.
3. Standard laboratory tests obtained in most emergency departments include:
   • Arterial blood gases (ABG), obtained initially and then serially to assess for status changes
   • Electrolytes and glucose levels
   • Complete blood cell count (CBC)

- Blood cultures
- Urinalysis

Diagnostic tests may include radiology, computed tomography (CT) scanning, and magnetic resonance imaging (MRI).

4. The airway management for a child with no cervical spine injury is as follows:
   - Position the airway in a manner that promotes good air flow
   - If secretions are obstructing the airway, suction the airway to remove them
   - If the child is unconscious or has just been injured, open the airway with the head-tilt/chin-lift maneuver
   - Place the fingertips on the bony prominence of the child's chin and lift the chin to open the airway; simultaneously, place one hand on the forehead and tilt the child's head back
   - If the airway is not maintainable, reposition the airway for appropriate air flow
   - Place the child immediately on oxygen at 100%, and apply a pulse oximeter to monitor oxygen saturation levels

5. Cardioversion is another means of applying electrical current to the heart besides defibrillation. It is used when the child has supraventricular tachycardia (SVT) or ventricular tachycardia with a pulse. Cardioversion may also be enhanced with medications. Cardioversion is delivered as synchronized—that is, the electrical current is applied on the R wave of the electrocardiogram (ECG).

6. Infants and young children are at greater risk for respiratory emergencies than adolescents and adults because they have smaller airways and underdeveloped immune systems, resulting in a diminished ability to combat serious respiratory illnesses. Young children often lack coordination, making them susceptible to choking on foods and small objects, which may also lead to cardiopulmonary arrest. In addition, sudden infant death syndrome (SIDS) is a leading cause of cardiopulmonary arrest in young infants.

Activity F

1. During the course of resuscitation, the nurse should assess the following to determine the child's response to the resuscitative effort:
   - Adequacy of chest rise
   - Absence or minimal presence of abdominal distention
   - Improved heart rate and pulse oximetry readings
   - Improved color
   - Capillary refill less than 3 seconds, with strengthening pulses

Activity G

1. **Answer: a**
   RATIONALE: According to PALS, the calculated minimum acceptable systolic BP for a five-year-old boy is 80; according to the formula 70 + (2 times age in years), that is 70 + (2 × 5) = 70 + (10) = 80.

2. **Answer: d**
   RATIONALE: Once the ABCs have been evaluated, the nurse will move on to "D" and assess for disability by palpating the anterior fontanel for signs of increased intracranial pressure. Observing skin color and perfusion is part of evaluating circulation. Palpating the abdomen for soreness and auscultating for bowel sounds would be part of the full-body examination that follows assessing for disability.

3. **Answer: a**
   RATIONALE: Inserting a small, folded towel under his shoulders best positions the infant's airway in the "sniff" position recommended by AHA's Basic Cardiac Life Support (BCLS) guidelines. A hand should never be placed under the neck to open the airway. The head-tilt/chin-lift technique and the jaw-thrust maneuver are used with children over the age of one year.

4. **Answer: a**
   RATIONALE: Obtaining central venous access is the priority intervention for a child in shock who is receiving respiratory support. Gaining access via the femoral route will not interfere with CPR efforts. Peripheral venous access may be impossible to obtain in children who have significant vascular compromise. Blood samples and urinary catheter placement can wait until fluid is administered.

5. **Answer: a**
   RATIONALE: Decreased skin turgor is a late sign of shock. Blood pressure is not a reliable method of evaluating for shock in children because children tend to maintain normal or slightly below normal blood pressure in compensated shock. Equal central and distal pulses are not a sign of shock. Delayed capillary refill and cool extremities are signs of shock that occur earlier than changes in skin turgor.

6. **Answer: d**
   RATIONALE: The appropriate tracheal tube size for the six-year-old child is 5.5 millimeters. According to the formula, divide the child's age by 4 and then add 4; in this case, divide 6 by 4 to get 1.5, and then add: 1.5 + 4 = 5.5 mm. Tube sizes of 6.0, 5.0, and 4.5 are inappropriate.

7. **Answer: a**
   RATIONALE: Because of the potentially devastating effects of drowning-related hypoxia on a child's brain, airway interventions must be initiated immediately. The child's airway should be suctioned to ensure patency. Other interventions, such as covering the child with blankets, inserting a nasogastric tube, and ensuring that the child remains still during an x-ray, are interventions that are appropriate once airway patency is achieved and maintained.

8. **Answer: a**
   RATIONALE: To assess the renal function, a chemistry panel test is performed on the client with poisoning. Urine and blood toxicology screens are also performed on the client with poisoning, but

these tests do not assess the renal functions. Serum electrolytes are performed on the client with near-drowning to assess the imbalance related to the development of shock.

9. **Answer: d**
RATIONALE: The left lower sternal border is the appropriate place for auscultating the tricuspid area. The second right interspace is the aortic valve, and over the second left interspace is the pulmonic valve; fifth interspace, midclavicular line is the mitral area.

10. **Answer: d**
RATIONALE: An oxygen flow rate of 10 L/minute is appropriate for infants and children. An adolescent, not a 9-year-old, would most likely require an oxygen flow rate of 15 L/minute for effective ventilation. All other options are valid when preparing to ventilate with a bag valve mask.

11. **Answer: a**
RATIONALE: The nurse should immediately start cardiac compression in the child. Only supporting a patent airway and adequate oxygenation takes precedence over cardiac compressions. Giving fluids is an intervention done later. Epinephrine is administered for treating bradycardia.

12. **Answer: d**
RATIONALE: Unilateral absent breath sounds are associated with foreign body aspiration. Dullness on percussion over a lung lobe is indicative of fluid consolidation in the lung, as with pneumonia. Auscultating a low-pitched, grating breath sound suggests inflammation of the pleura. Hearing a hy-

perresonant sound on percussion may indicate pneumothorax or asthma.

13. **Answer: c**
RATIONALE: To rule out accidental esophageal intubation, the nurse should auscultate over the abdomen while the child is being ventilated; there should not be breath sounds in the abdomen. Auscultating over the lung fields for equal breath sounds, observing for symmetrical chest rise, and inspecting the tube for presence of water vapor on the inside should be done to confirm the correct placement of a tracheal tube.

14. **Answer: c**
RATIONALE: Cold shock results in a decrease in cardiac output with an increase in SVR in septic shock. Septic shock is related to a systemic inflammatory response in which there may be increased cardiac output with a low SVR, known as "warm shock." Distributive shock is the result of a loss in the SVR. A relative hypovolemia occurs, most often with neurogenic injury–related shock and anaphylaxis. Cardiogenic shock results from an ineffective pump, the heart, with a resultant decrease in stroke volume.

15 **Answer: a**
RATIONALE: A complete blood cell count with differential is conducted to assess for a viral or bacterial infection in septic shock. A blood culture is performed to evaluate sepsis. A toxicology panel is performed if ingestion is suspected. C-reactive protein is used to evaluate infection.